Praise for
The Bipolar Disorder Survival Guide

"I used to spend way too much time searching the Internet for tips on managing my bipolar disorder. Now, whenever I need ideas about how to feel better, I just pick up *The Bipolar Disorder Survival Guide*. It is an incredible resource that gives me tons of new and effective coping strategies to try. Reading it, you'll feel like an expert is taking the time to really talk to you—it's clear that Dr. Miklowitz cares."
—CHRISTINE S., Houston, Texas

"A practical, straightforward book that will be a great help to those who have bipolar illness, as well as their families. I could not recommend this book more highly."
—KAY REDFIELD JAMISON, PhD, author of *An Unquiet Mind* and *Robert Lowell, Setting the River on Fire*

"This book is a true gift. As parents, watching our daughter's illness unfold was terrifying and heartbreaking. I only wish that Dr. Miklowitz's book had been available then to help guide us on this rollercoaster of a journey. It not only gives sufferers and their family members a better understanding of bipolar disorder, but also shows how to achieve stable moods and lead a full life."
—VICKY G., Santa Monica, California

"Dr. Miklowitz is an experienced therapist and skilled researcher whose decades of work with people with bipolar disorder shine through in this easy-to-follow book. If you or a loved one have bipolar disorder, I highly recommend this updated third edition."
—MARY A. FRISTAD, PhD, ABPP, Department of Psychiatry and Behavioral Health, The Ohio State University Wexner Medical Center

"The author's expertise, compassion, and experience are evident throughout. . . . Well worth reading and remembering."
—*NAMI Advocate*

"Recommended for patient education libraries and medium and large public libraries."
—*Library Journal*

THE BIPOLAR DISORDER SURVIVAL GUIDE

Also from David J. Miklowitz

THE BIPOLAR DISORDER SURVIVAL GUIDE

What You and Your Family Need to Know

THIRD EDITION

David J. Miklowitz, PhD

THE GUILFORD PRESS
New York   London

Copyright © 2019 The Guilford Press
A Division of Guilford Publications, Inc.
370 Seventh Avenue, Suite 1200, New York, NY 10001
www.guilford.com

The information in this volume is not intended as a substitute for consultation with healthcare professionals. Each individual's health concerns should be evaluated by a qualified professional.

Printed in the United States of America

This book is printed on acid-free paper.

Last digit is print number: 9   8   7   6   5   4   3   2   1

Library of Congress Cataloging-in-Publication Data is available from the publisher.

ISBN 978-1-4625-3498-2 (paperback) — ISBN 978-1-4625-3727-3 (hardcover)

Contents

Part III. Practical Strategies for Staying Well

Purchasers of this book can download and print enlarged versions of
select practical tools at *www.guilford.com/miklowitz2-forms*
for personal use or use with clients (see copyright page for details).

Preface

Bipolar disorder can be a great teacher. It's a challenge,
but it can set you up to be able to do almost anything
else in your life.

—Carrie Fisher

I first became interested in bipolar disorder in 1982 when, as a predoctoral psychology intern at the University of California, Los Angeles (UCLA), Medical Center, I supervised a bipolar support group with a fellow intern. The assignment was
a challenge, but I was immediately struck by how the members of the group—men
and women ranging in age from 19 to 50—had discovered, quite independently,
how to deal with their illness. They had learned to ask for medical and social support when the early signs of recurrences first appeared, to rely on their significant
others and friends for emotional support, and to separate themselves from the
disorder and fight its stigma. All of them understood that leading fulfilling lives
required more than just taking medications.

The experience inspired me to choose a PhD dissertation topic on bipolar disorder, specifically about family relationships among late adolescents and young
adults who had just come out of the hospital. In the decades since, I have cared for
or supervised the care of hundreds of people with bipolar disorder—both young
and old—and their families in the context of my research studies and clinical
practice. People have come to my office in a variety of clinical states, with unique
expressions of the disorder and beliefs about how it should be treated; specific factors in their genetic, biological, or family backgrounds that contributed to the disorder; and different understandings of what it meant for their future. Many have
had a love–hate relationship with the illness: They have cherished the intensity of
the emotional experiences that mania provides but have detested the low periods,
the disorder's unpredictability, and the emotional, practical, and financial damage
done to their lives.

My long-term collaboration (1979–1997) with the late Michael Goldstein, PhD, of UCLA resulted in the development of family-focused therapy (FFT), an intervention that assists people with bipolar disorder and their family members in coping during the periods after an illness episode. My experimental studies at the University of Colorado and those with my UCLA colleagues have shown that people who receive FFT and medications have lower rates of relapse and less severe symptoms than people who receive individual supportive care and medications. Their improvements can be observed for up to 2 years after they begin family treatment. Our most recent work has shown that teens with bipolar disorder benefit from FFT and medications as well, in terms of milder symptoms and better functioning after episodes of illness. These studies, funded by the National Institute of Mental Health, the Brain and Behavior Research Foundation, and various family foundations, have included over 1,000 people. The participants have varied in age, ethnicity, race, and socioeconomic status and included people experiencing their first manic or depressive episode as well as those who have been ill for most of their lives; people for whom the disorder poses only occasional life problems and those who are chronically in and out of hospitals; and people in a wide variety of living situations and family contexts.

I wrote this book to respond to a need voiced by virtually everyone with whom I have worked, along with their family members. People with the disorder wish for more understanding from their spouses/partners, parents, siblings, and coworkers. Their family members, in turn, want to know how best to help their relative with bipolar disorder without becoming angry, controlling, or overprotective. Both the patients and their family members ask the core question this book attempts to answer: How can people with the disorder achieve stable moods and lead more fulfilling lives while taking medications and dealing with the limitations the illness imposes?

What Can You Expect to Gain from Reading This Book?

This is a book about individual empowerment—recognizing the realities of your illness and taking steps to prevent episodes from occurring. It is my strong belief that people who do best with the disorder are those who have learned to recognize triggers for their mood cycles and learned how to minimize the impact of these triggers. They are people who stay close to their prescribed medication regimens and have trusting relationships with their physicians. They have regular therapists or go to support groups. They have come to appreciate their family members, who often have been the only ones to stand by them during and after illness episodes. They have learned as much as they can about the illness through books, articles, or conferences and regularly talk with and assist others who have the illness. They have learned to accept the disorder without limiting their personal goals because of it.

At that bipolar support group years ago, I was impressed by the members' ability and willingness to take care of each other as well as themselves. One group member regularly made trips to the local hospital inpatient unit to tell other patients about the advantages of obtaining medical and psychosocial treatment at the UCLA Mood Disorders Clinic. When a member of the group started to cycle into an episode, others were quickly able to recognize the early warning signs and offer assistance. Members were often blunt with each other but would say things that needed to be said.

I'd like to think of this book as performing the same function as that support group. It is my sincere hope that after reading it, you will feel less alone in your struggles, realize that there are effective treatments available, and have at your fingertips strategies to prevent mood swings from ruling your life. I hope this book will tell you the things that need to be said and that you'll use them to your benefit, even if you don't always want to hear them. Most of all, I hope you and your family members will become convinced that you can lead a full life and achieve many of your personal goals despite having the disorder. I wish you much success in your personal journey through the ups and downs of bipolar disorder.

A Word of Thanks

Many people deserve my heartfelt appreciation for supporting me in writing this book and providing friendship and mentoring over the past several decades. I feel especially grateful to my collaborators Ellen Frank, David Kupfer, and Boris Birmaher of the University of Pittsburgh School of Medicine, and Michael Gitlin from the UCLA Department of Psychiatry, for their clinical wisdom and encouragement of my research. The illness management tools outlined in this book—education, relapse prevention, effective communication and problem solving, relying on social supports, and social rhythm stabilization—emerged from our many collaborations.

Many teachers and close colleagues have been inspirational throughout my career and have strongly influenced how I think about clinical work, including Michael Goldstein, Ian Falloon, Keith Nuechterlein, Raymond Knight, W. Edward Craighead, Gary Sachs, Michael Thase, Steve Carter, Lyman Wynne, Robert Liberman, Angus Strachan, David Wellisch, Shirley Glynn, and Kay Jamison. My graduate students and postdoctoral fellows at the University of Colorado and UCLA were often the first to suggest clinical strategies for working with individuals or families, and their research has often influenced the direction of my own. They have included Eunice Kim, Tina Goldstein, Elizabeth George, Teri Simoneau, Dawn Taylor, Jeff Richards, Vicky Cosgrove, Kim Mullen, Jed Bopp, Chris Hawkey, Aimee Sullivan, Natalie Sachs-Ericsson, Jennifer Wendel, Kristin Powell, Aparna Kalbag, Patty Walshaw, Sarah Marvin, Lisa O'Donnell, Alissa Ellis, Danielle Keenan-Miller, Danielle Denenny, and many others. I am also grateful to Brittany Matkevich, Margaret Van de Loo, Nadia Takla, Natalie Witt, and Dana Elkun for their assistance with my research and clinical work. Colleagues with whom I collaborated at UCLA in the late 1980s hold a special place in my heart, including Margaret Rea, Martha Tompson, Jim Mintz, Jeff Ball, Robin Kissell, and Amy Weisman.

I have greatly enjoyed my friendship and research collaboration with psychiatrists David Axelson, Ben Goldstein, Kiki Chang, Manpreet Singh, Melissa DelBello, Robert Post, and Robert Kowatch. Special thanks go to my collaborators Chris Schneck, Alisha Brosse, and Aimee Sullivan for keeping the flame alive in Colorado. I feel very grateful to my friends and collaborators in the Department of Psychiatry at the University of Oxford, in the United Kingdom: Guy Goodwin, John Geddes, Andrea Cipriani, Chris Fairburn, and Mark Williams. Each has taught me something unique about mood disorders and their treatment.

I would like to extend special appreciation to several friends and colleagues who commented on the manuscript: Michael Gitlin, Melissa DelBello, Cheryl Chessick, Richard Suddath, Joseph Goldberg, Sheri Johnson, Amy West, and Sona Dimidjian. I am fortunate to have befriended and worked with Dr. Lori Altshuler (1957–2015), first during our training at UCLA and later as faculty colleagues.

Many thanks go to members of my family—my wife, Mary Yaeger; my daughter, Ariana; and my brother, Paul Miklowitz, and his family, Marija and Sabina—all of whom have brought me great joy and reminded me that life is not just about work. My late mother, Gloria Miklowitz, a children's author who published over 70 books, continues to be a source of inspiration during the difficult but rewarding process of writing. The memory of my father, Julius Miklowitz, a Caltech professor who taught me the value of research, hard work, and a life of learning, has guided me throughout my life.

Finally, I would like to express my sincere gratitude to two of the most talented, patient, and knowledgeable editors in the universe—Kitty Moore and Chris Benton of The Guilford Press. Their imprint appears throughout the book, including this latest edition. Without their encouragement, tenacity, support, and great senses of humor, this book would never have come to fruition.

Introduction
Bipolar Disorder: Where Are We Now?

This book has always been for and about people coping with bipolar disorder, in either themselves or a close relative. My primary purpose in this third edition is to bring readers up to date on a number of advances in the field—and new ways of thinking about treatment and self-management—since the second edition in 2010. Although some of these changes are major and some minor, most practitioners agree that people with bipolar disorder can expect a better outcome today than 10–20 years ago. More treatment pathways are open to you than ever before. Psychotherapy is increasingly accepted as an adjunct to conventional medications, data from randomized trials have shown new medical treatments to be effective, and practitioners are becoming more open to complementary and alternative medicines.

Unique Individuals and Personalized Care

Importantly, there has been a gradual shift in how people with mental health problems are approached by practitioners. There is an increasing awareness of the *uniqueness of the individual,* which shows up in how we diagnose bipolar disorder, the level and type of input we solicit from patients and their family members in treatment planning, and the push toward person-specific or "personalized" care— the matching of individual characteristics to effective treatments. It is now considered good clinical practice to have people with bipolar disorder (or their relatives) weigh in on major decisions about their treatment. The desire of the field for more consumer input is reflected in a number of ways: People with bipolar disorder and their family members now serve on university-based human subjects review boards, data safety monitoring committees, grant review panels, and focus work-groups charged with decision making about what types of care to offer in mental health practice settings.

Personalized care is a development that will almost certainly enhance individual outcomes over the long term. My own take has always been that people with bipolar disorder have the right (and perhaps the responsibility) to decide what's best for them rather than accepting the paternalistic stance that the doctor always knows best. I encourage people to consider the many factors that may influence how well they respond to treatment, such as whether anyone else in the family has bipolar disorder or whether their mood episodes have been both manic and depressed or just depressed. I have always advocated for people with lived experience to play a central role in their own illness management, but in the first two editions of this book the emphasis was on ensuring that they—and their families—had up-to-date research information on which to base their decisions. Now, in this new edition, I highlight what we know about predictors of response to the various treatment options you may be weighing, and how to individualize your use of available treatments to fit your health habits, lifestyle, or belief systems. As you go through the chapters, you'll see a number of health tips related to personalizing your care.

Bipolar Disorder as a Continuum

The importance of diagnosing and treating each person as a unique individual has emerged from the shift toward viewing psychiatric disorders through *dimensional models*. The National Institute of Mental Health has published a series of position papers and guidelines for the Research Domain Criteria (RDoC) system, which characterizes discrete illnesses in terms of shared underlying dimensions such as genetic vulnerability, emotional dysregulation, or cognitive impairment (Insel, 2009). Instead of classifying people into hard-and-fast categories like being bipolar or not, we are approaching them as being on a continuum of symptoms, functioning, and biological vulnerability. As a result, patients are more likely to get treated for the specific problems they're dealing with, even though they may fall short of the full criteria for bipolar disorder.

Take bipolar disorder and schizophrenia as examples. On the surface, these two disorders sound like completely different illnesses, the first being characterized by severe mood swings and the second by delusions and hallucinations. But RDoC emphasizes the fact that these disorders share about 40% of their genes (for example, Berrettini, 2003). Saying that someone is schizophrenic and not bipolar may lead practitioners to miss important areas of overlap such as depression, suicidality, problems in social awareness or cognition, sleep disturbance, or anxiety, all of which can occur in either disorder. Instead, if we say that a person has impairment in three dimensions—a mood dimension, a psychosis dimension, and a functioning dimension—we increase the likelihood that this person will receive treatments that are more targeted to his or her clinical profile.

Likewise, we should not assume that everyone who has been diagnosed with bipolar disorder got there by the same avenue. One person may have inherited bipolar disorder from a parent; another might have had a head injury; another may have a history of child abuse and loss experiences that contributed to difficulties in regulating moods and emotions. These variables should be factored into diagnosis and treatment to produce the best possible care for each unique individual.

Given its emphasis on categories and the presence or absence of well-defined and observable behaviors, the fifth edition of the *Diagnostic and Statistical Manual of Mental Disorders* (DSM-5; American Psychiatric Association, 2013) has not yet incorporated dimensional views of diagnosis. Nonetheless, there are signs of progress in the manual. For example, DSM-5 recognizes that patients with major depressive disorder can have co-occurring symptoms of hypomania or mania and that patients with mania/hypomania can have co-occurring symptoms of depression. One can now identify "subthreshold" mixed episodes in people with either major depression or bipolar disorder, whereas in prior editions of the DSM, having any mixed episode automatically meant you had bipolar I disorder.

As you can see, diagnoses that incorporate dimensions may lead to more fine-grained perceptions of how an illness takes shape in different people. For example, when you have major depression with only one or two manic symptoms, your doctor may think you have a bipolar spectrum disorder. You may not agree, but this is a debate worth having because it may affect medication choices, such as whether you should take antidepressants alone or in conjunction with a mood stabilizer.

Dimensional diagnoses have some negative implications for care as well. Most of medicine relies on distinct categories; diagnoses are not usually done by measuring what genetic abnormalities you do and don't have on a blood test. Not everyone agrees that lumping mild or subthreshold forms of an illness with more severe forms is a good idea. In fact, in the last two decades, bipolar disorder has suffered from "concept creep" (Haslan, 2016) as its boundaries have become broader and broader. Conditions that mimic bipolar symptoms, such as agitated depression or recurrent explosive outbursts in children (now called disruptive mood dysregulation disorder, or DMDD), have been attributed too readily to bipolar disorder. Psychiatric classification has fallen prey to other instances of concept creep, such as the expanding boundaries of autism spectrum disorders. The risk of dimensionalizing is that people will write off diagnoses like bipolar spectrum disorder as "fluff" or that doctors will overtreat mildly ill people with antipsychotic medications that are really intended for people with more significant symptoms.

Even when doctors think dimensionally, they have to identify a cutoff point above which they will treat you for a specific disorder and adopt the treatment assumptions that go with that diagnosis (for example, using mood stabilizers or second-generation antipsychotics [SGAs] before antidepressants or psychostimulants). However, we need to make sure your psychiatrist or therapist is not lumping you with people whose illnesses yours only resembles at a superficial level.

In this edition, my intention is to help you sort through new findings about bipolar disorder as a continuum so that you can approach the diagnostic (or rediagnostic) process with the background information you'll need. In the long run, thinking about both categories *and* dimensions may be optimal when you and your doctor are trying to find the most appropriate treatment.

Greater Emphasis on Resilience

The person-centered approach also shows up in our new definitions of treatment response. Many people with bipolar disorder and their family members say that *quality of life* or *degree of recovery* (ability to function at an optimal level despite the illness) is the most important outcome to them, even more important than staying free of recurrences. The person-centered approach includes a greater focus on *resiliency factors*—the individual or environmental attributes that help you get through the toughest times and still achieve your goals—rather than only on risk factors. This way of thinking is the basis of *positive psychology,* a person-centered approach to psychological health that emphasizes factors that promote good functioning and make life worth living (Seligman, 2002).

Consider the emphasis on maintaining a healthy lifestyle. In earlier editions of the book I stressed the importance of regular sleep–wake rhythms, but maintaining a healthy lifestyle also includes a regular exercise routine, a balanced diet, vitamins, and a balance of work (or volunteer) demands with time for friends or family. It might include time to meditate, write, or play or listen to music. These components of healthy living are of course recommended for everyone, but for those with bipolar disorder, maintaining a healthy lifestyle can mitigate the effects of stress on your risk of recurrences. In other words, the resilience view emphasizes factors that sustain us or contribute to our health rather than make us sick.

My view is that a greater focus on resilience and recovery encourages people to lead better and more meaningful lives with fewer limitations and to feel more in control of their fate. Hopefully, your doctor or therapist will adjust your treatment plan with you in ways that address factors unique to your individual situation, your values, and your goals rather than taking a "one-size-fits-all" approach. If recovery means having no or only mild symptoms while working at a job that does not satisfy you, or taking medications that are barely tolerable, we need a different definition of recovery and better treatments. I firmly believe that people with bipolar disorder lead happier lives when they do not carry the expectation that recovery means being free of all symptoms. A better definition of recovery is to lead a satisfying and fulfilling life despite symptoms of the illness and being able to work toward your life goals without sacrificing your mental or physical health.

Throughout the book, you'll notice that I encourage you to think about what outcomes are most valuable to you, even though these may change over time. Your valued outcomes may go well beyond symptom relief and include, for example, finishing school, getting promoted at work, having kids, or building stronger family or romantic relationships. Identifying what you want will help you determine whether treatments have been effective according to your own definitions of recovery.

Greater Societal Recognition of Bipolar Disorder

In the past decade, the news media have been awash in stories about people with bipolar disorder. Numerous celebrities (including Catherine Zeta-Jones, Demi Lovato, Sinead O'Connor, Patty Duke, and Carrie Fisher) have talked openly about having the disorder. These accounts are sometimes astonishing. For example, Suzy Favor Hamilton, an Olympic-level runner, writes about becoming a prostitute in Las Vegas during a lengthy manic period (Hamilton, 2016). Carrie Fisher described an extensive alcohol and drug abuse history that worsened when she became manic. We learn a great deal about resilience from these individuals. Their courage in telling their stories—despite knowing that disclosure would negatively affect their careers—has had the net effect of decreasing the societal stigma attached to bipolar disorder.

The widespread media coverage has also had some negative side effects. Bipolar disorder is sometimes described as a disorder of rich, self-involved people; an affliction that affects only artists; or a post hoc explanation for "acting out" or breaking laws. The widening of the bipolar spectrum to include celebrities who are impulsive, giddy, or overly exuberant, or who have very public meltdowns, has the potential to increase such misunderstandings. You may find yourself bristling as you compare yourself to more public personalities ("How do I cope with all of this without having a nanny and a lot of money?" or "I have all the same symptoms but none of the acting talent"). In this edition, I spend more time discussing the line between illness and ordinary moodiness. I hope these discussions help you, people in your family, and your close friends understand what it means to have bipolar disorder (for example, that you may not always be able to operate at full capacity) and what it doesn't mean (for example, that everyone with bipolar disorder is creative and that your talents will come to the fore only if you stop taking your medications).

The greater societal awareness of bipolar disorder has, unfortunately, not translated into accurate understanding. Many more people today can offer a reasonable, if sketchy, picture of what bipolar disorder is, but people with mental illness, including those with bipolar disorder, are still stigmatized as being unpredictable, violent, and untrustworthy. This misperception takes shape as ongoing discrimination: in a 2011 study of 1,182 people with bipolar disorder, 72% reported having experienced a moderate or high level of social discrimination (Brohan, Gauci, Sartorius, Thornicroft, & GAMIAN-Europe Study Group, 2011). Discrimination can affect your ability to get the job or promotion you want, lead to romantic breakups when a partner discovers you have bipolar disorder, or hinder your rights as a parent. In Chapter 13, you'll find an extensive discussion of the pros and cons of acquainting employers or coworkers with your disorder, different ways to present it, and knowing your rights in the occupational arena.

Greater Recognition of Cognitive Impairment

Cognitive functioning is one area where recognition of individual uniqueness, and the need for personalized care, has increased. We've always known that bipolar disorder comes with problems in thinking, attention, planning, vigilance, memory, and problem solving, but only in the last decade has it become clear that cognitive impairment is present even between mood episodes, during the "normal" or euthymic periods. We all have cognitive strengths and weaknesses, such as whether we routinely remember names, recall details of certain settings or conversations, or can attend to more than one thing at a time. But for those with bipolar disorder, the fact that cognitive functioning can affect mood and moods can affect cognition is particularly problematic. Cognitive problems and depression are the two strongest predictors of how people with bipolar disorder function in the community—such as whether they can hold a job, maintain relationships and friendships, or progress in school (Gitlin & Miklowitz, 2017).

Major advances in our understanding of cognitive impairments in bipolar disorder have come from neuroimaging (brain scan) studies. For example, when people with bipolar disorder engage in tasks involving the perception or regulation of strong emotions, there may be reduced activity in the prefrontal cortex (responsible for planning, foresight, decision making, and other "executive" functions of the brain) and excessive activation of the amygdala (a structure known to be involved in our emotional reactions to threat) (Townsend & Altshuler, 2012).

Medications often get blamed for cognitive impairments, and indeed, some medications (for example, topiramate or Topamax) can be mind-numbing in many individuals. Yet cognitive impairment is also a feature of the illness, and its severity may wax and wane alongside changes in mood states. In our efforts to make treatment more person centered, we need to take account of the various cognitive problems a person experiences at different stages of the illness. For example, cognitive-behavioral therapy (CBT) relies heavily on homework assignments, such as keeping track of your moods, thoughts, or self-statements; challenging your assumptions and replacing them with alternative ways of thinking; or keeping behavior, sleep, and mood charts. If you have significant difficulties with memory, attention, and planning, this may not be the right treatment for you.

As I've argued in previous editions, it is critically important to gauge how much you are able to handle after an illness episode. This capacity varies considerably from person to person. Your level of residual symptoms may suggest that you are getting better, but mentally you may not feel up to par (see Martha's story in Chapter 1). Moreover, people with bipolar disorder cannot always tell when their cognitive functioning is off-kilter. As a result, family members may get frustrated and blame you for not trying hard enough.

The good news is that researchers around the world are recognizing these problems, and in the last decade investigators have developed cognitive rehabilitation programs that aim to improve thinking, memory, work, and social functioning (for example, Torrent et al., 2013). These computer-aided programs usually involve practicing memory and attentional or problem-solving strategies in an individual or group setting (see Chapter 6). There are also new medications that enhance cognitive functioning and can be taken safely alongside mood stabilizers.

Cognitive impairments are quite frightening to people with the disorder and their family members. They fear that all cognitive impairments are permanent, or that they are becoming demented, or that how they are functioning now is how they will function for the rest of their lives. This is not the case; I will show you evidence that many people have improvements in functioning when their treatments are changed. Many handle high-level jobs despite the cognitive impairments associated with bipolar disorder.

Medical Treatments for Bipolar Disorder: Old, New, and Alternative

In the last decade, medical research on bipolar disorder has focused on developing novel treatments and enhancing the effects of treatments we already have (Geddes & Miklowitz, 2013). Medical treatments for bipolar disorder are being increasingly framed as combinations of conventional mood stabilizers like lithium, SGAs, antidepressants, antianxiety agents, psychostimulants (for comorbid attention-deficit/hyperactivity disorder, or ADHD), and sleep treatments. In parallel, more experimental trials have looked at combinations of medicines and even the order in which they're given, rather than simple "drug A versus drug B" studies. Studies are now incorporating quality of life or work and social functioning as important outcomes. Pharmacogenomic studies, in which medications are prescribed based on one's personal genetic profile, are in progress. Pharmacotherapy for bipolar disorder is much more sophisticated and person centered than it used to be.

Consider some of the changes that have been made in our treatment guidelines. In earlier editions of this book, I cited the often-stated view that the antidepressants known as selective serotonin reuptake inhibitors (SSRIs) should never be given to people with bipolar disorder unless these drugs are accompanied by mood-stabilizing agents like lithium or lamotrigine. The most recent research suggests that this principle does not always apply to individuals with bipolar II disorder. In fact, people with bipolar II disorder can be treated effectively with antidepressants alone, even those people who have not responded well to lithium (Amsterdam, Wang, & Shults, 2010). In bipolar II, rates of manic (or hypomanic) "switching" on antidepressants are no higher among people on antidepressants alone than among people who get an antidepressant with a mood stabilizer or a mood stabilizer alone (Altshuler et al., 2017). These findings have very real implications for your treatment: if you have bipolar II disorder and your depressions are severe and chronic, you may do well on an antidepressant.

There are new drugs on the market, some of which have been "repurposed" from use in another medical illness. Many of the newer agents are meant for people with treatment-resistant bipolar or unipolar depression, which usually refers to low mood states that do not improve with conventional antidepressants. An example of a repurposed medication is ketamine, a drug used in anesthesia and pain management. Ketamine—originally administered intravenously—has been found to bring people out of severe depressions quickly (Zarate et al., 2012). It is now available as a nasal spray in many quarters. However, there are concerns about ketamine, such as how long its effects last and its potential to become a drug of abuse.

Complementary and alternative treatments—which are not only medicines but can include herbal remedies or mindfulness meditation—are being greeted with more openness by practitioners and their patients than ever before, consistent with person-centered views of treatment. Drugs that affect neuroinflammatory pathways in the brain, such as omega-3 fatty acids (fish oil), are being tested as adjuncts to mood stabilizers; new data on transcranial magnetic stimulation and bright white light therapy are looking promising. But not everyone wants to take Chinese herbs, probiotics, or homeopathic remedies, or sit under lights to treat mood problems. How do we know what works? Investigators are making diligent efforts to test alternative treatments against (or in combination with) conventional medicines like lithium. Most alternative treatments have been tested in broad, unselected samples of people with depression (broadly defined) who may also have bipolar disorder, but the unique effects in the latter are not always clear.

Medical providers run the gamut from those who subscribe only to pharmaceutically derived medications and give little credence to complementary treatments to those who believe bipolar disorder can be treated *only* with complementary agents. The former view often goes with beliefs such as "homeopathic remedies are just placebo pills with cute names," whereas the latter view often goes along with "the pharmaceutical industry is evil" or "psychiatric medications are like poison to the brain."

My own take is that the increasing openness to complementary and alternative treatments is a positive development. Certain agents, such as omega-3, do appear to have beneficial effects on physical health, mood, and quality of life whether one has bipolar disorder or ordinary depression. You may feel better when taking them, even if only due to placebo effects. But we should not be blind to the disadvantages of alternative treatments either, such as when people mistake these agents for primary treatments (for example, "I don't have to take lithium if I'm taking fish oil") or believe that alternative treatments have no side effects (they do—for fish oil, they include nausea and an upset stomach). Many alternative treatments that are heralded as mood stabilizers or antidepressants have not been tested in placebo-controlled trials, raising the risk that outcomes could be worse than those obtained with conventional treatments. Finally, complementary treatments are a major industry, with companies pushing and profiting from them just as drug companies do from conventional pharmaceuticals.

Throughout the book, and especially in Chapter 6, be on the lookout for descriptions of various complementary and alternative treatments. My objective is for you to know the truth about these options and their current evidence base so that you can select from among the increasingly wide array of treatment options. You should not have to pay for a bushel of medications at the pharmacy and then go to the health food store for an equally daunting array of vitamins or supplements. Being an informed consumer makes for less burdensome (and probably more effective) treatment plans.

Advances in Psychosocial Treatments

If you have read an earlier edition of this book, you know that psychotherapy for bipolar disorder is my passion, particularly psychotherapy that includes family members. The past decade has seen a rapid increase in the number of studies testing specific psychosocial interventions in combination with medications, with individual, group, family, and even Internet approaches being evaluated. People with bipolar disorder want psychotherapy, and their family members often do as well. In fact, in our survey of 3,000 members of the consumer-based Depression and Bipolar Support Alliance (DBSA), over 50% said they (or their loved one) were getting both medications and psychotherapy.

Current approaches to psychotherapy recognize the uniqueness of an individual's history, as well as individual preferences for different types of treatment. As mentioned, one type of expertise derives from having lived through an illness and knowing what factors are important to your own stability. Sometimes people who have been through episodes of mania or depression become mutual support group leaders for DBSA or the National Alliance on Mental Illness and help others to cope with the disorder.

With personalized medicine, we choose treatments that match up with our risk factors: if family disturbances are most salient, family-focused therapy may be appropriate; if someone is struggling with sleep–wake irregularity, interpersonal and social rhythm therapy may be more appropriate. Another example: having a history of sexual abuse often results in posttraumatic stress disorder, for which cognitive-behavioral therapy is of paramount importance. A study of major depression found that mindfulness-based cognitive therapy (MBCT) was more effective in reducing recurrences among people with severe childhood trauma than in those without trauma histories (Williams et al., 2014).

The major drawback in the provision of evidence-based psychotherapy has been that these treatments are often unavailable or too expensive in the community. This is a serious problem, and although the situation is improving, you may find that you are limited by who is available to see you. Nonetheless, I will give you some online resources that will help you locate the services you need, as well as point you to websites and mobile applications that take the concepts of psychotherapies and translate them into self-care tools.

Bipolar Disorder in Children

The move toward personalized care is well illustrated by the recognition that many, if not most, people with bipolar disorder have their first symptoms in childhood or adolescence. We know that bipolar disorder can be present in children as young as age 5, although this is rare and there is not uniform agreement about what it looks like. An early onset of bipolar disorder is, sadly, associated with a more difficult course of illness in adulthood, with more periods of rapid cycling, time ill, and self-harm or suicidal thinking (Post et al., 2010). On the more optimistic side, intervening in the earliest stages of the illness has the potential to alter long-term course patterns. This new edition has a separate chapter on children (Chapter 14) that provides answers to many of the questions that parents frequently ask about pediatric bipolar disorder. If there is a family history of bipolar disorder in first- or second-degree relatives (grandparents, aunts, uncles) and mood swings in the child—indicated by inconsistent sleep, sudden bursts of energy, or outbursts of crying or laughing, for example—getting a full evaluation from a child psychiatrist or psychologist is one of the best things you can do. In the new chapter I talk about ways to find a good evaluator, what to ask about, and how you might present the evaluation to your child without scaring him or her.

If you have read widely about childhood bipolar disorder or communicated with people in other countries whose kids have it, you've almost certainly encountered varying opinions on the validity of this diagnosis. There is a lot of diagnostic sloppiness around the world, including in the United States. This is in part because diagnostic categories for children overlap considerably (for example, ADHD can look a lot like mania). When kids are mistakenly called bipolar and really have a different disorder, they may go for years with the wrong treatments or educational plans. Other youngsters are diagnosed with ADHD, anxiety, or oppositional defiant disorder when they really have bipolar disorder, once again resulting in ineffective treatments.

Many practitioners have learned to better distinguish bipolar disorder from disorders that look like it. But in some locales the clinical approach is still behind the times. As a parent, it's important to know the symptom criteria yourself (see the adult criteria in Chapter 2 and the information specific to children in Chapter 14) so that you don't accept a haphazard diagnosis. Insist on a full evaluation with a child psychiatrist or psychologist who is familiar with bipolar disorder and its comorbid conditions—it need not be his or her specialty.

One encouraging development has been the observation that some kids with bipolar disorder—even those who had full manic episodes in childhood—seem to be free of recurrences as they reach their late teens or early twenties (Birmaher et al., 2014; Geller, Tillman, Bolhofner, & Zimerman, 2008). Some young people experience major improvements in mental clarity and functioning as they age. So, if you are a teen or young adult who has just been diagnosed, being bipolar doesn't necessarily mean you have to take the medicines you are currently taking for the rest of your life. We do not know yet how many people have this outcome or how to predict it. But we do know that the long-term course of bipolar disorder varies considerably from person to person. Throughout the book, I will highlight strategies you can use to decrease your risk of recurrences.

• • • • • • • • • • • • •

The diagnosis and treatment of bipolar disorder have become increasingly sophisticated—and, most importantly, helpful to individuals with the illness—thanks to new awareness that each individual is unique and must be treated as such. Treatments continue to be refined to address a wide variety of needs beyond preventing recurrences of illness and managing symptoms. Keep in mind the themes discussed in this introduction as you go through the book to make the most of advances in the field as applied to your own treatment. I begin by explaining how this book may be of help, whether you are a person with the disorder or a family member.

PART I

The Experience and Diagnosis of Bipolar Disorder

CHAPTER 1

How This Book Can Help You Survive—and Thrive

• • • • • • • • • • • • •

Why Do You Need This Book?

- To understand the symptoms, diagnosis, and causes of your bipolar disorder
- To learn about effective medical and psychological treatments
- To learn self-management techniques to help you deal with mood cycles
- To improve your functioning in family and work settings
- To learn how treatment regimens and lifestyle strategies can be customized to your unique characteristics, symptoms, and life situation

• • • • • • • • • • • • •

Martha, 34, ended up in the hospital after storming out of the house where she lived with her husband and two school-age children and spending a disastrous night in a town over 2 hours away. Her problems had started about 2 weeks earlier, when she became unusually irritable with her husband, Eric, "slamming about the house," as he described it, and becoming easily provoked by the minor infractions of their children. She then began to sleep less and less and was increasingly preoccupied with many ideas for a tech start-up business she had been planning. Despite this intense focus, Martha was very easily distracted. She also began speaking very rapidly.

Her problems came to a head when she left the house in a fury shortly after dinner one night and impulsively took a bus to a gambling casino about

100 miles away. By her account, she met a man at a bar the same night and went to bed with him. The next morning she called her husband, crying, and explained what had happened. Needless to say, he was quite angry and drove to the casino to pick her up. He arrived at the agreed-upon place and time, only to find that Martha was not there. He returned home to find his wife disheveled, sleep deprived, and angry. After sobbing for several hours, she finally agreed to go with him to be evaluated at a local hospital. She was admitted to the inpatient unit and given a diagnosis of bipolar I disorder, manic phase.

Bipolar disorder is a mood disorder that affects at least 1 in every 50 people—and as many as 1 in 25 by some estimates—and puts them at high risk for the kinds of problems in their family, social, and work lives that Martha suffered. People with bipolar disorder are also at high risk for physical illnesses such as cardiovascular disease, alcohol and substance use disorders, and suicide. Fortunately, there is much hope. With medications, psychotherapy, and self-management techniques, it's possible to control the rapid shifts in mood from manic highs to severe depressive lows (called *mood disorder episodes*), prevent future episodes from occurring, decrease the impact of environmental triggering events, and cope well in the job and social world. These may sound like pie-in-the-sky promises, but they reflect decades of research as well as the rich and hopeful stories of people with the disorder.

Whether you have already been diagnosed with bipolar disorder, think you might have it, or are concerned about a family member or friend who has it, this book will help you understand the disorder, learn to manage it effectively, and teach others how to cope with it. In the following chapters you'll find up-to-date information on the nature of the disorder, its causes, its medical and psychological treatments, and the lifestyle changes you can make to manage the disorder. You'll also learn how to adapt these treatment or self-management strategies to your individual circumstances. The information should be relevant to you whether you have been treated on an inpatient basis, like Martha, or on a continuous outpatient basis, which is becoming more and more common.

Understanding the Facts about Bipolar Disorder:
Its Symptoms, Causes, Treatment, and Self-Management

The inpatient physician who saw Martha diagnosed her as bipolar very quickly and recommended a regimen of lithium, a mood-stabilizing medication, and risperidone (Risperdal), a second-generation antipsychotic (SGA) medication. After only a few days it was clear that she was responding well. But when her doctor made plans to discharge her, Martha had a litany of questions and worries about everything that was happening to her. Why was she being given "this death sentence" (her diagnosis) and "drugged and disposed of so quickly"?

Why was she being labeled manic, when most of what she had done, she felt, could be attributed to her personality or interpersonal style? "I've always been assertive and direct," she complained to her doctor, her husband, and almost everyone else she saw. "Since when is everything I do a mental illness?" Her doctor responded with sympathy but offered insufficient information to satisfy Martha. Under considerable pressure to get people in and out of the hospital quickly, he left her with a list of medications to take but little understanding of what had happened to her or what to expect once she got home.

If you were in Martha's position, in all likelihood you would find the hospital experience as confusing and frustrating as she did. In my experience, people with bipolar disorder and their family members usually are hungry for information about the disorder, particularly during or after a manic or depressive episode, even if the episode has not involved hospitalization. Of course, people with the disorder have an easier time assimilating information about it once they are over the worst of their symptoms. But even during the hospitalization, Martha and her husband would have benefited a great deal from some basic information: why her doctors suspected she had the illness, how the symptoms are experienced by the person with the disorder versus everyone else, the expected course of the illness over time, and what kinds of treatments would help. They would have benefited from knowing what to expect after she was discharged from the hospital, including her risks of cycling into new episodes. Without this information, it was difficult for Martha to put her experiences in context. As a result, she began to doubt the accuracy of the diagnosis and, by extension, the wisdom of complying with her prescribed treatments.

A major assumption of this book is that understanding the facts about your disorder will help you and your close family members accept, live with, and cope more effectively with it. Here are some important questions that often go unanswered because mental health providers simply don't have time or don't know the answers:

- ■ "What are the symptoms of bipolar disorder?"
- ■ "Who am I apart from my disorder?"
- ■ "Where does ordinary moodiness end and bipolar disorder begin?"
- ■ "Where did the illness come from?"
- ■ "How do I know when I'm becoming ill?"
- ■ "What triggers my mood cycles, and are the triggers different for the highs and lows?"
- ■ "What can I do to minimize my chances of becoming ill again?"
- ■ "How do I explain the illness to other people?"
- ■ "What can I expect from my future?"

By the end of this book, I hope you'll have gotten useful answers to these questions, together with a more complete understanding of bipolar disorder, a new grasp of who you are and how bipolar disorder fits into your life, and a wealth of illness management techniques. I also hope to leave you knowing where to turn when the future brings new challenges and you need additional information and advice.

> **Effective prevention:** Being able to put your illness in an informational context helps you prevent or at least minimize the damage associated with future recurrences and set appropriate goals for your immediate and long-term future.

Adjusting to the Aftermath of an Episode

Martha left the hospital with prescriptions for lithium and risperidone and an appointment to see a new doctor 2 weeks later. Upon discharge she agreed to follow the recommendations of the inpatient staff to continue taking her medications, but she knew little about what the medications were doing or exactly what was being medicated. She felt shaky, agitated, irritable, and mentally confused. She complained of physical pains that had no obvious source. These uncomfortable sensations were largely the result of continuing symptoms of her disorder, but in the absence of any information to the contrary, Martha assumed her confusion and pain were due entirely to the lithium.

She then noticed her mood start to drop, gradually at first. She felt numb, disinterested in things, tired, and unable to sleep even though she desperately wanted to. She began to spend more time during the day "sleep bingeing" to try to catch up from the night before. She awoke in the afternoon feeling worse and had difficulty with her usual responsibilities, such as making dinner or helping the children do their homework. She dreaded interacting with her neighbors. The idea of committing suicide crossed her mind for the first time. She felt guilty about the potential impact of her disorder on her children and wondered whether they would be better off without her.

Martha developed an upper respiratory infection, which kept her up late at night coughing. Compounding this stress, the neighbors were having work done on their house, and she was awakened from her fitful sleep by noise early in the morning. Her sleep became more and more inconsistent, and her daily and nightly routines—when she went to bed and when she woke up—began to change from day to day.

About a week after being discharged from the hospital, Martha's mood escalated upward again. Her thoughts began to race, and she started to think again about the tech start-up. Then, in what she later described as a flash, she decided that all of her problems—not just the mental confusion but also her cycling mood, her sleep disturbance, and her lethargy—were caused by lithium. Without checking with a physician or telling anyone, she lowered her lithium dosage. When she saw no immediate negative results, she discontinued it altogether. She stopped her risperidone next. Martha became severely irritable again, began to sleep less and less, and ended up back in the hospital only 3 weeks after her discharge.

Martha's story is all too common. Because the nature of the disorder was not explained fully to her, she thought of the episode as a sort of "nervous breakdown" requiring only temporary medication. She did not know that the illness could be recurrent. In Chapters 2, 3, and 4, you will become familiar with the expected course of bipolar disorder and the various forms that mood recurrences can take. This knowledge will help you feel more confident about sticking to a treatment and self-management plan that may help stave off recurrences.

Martha also would have benefited from knowledge of the factors that we believe cause the cycling of bipolar disorder: a complex interplay of genetic background, individual neurophysiology, and life stress, as discussed in Chapter 5. Many people who have bipolar disorder burden themselves with guilt and self-blame because they believe their mood disorder is caused solely by psychological factors or even sheer weakness of character. Martha could have avoided such self-blame if she had known that her dramatic mood shifts were associated with changes in the function of nerve cell receptors or activity in the limbic system of the brain. Her experiences would have made more sense to her in the context of her family tree: her mother had severe depression and her paternal grandfather was hospitalized once for "mental anguish" and "exhaustion."

Knowing about the biological causes of your disorder will also clarify why consistency with your medications is essential to maintaining good mood stability. Martha knew that she needed to take medications, but not why. Chapters 6 and 7 deal with medication treatments for bipolar disorder. Many drugs are available

---

PERSONALIZED CARE TIP:
Communicating with your physician

You will feel more effective in managing your disorder if you can openly communicate with your physician about which medications are most effective for you, their side effects, and the mixed emotions you may feel about taking them. Not everyone responds the same way to different medications. You may be having unusual reactions to a given medicine that could be corrected by adjusting your dosage or switching to a different drug. You may also harbor fears that the medications will cause long-term damage to your kidneys or that they will kill brain cells. These are all understandable concerns that your doctor should address.

nowadays, in various combinations and dosages. Doctors have to be constantly updated on which treatments to recommend to which patients, since the accepted treatment guidelines for this disorder change so rapidly.

Self-Management Strategies

Beyond taking medications and meeting with a psychiatrist, there are good and bad ways to manage your disorder. Self-management involves learning to recognize your individual triggers for episodes and adjusting your life accordingly. This book will teach you a number of self-management tools that will probably increase the amount of time that your moods remain stable. For example, Martha would have benefited from sleep–wake monitoring, or staying on a regular daily and nightly routine, including going to bed and waking at the same time, strategies described in Chapter 8. Likewise, keeping a mood chart (also covered in Chapter 8) would have provided a structure for tracking the day-to-day changes in her moods and revealed how these changes corresponded with fluctuations in her sleep, inconsistency with medications, and stressful events. Recall that Martha's worsening mood was precipitated by a respiratory infection and the appearance of neighborhood noise, which were stressful and disrupted her sleep–wake patterns. In addition to recognizing these events as triggers, Martha and her husband could have developed a list of early warning signs that would alert them to the possibility of a new episode of mania. In Martha's case, these signs included irritability and a sudden and unrealistic interest in developing a tech start-up. Chapter 9 provides a comprehensive overview of possible early warning signs of mania.

When Martha first started becoming depressed, certain behavioral strategies might have kept her from sinking further into depression, including behavior activation exercises and cognitive restructuring techniques, introduced in Chapter 10. She would have had the support of knowing that suicidal thoughts and feelings—a common component of the bipolar syndrome—can be combated through prevention strategies involving the support of close friends and relatives, counseling, and medications, as described in Chapter 11. She would have understood some of the differences between women and men during the depressed phase (for example, the role of the menstrual cycle), and how to manage some of the health complications that affect women who take mood-stabilizing medications, as discussed in Chapter 12.

Finally, many people with bipolar disorder worry that their children will develop the disorder. Raising children under these circumstances can feel like there is a sword hanging over your head. Martha worried constantly about Kirsten, her 14-year-old, who had hit adolescence with a vengeance, with unpredictable hours, irritability, withdrawal, sleep problems, and a deterioration in her academic performance. Was this a reaction to her mother's illness or the beginning of her own illness? In Chapter 14, you'll learn how to recognize early warning signs of bipolarity in your children as well as some useful strategies for obtaining a diagnosis and, if warranted, early interventions.

Coping Effectively in the Family and Work Settings

Martha spent 5 more days in the hospital but this time was discharged with a clearer follow-up plan. She met the physician who would see her as an outpatient to monitor her medications and blood serum levels. The inpatient social work team also helped arrange an outpatient appointment with a psychologist who specialized in the treatment of mood disorders. This time, she felt better about the hospitalization experience but was quite wary of what would happen once she was back at home.

After her discharge, Martha spoke with close friends about what had happened. They were sympathetic but said things like "I guess everybody's a little bit manic–depressive" and "Maybe you were just working too hard." When she disclosed to one friend that she was taking lithium, the friend said, "Don't get addicted." Although she knew her friends were trying to be supportive, these messages confused her. Was she really ill or just going through a tough time? Were her problems really an illness or just an extreme of her personality? Hadn't the physicians told her that mood-stabilizing medications were meant to be taken over the long term?

Martha's husband, Eric, seemed unsure of how to relate to her. He genuinely cared about her and wanted to help but frequently became intrusive about issues such as whether she had taken her medications. He pointed out minor shifts in her emotional reactions to things that formerly would have escaped his notice but which he now relabeled as "your rapid cycling." Martha, in turn, felt she was being told that she was "no longer allowed to have normal emotional reactions." She told him, "You can't just hand me a tray of lithium every time I laugh too loud or cry during a movie."

At other times Eric became angry and criticized her for the deterioration in her care of the children. Indeed, she didn't have enough energy to take them to their various activities or get them to school on time. She didn't feel up to the social demands of being a parent. "You aren't trying hard enough," Eric said. "You've got to buck up and beat this thing." At other times he would tell her she shouldn't take on too much responsibility because of her illness. Martha became confused about what her husband expected of her. What neither understood was that most people need a low-key, low-demand period of convalescence after a hospitalization so that they can fully recover from an episode of bipolar disorder.

Her children eyed Martha with suspicion, expecting her to burst into irritable tirades, as she had done prior to her first hospitalization. She began to feel that her family was ganging up on her. The family stress during the aftermath of her episode contributed to her depression and desire to withdraw.

Given the economic pressure her family was under, Martha decided to immediately return to her part-time computer programming job but felt unable to handle the long commute. When she arrived at work, she stared at the computer screen. "The programs I used to know well now seem like gobbledygook," she complained. She finally told her boss about her psychiatric hospitalizations. He seemed sympathetic at first but soon began pressuring her to return to her prior level of functioning. She felt uncomfortable around her coworkers, who seemed edgy and avoidant as they "handled me with kid gloves." The shifts in work schedules, which had been a regular part of her job before, started to feel like they were contributing to her mood swings.

Martha had significant problems reestablishing herself in her home, work, and community following her hospitalization. People who develop other chronic medical illnesses, such as diabetes, cardiac disorders, multiple sclerosis, or cancer, also can have trouble relating to their partner, children, other family members, friends, and coworkers. When you reenter your everyday world following a mood episode, even well-intentioned family members don't know how to interpret the changes in your behavior (for example, your irritability or lack of motivation). They often mistakenly think that you are acting this way on purpose and could control these behaviors if you only tried harder. As a result, they become critical, evaluative, and judgmental. They may also mistakenly think you can't take care of yourself and try to do things for you that you are more than capable of doing yourself. For example, they may try to actively manage your time, direct your career moves, telephone your doctors with information about you, constantly question you about your medications, or become vigilant about even the most minor changes in your emotional state.

In the workplace you may find your employer initially sympathetic but impatient. Your coworkers may be guarded, suspicious, or even scared. In addition, you may feel that you can't concentrate as well on the job as you did before you became ill. These difficulties are all a part of the convalescent period that follows an episode. In all likelihood, your concentration problems will diminish once your mood becomes stable. But it can be quite upsetting to feel like you're not functioning at the level at which you know you can.

As you are probably aware, bipolar disorder carries a social stigma not associated with medical illnesses. Even though bipolar disorder is clearly a disorder of the brain, and its genetic and biological underpinnings are well documented, it is still treated as a "mental illness." Many people still erroneously believe it is related to your personal choices or morals. As a result, you may feel alienated from others when they find out about your disorder.

On the hopeful side, there is much you can do to educate your family, coworkers, and friends about the nature of your illness. Certainly, people will respond to your disorder in ways that you will find uncomfortable, but their reactions will vary, at least in part, with how you present it to them. Chapter 13 is devoted to exploring ways of coping effectively in the family and workplace. You'll learn how to talk to your family, friends, and coworkers about your disorder so that they know how best to help you and don't force their misconceptions on you (as was the case for Martha). You'll learn specific strategies for communicating effectively and solving problems with your family so that disagreements about the disorder don't escalate into unproductive and stressful arguments.

> **Effective prevention:** One objective of this book is to familiarize you with the role of family and other social factors in contributing to, or ameliorating, the cycling of your bipolar disorder.

Martha: Epilogue

Martha's first year after her two hospitalizations was quite difficult, but now, several years later, she is doing much better. She found a psychiatrist with whom she feels comfortable. She is taking a regimen of lithium, lamotrigine (Lamictal), and a thyroid supplement. Her mood and behavior still shift up and down—for example, she reacts strongly to disagreements with her husband and still has periods of feeling down or unmotivated—but her symptoms are no longer incapacitating. In part due to her willingness to commit to a program of mood-stabilizing medications, she has not needed the intensive inpatient treatment she received initially.

Martha and Eric have improved their relationship. They regularly see a marital therapist, who has helped them distinguish how the disorder affects their relationship, how conflicts in their relationship affect the disorder, and what problems in their family life are unrelated to her illness. Together they have developed a list of the signs of her oncoming episodes and what steps to take when these signs appear (for example, calling her physician for an appointment to get her medications adjusted and, hopefully, prevent a hospitalization). Her children have become more accepting of her moodiness, and she has become more enthusiastic about parenting. For Kirsten, her 14-year-old, Martha engineered an evaluation with a child psychiatrist at the same facility where she got her treatment. The psychiatrist concluded that Kirsten had developed a mild depression, probably related to events in her family life and a boyfriend with whom things had not worked out. Individual therapy was recommended and was successful.

Martha has had frustrations in the workplace and finally came to the conclusion that "I'm just not a nine-to-fiver." She decided to try freelance work, which, although not as financially lucrative as her job, has reduced her stress and given her predictable hours.

Martha now has a better understanding of the disorder and how to manage it. For example, by keeping a mood chart she has learned to distinguish—for herself as well as for other people—between her everyday, normal mood swings and the more dramatic mood swings of her bipolar illness. She has learned to maintain a regular sleep–wake cycle. She recognizes that keeping her disorder well controlled is the key to meeting her own expectations of herself. She is now more comfortable trusting and enlisting the support of her husband and, especially, a close friend when she feels depressed or suicidal.

Martha recognizes that her disorder is recurrent but also feels that she is more in control of her fate. In summing up her developing ability to cope with the disorder, she said, "I've learned to accept that I've got something biochemical that goes haywire, but it's not the sum total of who I am. If I could change one thing about myself, it'd be other people's moods and how they affect me, even when it's their problem and not mine."

Above all, this book is about hope. If you've just been diagnosed with bipolar disorder, or even if you have had many episodes, you probably have fears about what the future holds. Martha's story—while perhaps representative of only one form of the disorder and one type of life situation—captures some of the ways that people learn to live with bipolar illness. *A diagnosis of bipolar disorder doesn't have to mean giving up your hopes and aspirations.* As you will soon see, you can come to terms with the disorder and develop skills for coping with it and still experience life to its fullest.

How This Book Is Organized

This book is divided into three sections. In the remaining chapters (2–4) of this section, "The Experience and Diagnosis of Bipolar Disorder," you'll learn about the symptoms and recurrent nature of the disorder from your own vantage point as well as that of your relatives and the physician who makes the diagnosis. You'll become familiar with the behaviors considered to be within the bipolar spectrum and learn what to expect from the diagnostic process. Chapter 4 offers you tips on how to cope with the diagnosis and addresses the question many people ask themselves: "Is it an illness or is it me?"

In Part II, "Laying the Foundation for Effective Treatment," Chapter 5 provides an overview of the genetic, biological, and environmental determinants of the disorder. You'll come to see how the disorder is not *just* about biology or *just* about environment, but an interaction of the two. Chapter 6 discusses medications for treating the biological aspects of the disorder (mood stabilizers, SGAs, antidepressants) and newer, alternative treatment approaches, including their effectiveness, how we think they work, and their side effects; and the role of psychotherapy in helping you cope more effectively with mood swings and their triggers. Chapter 7 deals with the issue of accepting and coming to terms with a long-term regimen of medications. For people with bipolar disorder—and many other recurrent illnesses—taking medications regularly and over the long-term poses many emotional and practical challenges. In this chapter you'll learn why taking medications consistently is so important and why some of the common arguments for discontinuing them (for example, "I don't need to take pills when I feel well") are erroneous.

Part III, "Practical Strategies for Staying Well," starts with tips to help you manage moods and improve your daily life (Chapter 8), strategies for derailing the upward cycle into mania (Chapter 9), and ways to recognize and handle depression (Chapter 10). I devote a special chapter to dealing with suicidal thoughts and feelings (Chapter 11), which, for many people with bipolar disorder, are a constant source of pain. You'll learn ways to get help from others when you're suicidal and some things you can do to manage these feelings on your own.

Chapter 12 contains a wealth of up-to-date information and advice just for women, on topics including how bipolar disorder affects and is affected by the reproductive cycle, how to have a healthy pregnancy and postpartum period in the context of mood symptoms and medications, and how bipolar disorder and its treatments affect women's health in unique ways. Chapter 13, "Succeeding at Home and at Work: Communication, Problem-Solving Skills, and Dealing Effectively with Stigma," is designed to help you handle the family, social, and work stress that usually accompanies the disorder and to educate others about the challenges you face. Finally, Chapter 14, "'Does My Child Have Bipolar Disorder?': How Would You Know and What Should You Do?," is brand new to this third edition. It explains how to get a good psychiatric evaluation for your child and what to do with the information once you receive it. In that chapter you'll learn about the current options for treatment (which are not only medicinal), as well as what we do and don't know about the future course for children who obtain early diagnoses. My hope is that you'll come away from this chapter with a clear set of steps you can follow to obtain help for your child.

CHAPTER 2

Understanding the Experience of Bipolar Disorder

Although bipolar disorder is very difficult to diagnose, the textbook descriptions of it make it sound like it shouldn't be so hard. After all, what could be more dramatic than shifting between extraordinarily manic behavior, feeling on top of the world and supercharged with energy, to feeling depressed, withdrawn, and suicidal?

Consider a surprising fact: On average, there is an 8-year lag between a first episode of depression or manic/hypomanic symptoms and the first time the disorder is diagnosed and treated (Post & Leverich, 2006). Why should it take so long for a person with the disorder to come to the attention of the mental health profession? In part, the answer is that the behaviors we summarize with the term *bipolar disorder* can look quite different, depending on your perspective. But even when people agree on how a person's behavior deviates from the norm, they can have very different beliefs about what causes the person to be this way. Consider Lauren, a 28-year-old single mother of three:

> Lauren describes herself as an "exercise junkie." In the past 3 weeks, a typical day went like this: Once she got the kids off to school, she rushed to the gym, where she worked out on an exercise bicycle for up to 2 hours. Then she downed a container of yogurt and went hiking for most of the afternoon. She would pick up her kids from school, make dinner for them, and spend the majority of the evening on the StairMaster. But she did not consult her psychiatrist until, by the end of the second week, she had become exhausted and unable to function. At this point she left the children with their grandparents and spent several days sleeping. She admitted to having had several cycles like these.

Now consider how Lauren, her mother, and her doctor describe her behavior. Lauren summarizes her problems as the result of being overcommitted. "It's incredibly difficult to take care of three kids, maintain a household, and try to stay healthy," she argues. "My ex-husband is of very little help, and I don't have many friends who can help out. Sometimes I push myself too hard, but I always bounce back." Her mother feels that she is "irresponsible and self-centered" and would "rather be exercising than taking care of her kids," and questions whether her children are getting enough guidance and structure. Lauren's doctor has diagnosed her as having bipolar II disorder.

Who is right? Lauren thinks her behavior is a function of her environment. Her mother describes the same behaviors as driven by her personality attributes. Her psychiatrist thinks she has a biologically based mood disorder. These different perspectives pose a problem for Lauren, because they lead to very different remedies for the situation. Lauren feels that others—particularly her mother—need to be more supportive and give her more help. Her mother thinks Lauren needs to become more responsible. Her doctor thinks Lauren needs to take a mood-stabilizing medication.

Almost every patient I have worked with describes his or her behavior differently from the way a doctor or family member would. Consider Brent, who has been having trouble holding jobs. He says he is depressed but feels it is due to being unable to deal with his hypercritical boss. As a result, he thinks he needs to switch jobs and find a more permissive work environment. His wife, Alice, thinks he is manic and irritable, not depressed, and that he needs long-term psychotherapy to deal with his problems with male authority figures. She also thinks he drinks too much and needs to attend Alcoholics Anonymous meetings. Brent's doctor thinks he is in a postmanic depressive episode and would benefit from a combination of medications and couple therapy.

Psychiatrists and psychologists usually think of bipolar disorder as a set of symptoms, which must be present in clusters (that is, more than one at a time) and last for a certain length of time, usually in "episodes" that have a beginning phase, a phase in which symptoms are at their worst, and a recovery phase (see the box on page 29). The traditional approach to psychiatric diagnosis described in Chapter 3 follows this line of reasoning. In contrast, people with the illness often prefer to think of bipolar disorder as a series of life experiences, with the actual symptoms being of secondary importance to the factors that provoked them. Family members or significant others may have a different perspective altogether, perhaps one that emphasizes the patient's personality or that views the deviant behavior in historical perspective (for example, "She's always been moody"). Although they are quite different, there is a degree of validity to all three points of view.

In this chapter you'll gain a sense of the different perspectives people take in understanding bipolar mood swings and how these different perspectives can lead to very different beliefs about which treatments should be undertaken. These perspectives include the personal standpoint, as described by patients who have the disorder; the observers' viewpoint, which usually means parents, a spouse, or close friends; and the doctor's viewpoint. Of course, there is also the viewpoint of society as a whole, which may be based on mental illness stigma or half-formed notions of what it means to be mentally ill. Any of these viewpoints can influence your own. Questions to pose to yourself when reading this chapter are:

- "How do I experience swings in my mood?"
- "Are they similar to the ways others with bipolar disorder experience them?"
- "How do I understand the causes of my behavior?"
- "How is my understanding different from the way others perceive me?"
- "How do I see myself differently from the way my doctor sees me?"
- "Do these different understandings mean disagreements about treatments?"
- "Are my choices being driven by societal expectations, which make me feel like I can't tell anyone about this?"

Understanding these varying perspectives will be of considerable use to you, whether you are on your first episode or have had many episodes, in that you will gain some clarity on how your own experiences differ from those of people without bipolar disorder. You may also come to see why others in your family or work or social environment seem so certain that you will benefit from medications, even if you don't agree with them.

Nuts and Bolts: What Is Bipolar Disorder?

Let's begin by defining the syndrome of bipolar disorder. Its key characteristic is extreme mood swings, from manic highs to severe depressions. It is called a mood disorder because it profoundly influences a person's experiences of emotion and displays of *affect* (the way one conveys emotions to others). It is called *bipolar* because the mood swings occur between two poles, high and low, as opposed to unipolar disorder, where mood swings occur along only one pole—the lows. Some people prefer the broader term *bipolar spectrum disorder,* which includes bipolar-like conditions that are less severe than traditional bipolar I or II disorder (for example, "unspecified bipolar disorder") but nonetheless cause suffering and interfere with functioning.

In the manic high state, people experience different combinations of the following: elated or euphoric mood (excessive happiness or expansiveness); irritable mood (excessive anger and touchiness); an increase in activity and energy levels; a decreased need for sleep; grandiosity (an inflated sense of themselves and their abilities); increased talkativeness; racing thoughts or jumping from one idea to

---

What Is a Bipolar Mood Episode?

- A set of symptoms that go together, with a beginning *prodromal* phase, a middle *acute* phase, and a final *recovery* phase.
- The *polarity* of a mood episode can be depressed, manic, hypomanic, or mixed.
- Episodes can last anywhere from a few days to several months.
- Some people switch polarities in the middle of an episode (for example, from depressed to manic or from manic to mixed).

---

another; changes in thinking, perception, and attention (for example, distractibility); and impulsive, reckless behavior. Manic episodes cause significant impairments in a person's work, social, or family life (for example, causing arrests or leading to traffic accidents). If someone has most of these symptoms but without impaired functioning, we use the term *hypomanic*. Manic or hypomanic episodes alternate with intervals of depression, in which people become intensely sad, blue, or "down in the dumps," lose interest in things they ordinarily enjoy, lose weight and appetite, feel fatigued, have difficulty sleeping, feel guilty and bad about themselves, have trouble concentrating or making decisions, and often feel like committing suicide.

Episodes of either mania or depression can last anywhere from days to months. Additionally, many people with bipolar depression (about 34%; McIntyre et al., 2015) experience depressive and manic symptoms simultaneously, in what we call *mixed episodes,* which I'll talk about in the next chapter. It is important to be aware of mixed episodes because they are usually longer and more severe than manic or depressive episodes and are often associated with use of alcohol and drugs (McIntyre et al., 2015).

Episodes of bipolar disorder do not develop overnight, and the severity of manias or depressions varies greatly from person to person. Many people accelerate into mania in stages. In 1973, two leaders in our field, Drs. Gabrielle Carlson and Frederick Goodwin, observed that in the early stages of mania, people feel "wired" or charged up and their thoughts race with numerous ideas (Carlson & Goodwin, 1973). They start needing less and less sleep and feel giddy or mildly irritable (*hypomania*). Later they accelerate into full-blown manias, marked by euphoria, anger, impulsive behaviors such as spending sprees, and intense, frenetic periods of activity. In the most advanced stages of mania, the person can develop mental confusion, delusions (beliefs that are irrational), hallucinations (hearing voices or seeing things), and severe, crippling anxiety. Not everyone experiences these stages, and many people receive treatment before they get to the most advanced stage.

People also spiral into depression gradually, although its stages are less clear-cut. For some, severe depressions seem to come out of nowhere, at times when they were otherwise feeling well. Some people have depressive episodes that are provoked by life events, such as losses of relationships. In others, major depression develops on top of ongoing, chronic periods of depression called *dysthymic* or *persistent depressive disorders* (see Chapter 10).

The periods in between manic and depressive episodes are symptom free in many people. For others, there are symptoms left over from previous episodes, such as sleep disturbance, ongoing irritability, or poor concentration. A 13-year study found that people with bipolar disorder spend an average of one-third of the weeks of their lives in states of depression, about 9% in states of mania, about 6% in mixed or rapid cycling states, and about 53% in *euthymic* or normal mood states (Judd et al., 2002). Most people experience problems in their social and work life because of the illness.

About 1% of the general population has bipolar I disorder, marked by swings from major depression to full mania. Another 1% has bipolar II disorder, in which people vary from severe depression to hypomania, a milder form of mania. New cases of bipolar disorder have been recognized in young children and in the elderly, but the average age at first onset is around 18 years, with a large proportion of people being diagnosed between the ages of 15 and 19 (Merikangas et al., 2007). Bipolar disorder is generally treated with a range of drugs, ideally given in combination with an evidence-based psychotherapy (see Chapter 6):

- Mood stabilizers such as lithium carbonate, valproate (Depakote), or lamotrigine (Lamictal)

- SGAs (also called atypical antipsychotics) such as quetiapine (Seroquel), risperidone (Risperdal), ziprasidone (Geodon), aripiprazole (Abilify), olanzapine (Zyprexa), or lurasidone (Latuda)

- Antianxiety agents such as clonazepam (Klonopin) or lorazepam (Ativan, Temesta)

- Antidepressants such as escitalopram (Lexapro), citalopram (Celexa), sertraline (Zoloft), paroxetine (Paxil), bupropion (Wellbutrin), venlafaxine (Effexor), and, most recently, ketamine (see Chapter 6 for a discussion of the risks associated with antidepressants)

Different Perspectives on Mania and Depression

As noted, the symptoms associated with bipolar mood disorder can be experienced quite differently by the person with the disorder, an observer, and a physician. The disorder affects *moods, behavior,* and *thinking.* Your moods, while usually clear to you, cannot always be observed by others. Likewise, you may not always be aware of your behavior or its impact on others, whereas others (family, friends, or doctors) may be acutely aware of it. When people look at the same set of behaviors or experiences through different lenses, you can imagine how much room there is for misinterpretation.

You may be quite articulate in describing what you are thinking and feeling. When in a manic phase, your thoughts may flow rapidly and life may feel exotic and wonderful. You may speak more than usual and more freely reveal your inner thoughts. Observers such as family members usually focus on your speech, which they may describe as too outspoken, boisterous, loud, or hostile; or your behavior, which they may describe as dangerous to yourself or others or impulsive in ways that negatively affect members of the family (for example, spending or investing your money suddenly). Your doctor is usually attuned to whether your mood, sleep, and behavior are significant departures from your normal state, taking into account how long they've lasted, how intense they are, and whether they cause impairment in your functioning (see the box on page 34).

In the following sections I describe mania and depression in terms of changes in mood, sleep, and behavior. I will focus on the personal experiences that really define episodes of bipolar disorder, which are summarized in the box on page 32.

PERSONALIZED CARE TIP:
Understand that other people see your moods and behaviors differently than you do.

Family and friends may react to changes in your behavior; you may focus on changes in your moods, thoughts, energy levels, or sleep; and doctors may be comparing your mood and behavior to what is normal for you or other patients they have seen. It doesn't mean they're right and you're wrong, but understanding these different perspectives can prevent disagreements that can lead to delays in your diagnosis and treatment.

You may agree that you have variable mood states, but your explanation for what causes these mood states may be quite different from the explanations of your doctor, family members, or friends. People with bipolar disorder often get angry when their doctors bring out a list of symptoms and ask them how many they have had and for how long. They find themselves reluctantly agreeing that they suffer from irritable moods but also know the triggers for these moods that other people may not see.

Experiences of Manic and Depressive Episodes

- Roller-coaster mood states (euphoria, irritability, depression)
- Changes in energy or activity levels
- Changes in thinking and perception
- Suicidal thoughts
- Sleep problems
- Impulsive or self-destructive behavior

Roller-Coaster Mood States

"How can I ever make plans or count on anything or anybody? I never know how I'm going to feel. I can be up and happy and full of ideas, but then the littlest things set me off. I'll drink a cup of tea and it doesn't match my expectation of how hot it should be, and I'll just react—I'll cuss, scream—I'm bitterly volatile . . . I'm afraid of my own moods."

—A 30-year-old woman with bipolar I disorder

Most people with bipolar disorder describe their moods as volatile, unpredictable, "all over the map," or "like a seesaw." Mood states can be irritable (during either depression or mania), euphoric, elevated or excessively giddy (mania), or extremely sad or even numb (depression).

How Your Mood Swings Look to Others

"When I'm mad, nobody better get in my face. I feel like crushing everything and everybody. Every little thing will provoke me. I hate everybody, I hate my life and want to kill myself in some really dramatic way. It's like a sharp-edged, pointed anger, like a burning feeling."

—A 23-year-old woman with bipolar II disorder

Family members, when describing the emotional volatility of their bipolar sibling, child, or parent, tend to emphasize the intimidation they feel in the face of sudden outbursts of rage that they don't feel they've provoked. Consider this interchange between Janelle, age 21, and her mother after Janelle had railed at her mother just minutes earlier.

Janelle: I wanna come back and live with you. I can handle it.

Mother: But you're not in a good place right now. Look how angry you just got.

Janelle: But you told me I wasn't ready to take care of myself! Of course I exploded!

Mother: And you're not. I can tell because you're overreacting to me, and that tells me you're probably not better yet.

It's hard to think of your mood swings as evidence of an illness, especially when every emotional reaction you have seems perfectly justified, given what's just happened to you. To Janelle, her angry outburst seemed an appropriate reaction to her mother, who had just questioned her competency. Her mother knows what her daughter is like when she's well and sees her irritability as a significant departure from this norm.

In contrast, the elated, euphoric periods of the manic experience can feel exceptionally good to the person with the disorder. Dr. Kay Jamison has written extensively about "exuberance," the wondrous feelings that can accompany manic episodes and states of heightened creativity, and how the desire to sustain these feelings can lead a person to stop taking medications (Jamison, 2005). Not all people with bipolar disorder experience their high moods as euphoria, however. For example, Beth, age 42, described her mood during manic episodes as "the sudden awareness that I'm not depressed anymore." Seth, age 27, described his manic states as "tired but wired." For some people, manic moods are just extreme states of irritability.

To your significant others, your euphoria or high mood may seem strange or clownish, and they may not share your enthusiasm, but they are unlikely to be as disturbed by it as they are by your irritability. To your relatives, especially those who have gone through one or more previous episodes with you, euphoric mood is worrisome to the extent that it heralds the development of a full-blown manic episode. Irritability is more troublesome, especially when it is trained on them or makes them fear conflicts or even violence.

Now consider how you experience depression. Would you describe it as an intense sadness, a numbing feeling, a feeling of being removed from others, a lack of interest in things you ordinarily enjoy? One man put it bluntly: "My depressions eat me alive. I feel like I'm in a fish tank that separates me from other people. It's all just hopelessness, and I don't see any future for myself." In contrast, a family member, friend, or lover might see your depression as self-inflicted. People who are close to you might feel sympathetic at first but then get irritated and annoyed. They may think you're not trying hard enough or could make this all go away if you had "the right mental attitude." You will probably experience these reactions as unpleasant, invalidating, and lacking in empathy.

What does the doctor look for? To determine whether the diagnosis is correct (if you are being diagnosed for the first time), or whether you are experiencing a recurrence of the disorder (if you've been diagnosed before), your doctor will evaluate whether your mood states are different, in terms of degree or intensity, from those of healthy people and from your own moods when you are feeling well. Do your moods—euphoric, irritable, or depressed—get out of hand and stay out of hand for days at a time? Do your mood swings cause problems in your social, work, and/or family life? The questions listed in the box at the bottom of this page are examples of questions your doctor may ask in evaluating whether your mood states are diagnosable from a clinical perspective.

Changes in Energy and Activity Levels

If someone asked you to describe your symptoms, you might not focus on your mood fluctuations. In fact, many people who are asked about their mood states answer with descriptions of their energy and activity levels. They're more conscious of what they do or don't do than of how they feel emotionally. They focus on the great increases in energy that they experience during the manic or mixed phases or the decreases in energy they experience during the depressive phases. In fact, DSM-5 lists increases in activity as a primary criterion for a manic episode, alongside elated or irritable mood.

One way to understand these fluctuations is to think of bipolar disorder as a dysregulation of drive states as well as of mood. Changes in normal motivational drives, such as those that govern eating, sleeping, sex, interacting with others, and achievement, are part and parcel of the bipolar pendulum. The normal drives that guide our behavior become intensified in mania and diminished in depression.

Questions a Doctor Might Ask to Distinguish Bipolar Mood Swings from Normal Mood Variability

- ■ "Do your mood swings cause problems in your social or family life?"

- ■ "Do your mood swings lead to decreases in your work productivity that last more than a few days?"

- ■ "Do your mood states last for days at a time with little relief, or do they change when something good happens?"

- ■ "Do other people notice and comment when your mood shifts?"

- ■ "Do your mood changes go along with noticeable changes in thinking, sleeping, and energy or activity levels?"

- ■ "Do your mood swings ever get so out of hand that the police have to be called or a hospitalization becomes necessary?"

If your answer to most of these questions is yes, then it is likely that your mood swings go beyond the normal range.

For example, people in manic episodes are driven toward rewards and often cannot stop themselves from getting entangled in schemes to achieve these rewards. When depressed, these drives are replaced by a withdrawn, amotivational, or apathetic state, with little pleasure from anything. Changes in drive states, of course, can have a tremendous impact on one's daily life and productivity.

Acceleration in Energy

"I feel like I have a motor attached. Everything is moving too slowly, and I want to go, go, go. I feel like one of those toys that somebody winds up and sends spinning or doing cartwheels or whatever . . . and to stop feels like being in a cage."
—A 38-year-old woman with bipolar I disorder

Consider the increases in energy level that accompany manic episodes. For Lauren, this surge took the form of an intense drive to accomplish a particular activity (exercising and getting in shape). For Cynthia it took the form of a strong desire for social contact and stimulation. When manic, she would call people all over the country whom she hadn't spoken to in years, double- and triple-schedule her social calendar, and become bored quickly with the company of others. Jolene's took on a sexual quality: Accumulating as many sexual partners as possible felt to her like a physical need. Neil felt the drive in relation to food: "I couldn't stuff enough things in my mouth. They [the nursing staff at the hospital] put this entire chicken in front of me and I, like, inhaled it."

Grandiose Behaviors

Quite often, increases in activity are accompanied by grandiose thinking or behavior. Grandiosity refers to behavior that most people would consider "over the top," dangerous, and unrealistic. It is usually associated with inflated (sometimes delusional) self-esteem or beliefs about one's powers or abilities.

"I walked into a real fancy restaurant with my mother and started jumping around and running, and there were these chandeliers on the ceiling. I thought I was Superman or something, and I leapt up to grab onto one of them and started swinging on it."
—A 21-year-old man describing his bipolar I manic behavior

Grandiose behaviors usually go along with high or euphoric feelings, but not invariably. You may experience an inflated sense of self-confidence and then feel impatient and irritable because others seem slow to go along with your ideas or plans. Grandiose behavior is detrimental not only because of its associated health risks but also because it leads to feelings of shame, which can compound your depression in the aftermath of a manic episode. In the case of the young man just quoted, the police were called in, a scuffle ensued, and a hospitalization followed.

Although he later related the incident with a degree of bravado, he admitted to feeling quite embarrassed by his public behavior.

In hypomanic episodes, which can occur in either bipolar I or II disorder, a person may have grandiose thoughts that are more muted than in full manic episodes. People in hypomania believe they are more intelligent, better looking, more clever, more creative, and less likely to make poor decisions than anyone else, but it does not reach the level of delusional thinking (for example, having special powers). They may believe that their actions will always lead to rewards and never other consequences.

Depressive Slowing

For every example already given, you can imagine what a counterexample would look like during the depressed phase. In depression, you may become unusually slowed down, like you're "moving through molasses." The most mundane of tasks feels like it requires tremendous effort. Your appetite is usually diminished, and taking a shower or brushing your teeth may seem unusually onerous. Typically, the last thing a depressed person wants is sex, and exercise has even less appeal. Socializing seems like an unpleasant chore that requires too much concentration and mental energy. It may also feel threatening, even if those you are meeting are your friends or neighbors. In depression, it can seem nearly impossible to initiate those tasks even if you desperately want to. In other words, depression is quite different from being lazy.

When drive states are heightened in hypomania and mania, important things can be accomplished and significant plans for personal advancement can be put into place. Unfortunately, the depressive aftermath of these heightened drive states can make the plans seem difficult or even impossible to accomplish. The inability to carry out plans that were hatched while manic can become a source of despair while depressed. A 19-year-old man with bipolar disorder described the switch from mania to depression like this: "I'm like a porpoise. I fly high up in the air and then I yell, 'I'm going down again!' And then I go underneath the water, and all the air, sunshine, and the ocean breeze just vanish."

What Do Others See?

Stephanie, a 20-year-old, had had several episodes of bipolar disorder. Her older sister described her manic, activated behavior this way:

> "She gets involved in these creative projects that we all want to support, like hand-painting dishes or making soap sculptures and trying to sell them. But then she seems to take it too far. She tries to sell them on Instagram and then she gets all riled up and frantic and stays up all night on the computer—and then she crashes and all the projects get dumped."

The rapid changes in energy and activity that accompany highs and lows are often a source of family conflicts. To observers, your activated behavior while initially hypomanic may look attractive or encouraging at first, especially if you are coming out of a depression. But it loses its charm as you become more and more manic and your behavior begins to look frenetic and purposeless. Observers (notably family members) are usually unaware of the feeling of purposefulness that you may be experiencing. They may become angry about your agitated, driven quality and apparent lack of concern for others. In the extreme manic states, family members become worried that you will hurt yourself or someone else. In parallel, they may become frustrated with your inactivity during depressed phases and give you "pep talks" that can contribute to your feelings of guilt or inadequacy.

To a doctor, your increases in activity are the surest clue that hypomania or mania has set in, but he or she will probably look for evidence that your behavior is consistently activated across different situations. The mere fact that you have taken on extra work projects is not enough to point to mania. So your doctor may ask you how many telephone calls you've made, how many hours you've worked, how much sleep you've gotten, how much money you've spent, how many social engagements you've arranged, or how much sexual activity or drive you've had. He or she may also base judgments about your state on how you behave in the interview room: whether you can sit still, whether you answer questions rapidly or interrupt a lot, whether your answers go off on tangents that are well beyond the question. He or she may look for *psychomotor agitation,* such as whether you wring your hands, pick at things, pace, or constantly fidget. Likewise, your physician will look for *psychomotor retardation* (being slowed down in your physical movements) and blank or "blunted" facial expressions during depressions.

A key point to remember here is that, to you, the increases in energy and activity that accompany manic or even hypomanic episodes may feel productive, creative, and purposeful. To others, including your doctor, they may seem pointless, unrealistic, or to signal a developing illness. During depressions, you may feel unable to do even the most basic of things, but others may unfairly accuse you of being lazy. These different perceptions will cause conflict between you and them, but it's important to hear out their perspectives while also explaining your own (see the section on active listening in Chapter 13).

Changes in Thinking and Perception

"My mind feels like I'm in one of those postcards of the city that are taken at night, with the camera moving. Lights feel like they have tails, the whole world is zooming—I love it. My mind is so full of thoughts that I feel like I'm going to burst."
                                        —A 26-year-old woman with bipolar I disorder

Manic and depressive moods almost always involve changes in your thinking. During mania this involves the speeding up of mental functions (racing thoughts) and the verbal expression of one thought after another in rapid-fire fashion (flight of ideas). Many experience the world differently: colors become brighter and sounds become intolerably loud. Mental confusion can accompany the most advanced stages of mania: the world begins to feel like a Ferris wheel spinning out of control.

During mania, your memory can seem extra crisp and clear. You may feel brilliantly sharp, easily able to relate one idea to another, and able to recall events in vivid detail. However, this apparent improvement in memory is often illusory; people experiencing mania think they remember better than they actually do. In fact, attention and concentration can become quite impaired during mania. You cannot keep your mind on any one thing because you are trying to process too many things at once. Your attention can become easily distracted by mundane things like random noises, the facial expressions of others, or the feeling of clothing against your skin.

As mania spirals upward, your thoughts can become increasingly jumbled and even incoherent. Others to whom you speak may be unable to understand you. They may try to keep you focused and ask you to slow down. You will probably find these interactions annoying and have the reaction that others seem slow, dumb, and uninteresting.

Some people with bipolar I disorder develop hallucinations (perceptual experiences that are not real) and delusions (unrealistic, mistaken beliefs) during mania. *Grandiose delusions* are especially common, such as thinking you are exceptionally talented in an arena in which you have had no formal training, that you have extraordinarily high intelligence, or that you have mental telepathy (the ability to receive information from others without speaking). In more severe delusional states, people believe they have special powers, that they are a major public figure, or that they receive messages from God, as this 19-year-old woman recounts.

> "[As I was cycling into mania], I got this idea in my head that I should throw a party for everyone I knew. As the days wore on, I believed that all my doctors—everyone who had ever treated me—were going to come. Before long, I thought Bruce Springsteen was coming, and so was Beyoncé, and I heard the voice of God telling me, 'Go to Dennis [ex-boyfriend]; he wants you.'"

Delusions and hallucinations are particularly scary to significant others, who view them as the most concrete sign of "craziness." Doctors will be especially attuned to these symptoms and will also be on the lookout for less dramatic signs of distorted thinking. Consider the following exchange between a psychologist and a 20-year-old man who was coming off the crest of his manic high. The man sat with a law book in his lap, arguing that he could pass the bar exam without going to law school and would sue anyone who challenged him:

Doctor: Have you had any unusual thoughts or experiences this past week?

Patient: No, not really.

Doctor: Any feelings like you have special powers or that you're a famous person? Last week you were thinking a lot about God and having—

Patient: (Interrupts.) Well, that was last week! *(Laughs.)* No, I don't think of myself that way, but I'm more like a young god, kind of like a teacher. *(Giggles.)* I think I have a lot to offer others.

The client above was still delusional. His thinking frequently got him into trouble with others, especially his parents, who were mostly concerned about his inability to hold a job. They were angered by his unrealistic beliefs in himself and his elaborate schemes for fighting the educational system.

In contrast, during depression it's hard to focus on even one thing. You will experience the slowing down of mental functions as difficulty concentrating or making simple decisions. Colors seem drab. Disturbances of memory are common: you may have difficulty recalling telephone numbers you use regularly, remembering appointments, or following a television program because of trouble holding earlier events in your memory.

Ruminations, in which a person thinks about a certain event again and again, are a frequent accompaniment to depression. Ruminations during the depressive phase are often self-recriminating. For example, when Margie became depressed, she was preoccupied with the thought "Was Paul [her boss] insulted when I didn't sit next to him at the meeting?" Similarly, Cameron recalled, "When I was manic I jokingly asked my friend if his wife was hot, and I couldn't stop thinking about how stupid that was when I got depressed." Depressive ruminations frequently include guilt or shame over past misdeeds, or feeling worthless, hopeless, or helpless. They can become all-encompassing and affect one's day-to-day functioning. When Patrice became depressed, she found herself "rehearsing like a mantra" statements like "I suck . . . I hate myself . . . I'm such a bitch."

Suicidal Thoughts

Ruminations often take the form of suicidal preoccupations—thoughts about the various ways one could kill oneself. These ruminations are most common during depressive or mixed episodes but can also be present during mania. Depending on how desperate a person feels, he or she may act on these thoughts or impulses, often with dire consequences.

Friends and family members will be particularly upset and scared by your suicidal thoughts, if voiced to them, and will usually do their best to help you deal with these thoughts, although they may not know what to say or do. Your therapist or physician is also likely to ask about them (for example, "Are you having any thoughts of hurting or killing yourself, as many people do when they're down?"). If you have never had suicidal thoughts before and have them now, you may feel afraid to express them. You may fear that the physician will hospitalize you immediately. This is certainly one treatment option, but not the only one. Others may include psychotherapy, modifications of your medication regimen, and/or various forms of community or family support.

Take the chance of discussing suicidal thoughts with your physician or therapist— you may find that some of these thoughts dissipate after you've shared them with someone else. You may also learn that mental health professionals are more helpful at such times than you would have expected. I will discuss suicidal feelings and actions in more detail in Chapter 11.

> **Effective prevention:** Telling your doctor—or a trusted friend or family member—about any suicidal thoughts you have may help alleviate those thoughts. Disclosing these thoughts may also prompt suggestions that you may not have considered.

Sleep Disturbances

Virtually all people with bipolar disorder experience disturbances of sleep in the period leading up to and during their episodes. When you get manic, you may feel no need to sleep. Sleeping feels like a waste of time, especially when so many things can get accomplished in the middle of the night! If you have hypomania, you may feel like you can get along with only 4 hours of sleep and still feel rested. During depression, sleep can feel like the only thing you want to do. When you are depressed, you may become hypersomnic, sleeping much more than usual (for example, 16 hours a day) and become unproductive and unable to function outside of the home. Alternatively you may have insomnia and find that sleep eludes you. You may lie awake at night tossing and turning, ruminating about the same problems over and over again, and then feel exhausted the next day. Sleep can feel frustratingly out of your reach.

Are sleep problems a symptom of bipolar disorder, or do they actually cause problems in mood? It appears that they are both symptom and cause. Most people have changes in mood when they have trouble sleeping, but people with bipolar disorder are particularly vulnerable to changes in the sleep–wake cycle (Harvey, 2011). I say more about sleep disruptions and mood states in Chapter 5.

Your doctor will probably ask you about sleep disturbances, with emphasis on whether the problem is falling asleep, waking up in the middle of the night, or waking up too early. A key question is whether you have *insomnia* (inability to fall or stay asleep, usually a sign of depression) or *decreased need for sleep,* meaning that you don't sleep much because you don't feel like you need it (a sign of mania or hypomania). Your doctor may ask you to keep track of your sleep if you have trouble recalling the nature of your disturbances. A spouse or partner may be affected by your sleep patterns—when one person can't sleep, the other often can't as well. Your own irritability, as well as that of your family members, can be a function of lack of sleep or inconsistent sleep habits.

Impulsive, Self-Destructive, or Addictive Behaviors

What do you usually do when you start to feel manic? When you are loaded with energy, you may feel like you have to have an outlet. Ordinary life moves too slowly. As a result, when people get manic, they often lose their inhibitions and behave impulsively. Many of these impulsive behaviors can be threatening to one's life or health, such as driving recklessly on the freeway, performing daredevil acts, or having unprotected sex with different partners. Martha's impulsive behavior (see Chapter 1) was a major cause of the marital problems she had after her manic episode.

Some people make unwise decisions, like spending a lot of money indiscriminately. Kevin was 34 and lived with his father. When manic, he convinced his father to liquidate part of his IRA, which Kevin invested wildly in various commodities. Most of the money disappeared. His family, understandably, was livid; his older brothers refused to talk to him anymore. Prior to this incident, Kevin had been making plans to move out on his own. But his father insisted he pay the money back before he agreed to help finance Kevin's attempts to become independent.

Carl, age 40, had bipolar II disorder and, when hypomanic, spent tremendous amounts of money on home improvements. He installed elaborate fireplaces, impractical bathroom fixtures, and eye-catching but gaudy paintings. His partner, Roberta, with whom he lived, became increasingly frustrated about their dwindling finances, and their conflicts intensified. In Roberta's view, Carl was unwilling to recognize his hypomania as the source of the problem.

Self-destructive behavior can take many forms. Many people turn to alcohol or drugs during manic or hypomanic episodes. Substance abuse is not an essential symptom of bipolar disorder, but it can become intertwined with mood symptoms in such a way that each worsens the other. Alcohol is often sought as a means of bringing oneself down from the high state and quelling the anxiety, confusion, and sleep disturbance that typically go with it. Some use cocaine, amphetamine, or marijuana to heighten and intensify the euphoric experiences of mania. During a depression, alcohol or drugs are usually craved as a means of dulling the pain, or what we call self-medicating. More than any other associated condition, drug and alcohol abuse makes the course of your bipolar disorder much worse (Yen et al., 2016). Mark, 36, who had bipolar II disorder complicated by alcohol dependence, described the role alcohol played in his depressions:

"When I'm down, drinking for me is like a security blanket. When I'm feeling my worst, the bottle is there in the closet, like an old friend. I don't think about what it's doing to my body, only that I need to numb myself out. Sometimes, just knowing there's a bottle in the cabinet is enough to make me feel better. I just can't stop myself. I keep blowing it."

Another person with bipolar disorder, Thad, 27, was less clear on why he drank when he was manic. While in the hospital, he summarized it like this: "I don't know what it is with me and booze. I know it's not funny, but whenever I get that way [high, manic], I just seem to need to tie one on."

Family members may be more bothered by your drug and alcohol use than your mood swings. They may even define your problems as alcohol or drug related and reject the bipolar diagnosis, thinking it is a way for you to justify continuing to drink. They may be incorrect about this, but you may need to undergo a thorough diagnostic assessment and life history to know for sure whether you have both (see Chapter 3).

Your doctor will probably be skeptical of the bipolar diagnosis unless there is concrete evidence that your mood swings occur when you do not use drugs or alcohol. Jeff, for example, had had several manic episodes before he developed problems with alcohol, and the bipolar diagnosis seemed justified. On the other hand, Kate's alcohol problems developed well before there was any evidence of mood swings, and her mood episodes—although characterized by irritability, sleep disturbance, lethargy, suicidality, and impulsiveness—were eventually attributed to the effects of alcohol intoxication.

Summary: Different Perspectives

As you already know or have just seen, people with bipolar disorder have very distinct experiences. Varying emotional states and changes in energy, judgment, thinking, and sleep characterize the swings between the poles. Family members or significant others are not likely to understand these widely fluctuating moods (unless they have bipolar disorder themselves) and are likely to focus on how your behavior affects them and others in your life. Most psychiatrists will be less interested in the meaning these experiences have for you than in the symptoms you've had that are consistent or inconsistent with the bipolar diagnosis, or that point to specific treatments (see Chapter 6).

These different perspectives may be a source of frustration for you, because you may feel like others don't understand you or aren't interested in your inner life. Likewise, your family members, and perhaps your doctor, will be frustrated if you seem to be oblivious to or unconcerned about the effects of your behavior on others. These disparate perceptions can be a source of conflicts over the treatment plan: You may feel that you've had profound experiences, but others only seem interested in labeling you as a sick person and demanding that you take pills. Many people with bipolar disorder, out of frustration over these issues, reject the notion that they are having symptoms and also reject the diagnosis and its associated treatments (see Chapters 3 and 4). Others are fortunate enough to be able to communicate effectively with their doctor and family members, who correspondingly make attempts to understand a perspective different from their own. The hope, of course, is that you will find a treatment regimen that will stabilize your mood without minimizing the significance that these personal experiences have held for you.

Whether you are having your first episode or have had many, the first step in obtaining optimal treatment is to get a proper diagnosis. Chapter 3 deals with this very important issue by answering the following questions:

- How is the disorder actually diagnosed by mental health professionals?
- What symptoms and behaviors do doctors look for?
- What can you expect during the diagnostic process?
- How will your doctor elicit information from you to determine the diagnosis?

In describing the diagnostic criteria, I'll touch on the important issue of *border conditions* and *comorbidities*:

- How do you know if you have bipolar disorder versus some other psychiatric illness?
- Does the diagnosis give a reasonable explanation for your behavior?
- If not, are there other diagnoses that fit you better?
- Do you have both bipolar disorder and a "comorbid" disorder?

CHAPTER 3

Into the Doctor's Court
Getting an Accurate Diagnosis

> The endless questioning finally ended. My psychiatrist looked at me,
> there was no uncertainty in his voice. "Manic–depressive illness."
> I admired his bluntness. I wished him locusts on his lands and
> a pox upon his house. Silent, unbelievable rage. I smiled pleasantly.
> He smiled back. The war had just begun.
> —KAY REDFIELD JAMISON, *An Unquiet Mind* (1995, p. 104)

You're not alone in feeling that mania and depression are very personal and intense experiences. Nor are you alone if you are wary of any stranger's ability to understand what you're going through, no matter how highly qualified as a medical professional. Many people experiencing bipolar symptoms postpone seeing a doctor for as long as possible because they already feel thoroughly misunderstood. Others have received multiple diagnoses from one or more professionals and have rejected these diagnoses as inadequate explanations for their experiences. Still others grudgingly accept a diagnosis of bipolar disorder but then express their resistance by refusing to comply with their treatment regimen. If you fit into any of these categories, I hope you'll reconsider the benefits of a professional diagnosis.

No diagnostic label can completely capture your unique situation. In fact, you may feel offended by the diagnostic label because it is incomplete, impersonal, or simply doesn't do justice to your life experiences. But these labels do serve a purpose. First, using standardized labels allows clinicians to communicate with each other. If I refer a client of mine to another mental health professional and say that "she has bipolar I disorder, with a current depressive episode and mood-incongruent psychotic features," I can be reasonably sure that this other doctor will know what to expect. This common language serves you well should you switch doctors, as so many of us do today.

Second, an accurate diagnosis is important to selecting the right treatment. If you are misdiagnosed as having depression alone, for example, your doctor might recommend a standard antidepressant medication such as fluoxetine (Prozac), sertraline (Zoloft), or bupropion (Wellbutrin) without a mood stabilizer like lithium (see Chapter 6). If you actually have bipolar I disorder, this treatment regimen could cause you to swing into mania or hypomania. Likewise, if you were diagnosed as having bipolar II when the real problem is ADHD, you might not benefit from the SGAs you've been given. An accurate diagnostic label helps doctors treat the whole syndrome that is affecting you rather than just the symptoms you are reporting right now.

Diagnoses also help you prepare for the challenges the future might hold. Will you have another episode? Will you be able to go back to work? How will you know when you're getting sick again? Being confident of the diagnosis makes you more likely to benefit from the volumes of information that researchers and clinicians have gathered from thousands of people with bipolar disorder. You will be more convinced of the importance of taking mood-stabilizing or antipsychotic or antidepressant medications to prevent future episodes, but you may also learn that those medications have to be chosen carefully and in a particular order, with dosages increased in a schedule that works for you. If you've just had your first episode of depression or mania, you may feel able to go back to work right away, but the experiences of many people who needed a period of convalescence before going back to work will provide some important guidance.

> **Effective prevention:** An accurate diagnosis—including whether you actually have bipolar disorder, the type you have, and whether you have any comorbid disorders—leads to a clearer prognosis (the ability to predict what course your disorder is likely to follow), which may help minimize the life disruptions associated with mood disorder episodes.

The Criteria for a Diagnosis of Bipolar Disorder

Psychiatrists and psychologists rely on the *Diagnostic and Statistical Manual* to make diagnoses. Note the term *manual* in the title: A clinician should be able to pick up the manual and decide whether a patient meets the criteria for a specific psychiatric illness. Applying these diagnostic criteria reliably (that is, being able to tell one disorder from another) cannot be done quickly or haphazardly: it requires considerable training, experience, and skill on the part of the mental health professional.

The first edition of the DSM was published in 1952; other editions were published in 1968, 1980, and 1994 (with text revisions in 1987 and 2000). DSM-5 was published in 2013. Each version has been informed by the research and observations of many investigators and clinicians and by experiences elicited from numerous patients with psychiatric disorders. No diagnostic manual is perfect, and not everyone agrees with the premises of the DSM. In my opinion, DSM-5 is a critical and useful manual, and no one has created another diagnostic system that provides a reasonable alternative. Keep in mind, though, that the disorders and symptoms in DSM-5 (for example, whether you have insomnia or not) are really dimensions, with people falling along a continuum of bipolarity or sleep disturbance. I'll say more about this shortly.

Your doctor will first identify which symptoms you have (for example, irritability, increased activity), how severe these symptoms are, and how long they have lasted. From your particular pattern of symptoms, he or she will then determine if you are currently in an episode of depression, hypomania, or mania, and if so, whether the diagnosis of bipolar disorder—as outlined in DSM-5—fits you. If it does, your doctor will then be concerned with which kind of bipolar disorder you have: Is it bipolar type I or II? Unspecified bipolar disorder? Are there mixed features? Is your episode mild, moderate, or severe? Are you currently in full or partial remission?

Bipolar I Disorder

The box on page 47 describes the major subtypes of bipolar disorder listed in DSM-5. For bipolar I disorder, you must have had at least one manic episode characterized by a sustained period of elated, euphoric, or irritable mood, increased activity or energy, and three other associated manic symptoms (grandiose thinking, decreased need for sleep, pressured speech, racing thoughts or rapidly flowing ideas, increases in activities that are either aimed at some goal or are agitated and purposeless, distractibility, or impulsive behavior) that lasted a week or more or were interrupted by emergency treatment. The symptoms must cause impairment in functioning such as problems at work, at school, or at home. If manic symptoms co-occur with three or more symptoms of depression, the episode is referred to as "mixed." Note how these symptoms capture the essence of the subjective experiences of mania described in Chapter 2: the roller-coaster mood states, increases in activity and drive, changes in thinking and perception, and impulsive or self-destructive behaviors.

If this is the first time you're encountering these criteria, you may find yourself reacting negatively to how reductionistic the symptom labels are: what you see as clear insights and the energy to get important things done may be labeled by DSM-5 as grandiosity, for example. Your reactions are certainly understandable.

These symptom labels are shorthand for very complex life experiences and mood states, much like the diagnostic label itself.

In most cases, a person with bipolar I disorder will also have had, at some point in life, a *major depressive episode*: a minimum 2-week period with at least five symptoms of major depressive illness (low mood, loss of interests, weight loss or appetite change, lack of energy or fatigue, agitated or slowed movements, difficulty concentrating, low self-worth, sleep problems, suicidal thoughts or actions) with significant difficulty in everyday functioning.

The DSM-5 Subtypes of Bipolar Disorder

Bipolar I disorder

- At least one lifetime episode of mania
- Although not required for the diagnosis, at least one lifetime episode of major depressive disorder

Bipolar II disorder

- At least one lifetime episode of hypomanic disorder
- At least one lifetime episode of major depressive disorder

Unspecified bipolar disorder (formerly not otherwise specified, *or NOS)*

- Rapid alteration between manic and depressive symptoms that meet the severity criteria for mania or depression but fall short of the duration criteria (episodes of hypomania lasting fewer than 4 days; depressive episodes lasting less than 2 weeks). This category also covers people with multiple manic episodes (with impairment of functioning) that fall one symptom short of the required number of symptoms.

Episode designations

- The full diagnosis requires a "polarity" designation of your current episode (manic, hypomanic, depressed) plus two "specifiers." The first is whether *mixed features* are present (that is, at least three symptoms from the opposite polarity, such as racing thoughts that accompany a depressive episode). The second specifier is an *anxiety/ distress* feature: whether you have severe subjective apprehension, nervousness, or anxiety in conjunction with your depression or mania. People with comorbid anxiety sometimes do not respond to mood stabilizers alone and may require other medications or therapies to stabilize fully.

If you've never had a major depressive episode but you've had mania, your doctor will still diagnose you with bipolar I disorder, based on the assumption that a depression will eventually occur if your disorder is not treated adequately. Indeed, there are people who have had only manic or mixed episodes ("unipolar mania"), but it is rare: in a 20-year follow-up of 27 people who had had a manic episode but no periods of depression, 20 developed a major depressive episode in the interim, suggesting that most people with unipolar mania have just not had a depressive episode yet (Solomon et al., 2003).

Bipolar I Course Features

People with bipolar I disorder can experience episodes of mania and depression in different sequences. Some people have manias followed by depressions followed by periods in which their mood returns to normal (*euthymic* mood). Other people have depressions followed by manias, which are then followed by euthymic mood. Some people with bipolar I have recurrent hypomanic episodes, but in contrast to bipolar II disorder, these hypomanic episodes may escalate into full manic episodes if not treated. Other people with bipolar I or II disorder have rapid cycling states, which I'll discuss further later.

In DSM-5, mixed features are not a type of episode as they were in the previous edition (DSM-IV-TR; American Psychiatric Association, 2000). They are a dimension along which depressed people with different amounts of mania or hypomania can be compared. What this means is that, even if your diagnosis ends up being major depressive disorder, you may meet criteria for a mixed features specifier if you have three or more symptoms of mania or hypomania.

It can be difficult to tell if you have major depression only or major depression with mixed features. Irritability, distractibility, and psychomotor agitation can occur in either state. Some people describe depression with mixed features as a "tired but wired" feeling. You can feel extraordinarily pessimistic and hopeless, fatigued, and unable to concentrate, but still feel "revved," anxious, irritable, driven, and sleep deprived, with your thoughts moving very rapidly. Others feel manic, elevated, and full of ideas and energy but also become preoccupied with death or feelings of worthlessness, lose their appetite, and complain of terrible problems falling and saying asleep.

Bipolar II Disorder

In the introduction to this edition, I noted that some writers think of bipolar disorders on a spectrum or dimension, with bipolar I having the most severe manic symptoms, bipolar II the next most severe, and unspecified bipolar disorder the least severe. According to this view, bipolar II is a point along a continuum of bipolarity, rather than a separate category as it is in DSM-5 (Phelps, 2012). The spectrum conceptualization could help identify subthreshold forms of bipolar disorder that may not respond well to antidepressants, but it's unclear that these subtypes directly parallel illness severity or degree of impairment. In fact, one study found that children with unspecified bipolar disorder had more impairment over time compared to those with bipolar I or II (Birmaher et al., 2006).

In bipolar II, a person alternates between major depressive episodes and hypomanic episodes. Hypomanias are milder forms of mania that may not last as long as full manias (the minimum requirement for the diagnosis is 4 days), but the number of symptoms required is the same (that is, elated or irritable mood, increased activity, and three other symptoms). People with hypomania experience the first of the three stages of mania described in Chapter 2, but they do not go beyond this: they have sleep problems, irritability, increased activity, and an inflated sense of themselves, but not to the dangerous or psychotic levels of the fully manic person. Generally, hypomanic episodes do not cause big problems in your work, family, or social life, but you may still experience some interpersonal difficulties when in this state (for example, more arguments with your spouse or kids or more confrontations with coworkers). Hypomanias do not require hospitalization.

Hypomanic episodes can be quite enjoyable to the person experiencing them. In general, others will be baffled and put off by your energetic, hypersexual, intrusive, and driven quality when hypomanic (for example, they may tell you to "chill out"). Your family members or friends may also be relieved by what they perceive to be the disappearance of the depressive states that often precede the energized one. Consider Heather, who had bipolar II disorder:

> Heather, age 36, was a professional conference coordinator. She described herself as almost always depressed. When she went through her divorce, contact with her soon-to-be ex-husband "felt like a drug I needed—it was the only thing that kept me alive." She became suicidal at that time. But soon after, she began planning a conference for a group of architects and started dating one of them. The work and the new relationship "wired me . . . I got my energy back. I stopped sleeping and staying in my condo so much of the time . . . went walking my dog at 2 A.M., sent out emails at all times of night. People told me I seemed much better, like I had my old self back, but I knew I was going overboard."

The treatment decisions you make with your doctor are likely to be different for bipolar II and I. Most current guidelines suggest you take a mood stabilizer or SGA for either condition. However, there is evidence that some people with bipolar II depression can be treated with an antidepressant alone (Amsterdam et al., 2010). Ten years ago, most practitioners considered this unthinkable because of the potential of antidepressants to cause rapid cycling of moods. The most recent research, however, indicates that the short-term outcomes of people with bipolar II depressions who received antidepressants alone do not differ from those of people who received lithium alone or antidepressants plus lithium (Altshuler et al., 2017; see Chapter 6).

People with bipolar II are more likely to develop rapidly cycling moods than those with bipolar I disorder, indicating that it can be more difficult to find an optimal medication regimen (Schneck et al., 2008). Chronic periods of depression appear to be the major difficulty experienced by people with bipolar II disorder, with one study finding that patients spent 37 weeks depressed for every 1 week they spent hypomanic (Judd et al., 2003).

Keep in mind what different bipolar subtypes may mean for your treatment. If you have bipolar II, you still need to be careful about your high periods: hypo-manias, while fun and exciting, can herald the development of severe depressions or more rapid mood cycles. The strategies I recommend for maintaining wellness and recognizing the beginning of new episodes (Chapters 8 and 9) will be just as relevant to your health.

Unspecified Bipolar Disorder

DSM-5 has a "hedge" category called unspecified bipolar disorder. This cat-egory usually is reserved for people who have had several manic episodes that do not meet the full duration criteria. Some definitions require you to have had a major depressive episode as well. For example, Shelley, 31, had had three hypo-manic episodes with irritability, decreased need for sleep, distractibility, and pres-sure of speech that each lasted 1–2 days; her single depressive episode came after the birth of her first child.

Estevan, age 46, had lengthy, unremitting periods of depression that his doctor originally labeled as dysthymic disorder. His diagnosis was changed to unspecified bipolar disorder when he had two brief (2-day) manic episodes marked by irritable mood, grandiosity, and decreased need for sleep, along with a sudden deterioration in his functioning. Both episodes remitted quickly but, sadly, were followed by a return of his depressive state.

Unspecified bipolar disorder is most frequently used to describe children or adolescents whose cycling pattern looks much like an adult bipolar I cycle, but whose episodes are frequent and very short (for example, lasting only a day). Although this symptom pattern may sound like it could characterize almost any child, it is actually fairly rare: the child has to meet full mania or hypomania criteria and show clear changes in functioning for this single day. Children also have to have had multiple episodes like this, not just one. About 58% of kids who have the unspecified bipolar diagnosis and are genetically susceptible to bipolar disorder (that is, they have a first- or second-degree relative with bipolar disorder) "convert" to bipolar I or II disorder in 4–5 years. They also experience substantial impairments in their school and social functioning even before the conversion occurs (Birmaher et al., 2009). So, unspecified bipolar disorder can be used to help identify people who are at risk for developing the full syndrome with associated problems in functioning.

Rapid Cycling

Rapid cycling is a "course specifier" in the DSM-5 system, meaning that it can accompany the bipolar I, II, or unspecified subtypes. In rapid cycling, people quickly switch back and forth from mania or hypomania to depression or mixed mania/depression, with four or more distinct episodes in a single year. In other words, you have many episodes in a short period of time. Some people even have ultra-rapid cycling, in which they have at least one episode per month, or ultradian rapid cycling, which means switching from one mood pole to the other several times in 1 week or even within a single 24-hour period.

If you have rapid cycling, you may have symptoms that don't fit neatly into the mood disorder criteria, such as severe anxiety or migraine headaches (Gordon-Smith et al., 2015). As a result, you may have to go through quite a bit of trial and error with your doctor before finding the right combination of medications. Your doctor should help you rule out other factors that could contribute to your frequent mood swings, such as thyroid abnormalities. The good news is that rapid cycling appears to be a time-limited phenomenon: people do not rapidly cycle their whole lives (Coryell, 2009; Schneck et al., 2008). I'll talk more about frequent cycling in Chapter 6 on drug treatments.

The Progression of Bipolar Episodes

Many people—including those who have not yet been diagnosed with bipolar disorder and those who have but are in doubt about it—find the diagnostic criteria quite confusing. Many clinicians do as well! You may wonder whether having only one or two manic or depressive symptoms qualifies you for the diagnosis or what it means if you had one symptom in January, none in February and March, and a different symptom in April. You and others around you may wonder whether your rapid mood swings are just features of your personality.

One of the keys to making the diagnosis of bipolar disorder is to think in terms of clusters of symptoms that cycle together in discrete episodes. There must be evidence that you have had time-limited mood episodes that alternate with periods of healthy functioning or that alternate with intervals of the opposite pole of the illness (for example, manic episodes that are followed by depressive episodes). As I mentioned in Chapter 2, episodes are intervals when your mood, activity level, thinking patterns, and sleep all change at the same time (see the graph on page 52). Additionally, episodes usually have a prodromal buildup phase, an active

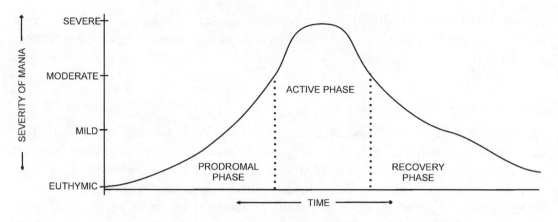

The phases of a manic episode.

or acute phase, and a residual or recovery phase. Consider Tom, a 46-year-old with bipolar I disorder:

> Tom described a 6-month-long depressive episode that progressed into a mixed episode. As his depression developed over several weeks (prodromal period), he experienced increasing sadness and loss of interest in his usual activities, but a mild paranoia with anxiety also developed. He began to feel that no one in his family was on his side and that they were talking about him behind his back. As he progressed into a full mixed episode, his depression worsened and so did his anxiety and paranoia, but he also developed an irritability and anger that he expressed inappropriately. In one case, he broke some dishes; in another, he kicked in a door. He had an altercation with the neighbors which he left cursing. His family members became scared of him. His sleep deteriorated, and his thoughts took on a rapid, ruminative quality ("I think about death and that there's no future—doesn't seem like there's anything I or anybody can do"). As he recovered from this episode—a process that took several months and required an increase in his lamotrigine dosage and the addition of an SGA—he felt less hopeless, his thoughts slowed down, and he became easier for others to communicate with. Nonetheless, he continued to feel anxious, sad, and easily irritated by others. In his sessions with his therapist, he began to see how his behavior affected his family and that at least some of his paranoid feelings were unfounded.

Notice how, in Tom's case, a single episode progressed in stages. Some symptoms (his hopelessness and paranoia) changed more rapidly than others (his sadness and anger). The length of bipolar episodes varies from person to person.

It may not always be possible to tell when you are finished with an episode (that is, you are in the recovery phase) or developing a new one. If you have already had a number of episodes, you probably are more attuned than most people to what it feels like to be ill versus well. But if you're in your first episode, you may be unclear as to when you're back to normal or what it feels like to be getting sick again. As you'll see when we discuss self-management techniques, knowing your prodromal phase symptoms (the signs that an episode of mania, hypomania, or depression has begun) and when to get treatment for these symptoms helps protect you against further escalation of the disorder.

Diagnostic Self-Evaluation as a Starting Point or a Backup Check

The self-administered checklist that follows is a starting point in determining whether your diagnosis is correct. If you have never seen a psychiatrist but think you might need to, the checklist will orient you to the kinds of mania or hypomania symptoms your doctor will ask about. If you've already received the diagnosis of bipolar disorder and are suspicious of it, the list provides you and your doctor with a backup check. The Mood Disorder Questionnaire is not a diagnostic instrument: just because you check off the items does not mean that you have the disorder, only that you may have had symptoms of mania that you and your doctor will want to discuss. Likewise, if none of the symptoms sound familiar, you may still have the disorder, but you and your doctor will want to discuss other diagnoses as well.

The checklist does not include the depressive pole of the illness (the symptoms of major depressive disorder described earlier, such as intensely sad mood, loss of interests, insomnia, or fatigue) because, technically, to be diagnosed with bipolar I disorder you do not need to have had a depressive episode if you have had one manic (or one mixed) episode.

In filling out the checklist, and in discussing the symptoms with your physician, keep in mind that these symptoms must co-occur during the same period of time. Having had racing thoughts at one time in your life and decreased need for sleep during another period is not the same thing as having a manic or hypomanic episode.

What the Doctor Will Want to Know: Steps toward Diagnosis and Treatment

Many of my patients have come to me feeling that their initial diagnosis was made too hastily. Either they became victims of the managed care rush to make diagnostic and treatment decisions or they were never asked about elements of their life story that, to them, seemed critical to an understanding of their mood problems.

Mood Disorder Questionnaire: A Self-Administered Checklist

Has there been a period of time when you were not your usual self and you:

	Yes	No
Felt so good or so hyper that other people thought you were not your normal self or you were so hyper that you got into trouble?	_____	_____
Were so irritable that you shouted at people or started fights or arguments?	_____	_____
Felt much more self-confident than usual?	_____	_____
Got much less sleep than usual and found you didn't really miss it?	_____	_____
Were much more talkative or spoke much faster than usual?	_____	_____
Had thoughts racing through your head or couldn't slow down your mind?	_____	_____
Were so easily distracted by things around you that you had trouble concentrating or staying on track?	_____	_____
Had much more energy than usual?	_____	_____
Were much more active or did many more things than usual?	_____	_____
Were much more social or outgoing than usual, for example, telephoning friends in the middle of the night?	_____	_____
Were much more interested in sex than usual?	_____	_____
Did things that were unusual for you or that other people might have thought were excessive, foolish, or risky?	_____	_____
Spent excessive money that got you or your family into trouble?	_____	_____
If you checked yes to more than one of the above, have several of these ever happened during the same period of time?	_____	_____

How much of a problem did any of these cause you (being unable to work; having family, money, or legal troubles; getting into arguments or a fight; etc.)? Please check one response only.

No problem _____   Minor problem _____

Moderate problem _____   Serious problem _____

Adapted by permission from Hirschfeld et al. (2000). Copyright © 2000 Robert M. A. Hirschfeld, MD.

Whether you have already been diagnosed and wish to review whether your case has been handled correctly, or you are preparing for your first evaluation, understanding the sequence of steps in the diagnostic and treatment process will help. These steps include the diagnostic referral, reviewing your prior medical records, and the diagnostic interview.

As I review the steps in the diagnostic process, keep in mind that your doctor will base your diagnosis largely on the symptoms you have recently experienced. How you developed these symptoms (also called the *etiology* of your disorder) is a different question. You may feel that these symptoms are not the product of imbalances in the brain as much as current stressors (for example, having just broken off a relationship) or childhood issues (traumatic events such as physical or sexual abuse or prolonged separation experiences). If your doctor is doing his or her job, these psychological issues will be addressed later in treatment, after the diagnosis has been established and after the two of you have agreed on a medication treatment plan. If your doctor does not do psychotherapy, ask him or her for a referral so that you receive simultaneous treatment with a therapist. In Chapter 6, I talk more about the kinds of psychotherapy that may be most helpful after an episode.

Step 1: The Diagnostic Referral

The first step in getting a proper diagnosis is to find the right doctor. If you have private insurance, you may be able to see someone who specializes in mood disorders. If it is unclear whether a doctor is a specialist, you should feel free to ask. You can also obtain information about who in your area treats persons with mood disorders from the American Psychiatric Association (888-35-PSYCH; *apa@psych. org*) or the Castle-Connolly "America's Top Doctors" website (*www.castleconnolly. com/doctors/results2.cfm*). If you are seeking a therapist who knows something about mood disorders, the provider referral list of the Association for Behavioral and Cognitive Therapies (*www.abct.org*) is a good place to start.

If you have a managed care plan, Medicare, or no insurance, you may not have a lot of choice about whom you see. Hopefully, your plan will direct you to a mental health professional who has at least some experience in mood disorders. But this may require some detective work on your part. Nancy, for example, thought she might have bipolar disorder and wanted to see a psychiatrist but was confused by the number of doctors she found online who purportedly treated mood problems. She called several but could reach only their receptionists, who gave her information like "Dr. Rosen sees mainly adults" or "She has a general psychiatry practice." She finally discussed the matter with her general practitioner, who referred her to a psychiatrist in town who was covered by her insurance plan and, although not a specialist, was known to have experience in the treatment of mood disorders.

In the sections below, "your doctor" refers to the mental health professional who is conducting your diagnostic evaluation, whether or not he or she is actually an MD. In today's managed care environment, your initial evaluation may not be done by a psychiatrist. Many insurance plans have an intake worker who determines the need for follow-up psychiatric care. However, this does not mean your care will be inferior. Mental health professionals from other disciplines (for example, psychology, social work, nursing) are often well trained in diagnostic methods. There is a good chance that this intake worker will refer you to a psychiatrist if there is any suspicion that you have bipolar disorder, and he or she will almost certainly do so if you have had prior manic episodes. But if you don't feel that this initial evaluation was adequate or led to appropriate follow-up care, be assertive with your health care program in asking for follow-up appointments or second opinions.

Step 2: Reviewing Your Records

The doctor you do see will probably want to review any prior medical records that other doctors have for you. The records usually contain previous diagnoses (which may or may not include bipolar disorder), your previous medications (including how well you responded and if you experienced side effects from them), relevant blood tests, and information about your medical, social, and family history.

Your doctor will ask you to sign a HIPAA "release of information" form, which allows him or her to gain access to your records. Of course, you can refuse to sign this release, but refusing is not in your best interest. Even if you feel your previous psychiatric care was flawed, it will help your doctor to know about these flaws, as well as what treatments were tried and why they were discontinued. Your new doctor will not necessarily recommend the same treatments you've had in the past.

If this is your first visit to a mental health professional, you may not have prior medical records. If you have had other psychiatric consultations, you may wonder why your new doctor needs to conduct a new diagnostic evaluation and can't simply review your medical records. There are many reasons that medical charts alone are inadequate for determining your diagnosis, treatment, or prognosis. First, medical charts are often sketchy. They contain comments like "patient complains of depression" without specifying the severity of this depression, whether other symptoms co-occurred, or whether the depression occurred for a length of time or in discrete episodes. Chart notes are often written by professionals focused on other aspects of your medical or psychiatric care (for example, an endocrinologist evaluating thyroid functioning) rather than your bipolar disorder. So think of the prior medical records as supplemental information that may help your doctor clarify the diagnosis and treatment plan. The majority of his or her judgments will come from the face-to-face diagnostic interview.

Step 3: What to Expect from the Diagnostic Interview

The diagnosis of bipolar disorder is established through a clinical interview, in which you will be asked whether you have experienced certain symptoms over a given period of time and over your lifetime. If your doctor conducts a comprehensive interview, he or she will ask not only about your mood disorder symptoms but also whether you have ever had psychotic symptoms (for example, hallucinations), drug or alcohol abuse, anxiety symptoms, ADHD symptoms, or other problems.

Filling out the self-administered checklist from page 54 may help your doctor obtain some of this information more efficiently. Because the checklist is based on the DSM, it may parallel some of the questions your doctor will ask. You can provide it at the beginning of the first interview as a way of ensuring follow-up on certain symptoms that may concern you.

During this interview, your doctor will probably want to know not only which symptoms you've experienced but also which symptoms typically go together with other ones (that is, in discrete episodes), the severity of these symptoms, and their duration. Your doctor has a threshold in mind for how severe and how impairing a symptom must be before it is considered part of the bipolar syndrome. For example, when asking about "loss of energy or fatigue," your doctor will want to know such things as whether you've been unable to go to work because of fatigue or whether you have trouble studying for classes or doing housework. When asking about insomnia, he or she may want to know how many nights of the week you have trouble sleeping and whether your lack of sleep impairs your ability to drive, concentrate at work, play sports, or conduct any of your usual activities. In many ways bipolar symptoms are just exaggerations of normal mental, behavioral, and emotional processes, and some degree of variability in mood, sleep, or activity level is part of the human condition. Your doctor has to establish whether your symptoms meet accepted criteria for severity and impairment.

Interviews can be quite subjective, and there is always the possibility that the way the doctor asks you the questions, and the way you answer them, will affect the final diagnosis. Consider the following interchange between a doctor and Rego, a 30-year-old man with bipolar disorder. Notice that this doctor probes carefully for certain symptoms, and Rego, correspondingly, gives useful examples of his experiences and behavior.

Doctor: Did you ever have a weeklong period when you felt very happy or very irritable?

Rego: No, not really.

Doctor: Or when you felt very grouchy or easily provoked?

Rego: No.

Doctor: How about feeling charged up and full of energy?

Rego: Yes.

Doctor: What was that like?

Rego: Well, in March I was running at full tilt, full of, like, all sorts of ideas. I thought I could develop a weather-monitoring system that could be operated from my basement.

Doctor: How were you sleeping at the time?

Rego: Not at all! I didn't need to, and I got resentful when people told me I should.

Doctor: Resentful? Tell me more.

Rego: Well, nobody appreciated what I was trying to do. Everybody seemed like they were moving slowly. One time, I practically bit this guy's head off for calling me when I was in the middle of a project. And I yelled at my kids a bunch of times because they kept interrupting me.

In this example, the doctor has found evidence of irritable mood and other manic symptoms in this patient's history. Had the doctor not done this probing, evidence of the manic syndrome might not have emerged.

The diagnostic interview will take at least an hour or two. If you have a particularly complicated set of symptoms, your doctor may request several sessions to be reasonably sure of the diagnosis. A long interview can be tedious, especially if you've been through one before, but in most cases you'll find that your and the doctor's time has been well spent. The information you provide will inform a careful diagnosis, which will almost certainly translate into better treatment.

Does the Diagnosis Fit?
Could You Have Another Disorder Instead?

If you are having your first problems with depression or mania, and possibly even if you have had numerous episodes of mood disorder, you will probably want to discuss the accuracy of the diagnosis with your doctor. Does the diagnosis give a reasonable explanation for the kinds of problems you've had with your mood states, behavior, and relationships with other people? Could you have another disorder instead? You may wonder whether the mood swings you experience are really a part of your personality (see Chapter 4). You may believe that you have a different psychiatric disorder or no disorder at all. Alternatively, you may believe, rightfully, that you have another condition in addition to bipolar disorder.

Bipolar disorder can be difficult to tell apart from other disorders that share features with it. In this section, I discuss the problem of misdiagnosis. I also discuss the disorders that are often confused with bipolar disorder and how they differ from it. Sometimes these disorders are diagnosed alongside bipolar disorder (*comorbidity*).

What Can You Do If You Think You've Been Misdiagnosed?

There are many reasons that bipolar disorder can be hard to distinguish from other disorders. First, moods can vary for any number of reasons, which can include hormones, personal stress, sleep problems, personality disturbances, diseases of the brain, or ingestion of drugs or alcohol. Second, people with the disorder often have trouble describing their mood states to others and giving accurate histories of their disorder. Third, mental health professionals are not always adequately trained to recognize the subtle forms of the disorder (for example, mixed states, rapid cycling, mania with anxiety, hypomania).

Diagnostic confusion can also occur because of the diagnostic criteria themselves. Certain symptoms are characteristic of more than one disorder. Psychotic experiences (for example, grandiose delusions) can occur in disorders other than bipolar disorder, such as schizophrenia. Problems with distractibility occur in mania and in ADHD. Sleep disturbance and irritability can occur in depression, anxiety disorders, or psychotic disorders. Mood variability—rapid and short-term mood changes—is a key feature of borderline personality disorder as well as bipolar disorder.

Try to be as patient as you can with the diagnostic process. The common use of DSM-5 and improved training in the recognition of mood disorders make diagnoses more reliable than they used to be. Nonetheless, errors inevitably occur. Your physician may need to observe you during an episode and once you have recovered to be sure of your diagnosis. If you have strong doubts about the diagnosis you have been given, getting a second opinion is a good idea.

PERSONALIZED CARE TIP:
Interviewing your doctor

If you're not convinced the diagnosis is correct, ask him or her the following questions:

- What is the rationale behind the doctor's opinion?
- What diagnostic criteria does the doctor think apply to you?
- Is the doctor considering other diagnoses, and if not, why not?
- Do you think you have a mood (depressive or bipolar) disorder? If not, explain why not.

If you do seek a second opinion, be prepared to be asked some of the same questions about your symptoms that you were asked the first time. Tell the new psychiatrist why you think you have some disorder other than bipolar and, specifically, why you don't think the diagnostic criteria for bipolar disorder fit. Alternatively, if you think that bipolar is the correct diagnosis but you've been diagnosed with something else, tell the new physician why you believe this. Bring along a close family member, significant other, or trusted friend. This person can offer a different perspective on your symptoms and life experiences, which may be quite useful to the mental health professional who makes the diagnosis.

Most of all, it's important to work collaboratively with your doctor. Relate what you can about your history and report events and symptoms as accurately as possible, even if what you are reporting is sometimes embarrassing or painful to talk about. Try to see things from the doctor's perspective even though his or her questions may sometimes seem like they're missing the mark.

Comorbid Disorders

The term *comorbidity* refers to the co-occurrence of two or more psychiatric disorders in the same person (and usually at the same time). Many people have more than one DSM-5 psychiatric disorder. In clinical practice, people are often given multiple diagnoses, sometimes because they have more than one disorder and sometimes because the clinician isn't sure which diagnosis best applies and therefore diagnoses more than one. A carefully designed large survey of psychiatric disorders in the general population—the *National Comorbidity Survey Replication*—concluded that 45% of people with one psychiatric disorder report two or more disorders (Kessler, Berglund, Demler, Jin, & Walters, 2005). People with bipolar disorder most frequently reported comorbid ADHD, anxiety disorders, or alcohol or drug abuse disorders.

What does it look like when a person has two or more comorbid disorders? Consider Elena, a 49-year-old woman who has bipolar II disorder and ADHD.

Elena had several long-lasting depressive episodes, during which she had had difficulty holding a job. Her hypomanic periods were characterized by irritability, racing thoughts, increases in energy, and sleep disturbance. Her husband, Chris, was understanding of her depression but became enraged at the fact that when he tried to talk to her about her job situation, Elena's eyes would glaze over and she seemed not to be listening. Chris also complained that she made a lot of careless mistakes: when she sent her résumé to prospective employers, there was often a page missing or the printing was slanted. She also frequently forgot appointments with her doctors and prospective employers. Her forgetfulness and inattention seemed to characterize her behavior most of the time, even when she wasn't depressed.

In Elena's case, the codiagnosis of bipolar disorder with ADHD led her physician to recommend a regimen that included a mood stabilizer and dextroamphetamine (Adderall), a drug designed to improve attention and concentration.

The box on page 62 lists disorders that are often comorbid with bipolar disorder or confused with it diagnostically. ADHD, borderline personality disorder, anxiety disorders, and cyclothymic disorder can all be codiagnosed with bipolar disorder. The others require that the clinician make a decision between these diagnoses and bipolar disorder.

Attention-Deficit/Hyperactivity Disorder (ADHD)

Do you have ongoing difficulties with . . .

- Paying attention to details?
- Making careless mistakes in work or other activities?
- Listening to others?
- Organization?
- Distraction?
- Forgetfulness?

ADHD is usually a childhood-onset disorder characterized by difficulty attending to tasks. A child who has ADHD with hyperactivity or impulsivity will fidget, blurt out answers to questions, continually jump out of his or her seat, and talk excessively. Notice how similar these symptoms are to mania! Distinguishing childhood-onset bipolar disorder from ADHD, or distinguishing adult bipolar disorder from the continuation of ADHD first diagnosed in childhood, can be extremely difficult. And it is possible to have both. Studies put the estimate of comorbid ADHD at between 9.5 and 48% in bipolar adults, a wide range that tells us that geographic location, assessment methods, and differences in study samples (for example, whether patients of any economic class are included) are likely to be important (Harmanci, Çam, & Etikan, 2016; Kessler et al., 2006).

Even among adults, distinguishing bipolar disorder from ADHD is important, because the primary drugs for treating ADHD are stimulants such as methylphenidate (Ritalin) or amphetamine/dextroamphetamine. These drugs are not usually given to people with bipolar disorder unless accompanied by a mood-stabilizing agent like lithium or valproate. There is currently debate about whether stimulants can cause mania in a person vulnerable to bipolar disorder. You'll learn more about these medications in Chapter 6.

Pediatric studies have estimated that as many as 90% of children and 30% of adolescents with bipolar disorder also have ADHD, although not everyone agrees on these figures (Pavuluri, Birmaher, & Naylor, 2005). Mental health professionals have a habit of codiagnosing bipolar disorder and ADHD, particularly in children, even though they may be using the same symptoms to justify each disorder. Unfortunately, this habit leads to imprecision. It is possible to have both bipolar and ADHD, and many people do, but there are also ways to tell them apart.

First, the cognitive problems associated with ADHD do not change much from day to day or week to week, unless the person is taking Ritalin or a similar psychostimulant medication. People with ADHD have fairly constant problems with attention, distractibility, and organization, regardless of their mood state. In contrast, people with bipolar disorder may become impulsive and have difficulty attending, but mainly when they are in the midst of a manic, mixed, or depressed episode. For example, Teri, age 37, had bipolar II disorder and worked successfully as a graphic artist during her periods of mood stability. Only when she was depressed was she unable to concentrate on her design layouts. Nick, age 52, with bipolar I disorder, was a successful computer programmer who was known among his colleagues for his ability to stick with difficult problems and solve them. But when he had mixed episodes, he would become unfocused and distractible, jumping from one task to another without gaining closure on any of them.

ADHD is not accompanied by the extreme high and low mood states that are the hallmark of bipolar disorder. It is not typical for people with ADHD to experience elated highs, goal-directed behavior, hypersexuality, decreased need for sleep, or grandiosity (Geller et al., 1998), or to experience deep depressions with suicidality, feelings of worthlessness, fatigue, and loss of interests alternating with periods of mood stability. People with both bipolar disorder and ADHD are at an increased risk for suicide, possibly due to the increased impulsiveness associated with the two conditions (Lan et al., 2015).

Psychiatric Disorders
Often Confused with Bipolar Disorder

- Attention-deficit/hyperactivity disorder (ADHD)
- Borderline personality disorder
- Cyclothymic disorder
- Schizophrenia or schizoaffective disorder
- Recurrent major depressive disorder
- Anxiety disorders
- Substance-induced mood disorder

ADHD is usually associated with difficulty in school settings. When you were in school, were you generally able to keep your mind on class activities? Have you functioned well in tasks that require concentration and sustained effort since then? If the answer to both of these is yes, it is unlikely that you have ADHD, although a thorough answer requires cognitive testing. If you think you might have ADHD, raise the possibility with your doctor and ask for a separate neurological evaluation of that condition. There is some evidence that ADHD can show up for the first time in adulthood, but in only about 7% of people; the other 93% have had ADHD since they were children or adolescents (Lopez, Micoulaud-Franchi, Galera, & Dauvilliers, 2017).

In addition to medications for ADHD, you can enroll in "cognitive rehabilitation" programs in your area that help you develop strategies for improving your attention and concentration (see the Resources). If you'd like more information on ADHD, take a look at the National Institute of Mental Health's website (*www.nimh.nih.gov/health/publications/attention-deficit-hyperactivity-disorder/complete-index.shtml*).

Borderline Personality Disorder

Do you have . . .

- Difficulty defining for yourself who you are or who you want to be?
- A history of very intense and unstable relationships with people?
- A history of making great efforts to keep people from abandoning or leaving you?
- Frequent periods of feeling empty or bored?
- Difficulty controlling angry outbursts?
- A history of impulsive or reckless behavior that involves sex, spending money, substance abuse, or eating?
- A history of self-destructive acts (for example, self-cutting)?

Personality disorders are long-lasting patterns of disturbance in thinking, perceiving, emotional response, interpersonal functioning, and impulse control. The hallmarks of borderline personality disorder are instability in mood, relationships, and one's sense of self or identity. People with borderline personality disorder feel chronically empty and bored, have terrible trouble being alone, and frequently make suicidal gestures or threats. They tend to have remarkably reactive moods and quickly become intensely sad, anxious, or irritable in response to events involving close relationships. These mood states last for only a few hours or, at most, a few days. Borderline personality disorder generally continues throughout adulthood unless the individual seeks treatment.

Carla, age 27, called her boyfriend up to 10 times a day. When she did, she often raged at him for "not being there for her" and, if she couldn't reach him, accused him of being with another woman. When alone, she would feel like she was disappearing, and feel intolerable cravings to smoke, binge eat, drink alcohol, vomit, or cut herself with glass. She tried to hurt herself in minor ways several times, but never severely enough to threaten her life. These problems had continued for several years, despite the fact that she was in psychotherapy and had tried various forms of antidepressant medication.

There are several parallels between borderline personality disorder and bipolar disorder, particularly bipolar II disorder and its rapid cycling forms, but there are also discernible differences. In borderline personality disorder the changing mood states are usually very short-lived and a reaction to being rejected or even just slighted by people with whom the person is closely affiliated. In fact, the disturbances in people with borderline personality are often visible only when one observes their romantic relationships. They tend to idealize and then devalue those with whom they become close, and they go to great lengths to avoid what they experience as abandonment.

People with borderline personality disorder do become depressed and often meet full criteria for a major depressive episode at some point in their lives. This is one of the reasons that telling it apart from bipolar II disorder is so difficult—the person may have had times of being excessively angry, restless, anxious, and depressed, which can look like a mixed episode. But people with true borderline personality disorder do not become manic and very rarely become hypomanic, with a 4-day or greater period of activation. If you think some of the preceding features fit you, it is possible you have bipolar disorder comorbid with borderline personality disorder.

Why is it important to know if you have borderline personality as well as (or instead of) bipolar disorder? Currently, there are no agreed-on drug-treatment guidelines for people with borderline personality or those with both borderline and bipolar disorders. People with both disorders tend to have more trouble finding the right combination of medications than people with bipolar disorder only. This is in part because their doctors may not have done a careful diagnostic assessment. On the other hand, if you have been misdiagnosed with borderline personality disorder when your real diagnosis is bipolar II disorder, you might do better with medications like lamotrigine (Lamictal) or quetiapine (Seroquel) than with medications you may have been given—typically, antidepressants like fluoxetine (Prozac) (John & Sharma, 2009).

If you think you might have borderline personality disorder, it is especially important to consider certain structured forms of psychotherapy in addition to medications. Various treatments have research support for borderline personality disorder, most notably *dialectical behavior therapy* (DBT), which combines cognitive and behavioral strategies with Zen Buddhist mindfulness practices (Linehan & Wilks, 2015); and mentalization-based therapy, which explores our tendency to misread our own or others' emotions (Bateman & Fonagy, 2010).

Cyclothymic Disorder

Do you have . . .

- Short periods of feeling active, irritable, and excited?
- Short periods of feeling mildly depressed?
- A tendency to alternate back and forth between the two?

To make matters even more complicated, you can have a fluctuating form of mood disorder marked by short periods of hypomania alternating with short, mild or moderate periods of depression. To have cyclothymic disorder, you must have alternated between high and low periods for at least 2 consecutive years and never been without mood disorder symptoms for more than 2 months at a time (American Psychiatric Association, 2013). How is this different from bipolar II disorder or unspecified bipolar disorder? Consider the following vignette:

> Katherine was a 30-year-old woman who, since adolescence, had experienced a pattern of alternating between 2- to 3-day periods during the week in which she cried a lot and felt sad and less interested in things and weekends in which she would feel irritable, energetic, and talkative. She had never been hospitalized for either her depressive or hypomanic symptoms, nor had she been suicidal or unable to concentrate, or lost significant amounts of weight. Her boyfriend sometimes complained about her moodiness and rage. Although it was more difficult for her to work when she was depressed, she had never lost a job because of it.

Katherine received a diagnosis of cyclothymic rather than bipolar disorder. Had her depressions been worse and/or required hospitalization, her diagnosis might have been changed to bipolar II disorder with cyclothymic disorder. One can be diagnosed with both!

The psychiatrist Hagop Akiskal from the University of California, San Diego, views cyclothymia as a disturbance of temperament that predisposes people to bipolar disorder (Akiskal et al., 2006; see also Chapter 4). In fact, cyclothymia has a lot in common with bipolar I and II disorders in terms of its pattern of inheritance and its presumed biology. Cyclothymia is listed in DSM-5 as a mild form of bipolar disorder. About one in every four children and adults with cyclothymia progresses to bipolar I or II disorder (that is, they develop full-blown manic episodes, longer hypomanias, or major depressive episodes) over periods of 2 to 4 years (Kochman et al., 2005; Axelson, Birmaher, Strober, et al., 2011).

Why do psychiatrists bother with these distinctions among mild and moderate forms of bipolar disorder? We go back to the idea that bipolar disorder may exist along a continuum (Phelps, 2012). Cyclothymic disorder and unspecified bipolar disorder are both predisposing factors for more severe presentations of bipolar I or II disorder (Van Meter & Youngstrom, 2012). The presence of cyclothymic disorder, especially if the person also has a family history of bipolar disorder, may herald the need for early intervention (for example, taking a low dose of mood-stabilizing medications or learning coping strategies to regulate responses to stress) to reduce the likelihood of a full mania onset.

There are very few studies on the ideal treatments for cyclothymia. As a result, psychiatrists tend to treat people with the disorder similarly to individuals with bipolar I or II, with mood stabilizers like lithium, lamotrigine, or valproate. Nonetheless, people with cyclothymia often function without medication because their disorder is generally less severe and less impairing. For some, the label *cyclothymia* feels less frightening than *bipolar II disorder,* even though they have many similar features.

Schizophrenia

If you are a person with schizophrenia, you will experience some of the following symptoms:

- Delusions, such as believing that you are being followed, your thoughts are being controlled by an outside force, your thoughts are being stolen or altered in some way, or that someone (or some organization) wants to hurt you

- Hallucinations, in which you hear a voice or see a vision (or in rarer cases have taste or smell sensations that others don't have)

- Lack of motivation, apathy, and disinterest in seeing anyone

- Loss or "blunting" of emotions

- Jumbled or confused communication and thinking

It can be quite difficult to distinguish bipolar disorder from schizophrenia, especially when a person is first seeking treatment or has a first hospitalization. People with schizophrenia do not have multiple personalities, as is commonly believed. Instead, they have delusions (mistaken, unrealistic beliefs) or hallucinations (sensory experiences like voices, without a real stimulus). They can experience severe depressions, but often their biggest problem is being cut off from their emotions (flatness or blunting of affect). People with bipolar disorder can also have delusions and hallucinations; these are typically (but not invariably) of a manic, grandiose type (for example, "I have finely tuned extrasensory perception") or of a depressive sort (for example, "I am to be punished for my bad deeds").

According to DSM-5 criteria, you have bipolar disorder instead of schizophrenia if, during your episodes, you experience severe swings of emotion and energy or activity levels, and your delusions or hallucinations (if they occur at all) do not appear until after the onset of your mood swings. If your delusions and hallucinations develop before your mood swings and/or persist after your depressive or manic symptoms clear up, you would more likely be diagnosed with schizophrenia or *schizoaffective disorder*, a blend of the schizophrenia and mood disorder categories.

These distinctions are important in relation to your prognosis. The long-term outcome of schizophrenia—in terms of symptom severity, number of hospitalizations, ability to work, and other quality-of-life indicators—is worse than that of schizoaffective or bipolar disorder (Goghari & Harrow, 2016; Harrow, Grossman, Herbener, & Davies, 2000). There are also implications for treatment. If your diagnosis is schizophrenia or schizoaffective disorder, your physician will probably start you on drugs like ziprasidone (Geodon) or risperidone (Risperdal) before introducing lithium or other mood stabilizers (see also Chapter 6). These are SGAs with mood-stabilizing properties. If the doctor feels your bipolar diagnosis is accurate but you have psychotic symptoms or severe agitation, he or she may recommend one of these drugs along with a mood-stabilizing agent. Consider the experiences of Kurt, age 19:

> Kurt believed there was a "gang of nine" that roamed the planet and was looking for him. He described his "self" as a shell that was gradually deteriorating and would eventually be taken over by this gang. When he became preoccupied with the gang of nine, he would become revved up, irritable, easily provoked to tears, speak a mile a minute, and stop sleeping. He was hospitalized because his thinking became increasingly bizarre and his parents became afraid of him. When his older brother visited him in the hospital, Kurt ran up to him, threw his arms around him, began crying, and screamed, "Thanks for saving me!" After hospital treatment with risperidone, he calmed down considerably and began sleeping again. But he continued to believe a gang was following him and that its members were waiting for him to be discharged from the hospital.

Notice that Kurt's primary disturbance is in his thinking processes rather than his mood. He continued to be preoccupied with his beliefs even after his mood and sleep problems improved. He was given the diagnosis of schizoaffective instead of bipolar disorder. These diagnostic distinctions are among the most difficult to make reliably. Often, people with these unclear patterns of symptoms have to be observed across several episodes and have to try many different medications before their diagnosis becomes clear.

Recurrent Major Depressive Disorder

Have you had major, severe periods of depression that have come and gone, but no obvious signs of mania or hypomania? It may seem simple to distinguish people with only recurrent depressions (unipolar depression) from those who have both depressions and manias, but it is actually quite difficult. In the most common situation, a person has had repeated episodes of major depression and then undergoes a brief period (a few days) of feeling "wired," "up," and "ready to take on the world." Is this bipolar II disorder? Or simply the high most of us would feel after coming out of a long depression?

A true hypomanic episode involves an observable change in a person's behavior. A hypomanic person sleeps less, feels mildly or moderately elated or irritable, and has racing thoughts or becomes talkative. If this state lasts for days at a time, and others have commented on it, a hypomanic episode (and bipolar disorder) is suspected. In contrast, a person who simply feels good and more energetic after being depressed, but who has few or none of the other symptoms in the hypomanic cluster, probably has *major depressive disorder.*

Some people have major depressive episodes with agitation, which can look a lot like a bipolar mixed episode. Bethany, age 37, had major depressive episodes in which she became anxious, restless, and unable to sit still. Her main feeling was one of dread rather than the optimism or confidence usually characteristic of hypomania or mania. Her doctor diagnosed her with major depressive disorder.

If you have major depressive episodes that alternate with short hypomanic periods, and there is a history of bipolar disorder in your family, *unspecified bipolar disorder* may be the appropriate diagnosis instead of major depression with agitation. As mentioned earlier, if your doctor cannot be certain whether you have unipolar depression or bipolar disorder, and especially if bipolar runs in your family, he or she will probably recommend that you take a mood stabilizer before taking an antidepressant.

Anxiety Disorders

Anxiety disorders may co-occur in as many as 75% of patients with bipolar I or II disorder, with lifetime histories of panic attacks being the most common (Merikangas et al., 2011). Anxiety disorders are a broad category that includes posttraumatic stress disorder (anxiety, emotional numbness, and intrusive memories related to a traumatic event), generalized anxiety disorder (a constant state of worry and apprehension, along with physical signs of anxiety), panic disorder (sudden bursts of anxiety and terror and feelings of impending doom, with a strong desire to escape), obsessive–compulsive disorder (intrusive thoughts that are neutralized by performing a ritualistic activity, such as cleaning, washing, or checking repeatedly), social anxiety disorder (severe anxiety when one is a focus of others' attention), and other conditions.

It may sound strange that doctors would confuse mania or depression with anxiety attacks, but it happens all the time.

Fiona, age 33, had bipolar II disorder and generalized anxiety disorder. In between her mood episodes, she had mild depressive symptoms such as a sluggish feeling, irritability, and occasional suicidal thoughts. She had nearly constant anxiety. She worried about failing at her job, with predictions of catastrophe: that little mistakes she made would be the cause of her downfall and would lead to her being fired, and ultimately homeless. Her anxious ruminations could take her well into the night. She acknowledged feeling apprehensive most of the day, even when nothing felt like a direct threat to her. During her acute depressive episodes, her worries became worse, but they were still there and could be quite crippling even when she wasn't particularly depressed. Her anxieties let up during her short hypomanic periods, when she felt productive, goal-driven, energetic, and elevated in mood.

Fiona would not have been diagnosed with a comorbid anxiety disorder if her anxieties occurred only during her mood episodes. As noted earlier, there is a course specifier—anxious distress—that is diagnosed alongside mood episodes. In contrast, Fiona felt anxious even when she was relatively free of mood symptoms. If, like Fiona, you have a full comorbid anxiety disorder, or you and your doctor agree that an anxiety disorder is a more appropriate diagnosis than bipolar disorder, the doctor is likely to recommend that you take an SSRI antidepressant, of which Prozac, Lexapro, and Zoloft are common examples. He or she may also recommend cognitive-behavioral therapy (CBT), which has a strong research record in treating anxiety. In Chapter 6 I'll discuss the pros and cons of antidepressants in bipolar disorder.

Substance- or Medication-Induced Bipolar Disorder

Are all of the following true for you?

- You have had episodes of depression and mania.
- These symptoms developed after you took a street drug, drank a large quantity of alcohol over several days or weeks, or began taking an antidepressant, a stimulant, or some other prescription medication that affects moods.
- Your mood symptoms subsided shortly after you stopped drinking alcohol or taking the drug.
- You have not had other manic or depressive episodes, except those brought on by alcohol or drugs.

Manic and depressive symptoms can be mimicked by certain drugs of abuse. Cocaine, amphetamine ("speed"), methamphetamine, heroin, Ecstasy, and LSD have all been known to create manic-like states, often with accompanying psychosis. Amphetamine, in particular, has been known to produce irritable, hyperactivated, paranoid, and delusional states. It is unlikely that alcohol abuse or dependence will directly cause a manic episode, but it can certainly contribute to a spiraling depression.

DSM-5 uses the label *substance/medication-induced mental disorders* to distinguish mood disorders brought on by external substances from those that are due to a person's inherent physiology. Mood disorders that are the direct function of drugs, alcohol, or medications are usually short-lived, disappearing more quickly (usually in 4 weeks or less) than non-substance-related mood disorders, and are usually treated through detoxification and chemical dependency programs (or stopping the relevant medication). Sometimes substance-related mood disorders abate without treatment. However, substances can contribute to the onset of the first episode of bipolar disorder, which then takes on a course of its own. It is not uncommon for people with bipolar disorder to say that their first manic episode began shortly after they began experimenting with street drugs.

As I discussed in Chapter 2, you can have both a mood and a substance abuse disorder, with one influencing the course of the other. Mood swings make you more likely to take drugs or alcohol, and drugs or alcohol can worsen your mood swings. About 50% of people with bipolar I disorder and about 37% of those with bipolar II disorder have had an alcohol or substance use disorder at some point in life—a rate that is much higher than the general population rate of 10–20% (Kessler et al., 2005; Merikangas et al., 2011). So, even if you originally sought treatment for depression, your doctor may diagnose a substance/medication-induced depression and recommend that you take part in a 12-step program (for example, Alcoholics Anonymous) or individual therapy designed to help you overcome chemical dependency problems.

Ideally, your doctor will help you assess the sequence of your mood symptoms and drinking or drug use: Do you usually get depressed and then drink? Does it ever happen that you drink and then get depressed? Do you use cocaine or marijuana and then get manic or hypomanic, or is it the reverse? Usually, the doctor will not be able to tell for sure if you have bipolar disorder until you have remained sober or drug free for a period of time. Again, your close relatives and significant others may be of help here. For example, your spouse may be able to recall how and when your behavior started to shift in relation to when you took certain substances.

An important consideration is whether your manic, hypomanic, mixed, or rapid cycling states have developed after taking an antidepressant. Karine, in the example that follows, showed symptoms that strongly mimicked a mixed episode, but her symptoms stopped once the antidepressant was withdrawn. If you do become manic or hypomanic because of antidepressants, you may indeed have bipolar disorder, but more evidence will be required.

> Karine, age 48, had been severely depressed and anxious for about a month after the death of her father. She had never had a manic or a hypomanic episode. Her physician put her on an antidepressant, but it did not make her depression better; in fact, her anxiety got worse. Her physician then gave her a different kind of antidepressant.
>
> > "At first, I felt great. I could focus on things like never before. I no longer needed cigarettes to keep my mind on my work. But then my mood started to go up and down like a seesaw. My sleep got worse and worse—I woke up almost every hour. I felt wired, but then my depression came back. I started feeling really irritable and worried, and I couldn't stop my ruminations, which were like a DVD playing on fast-forward. I had to take Ambien (a sleep medication) nearly every night. I couldn't stand it."
>
> Her physician took her off the antidepressant gradually. Her mood continued to fluctuate for a few weeks but then returned to a milder state of depression. She was eventually treated successfully with lamotrigine (Lamictal) and CBT. Her rapid cycling was considered an instance of substance-induced depressive disorder, although she was also believed to have "uncomplicated bereavement," a form of major depression that is a reaction to a loss experience. She was never given the diagnosis of bipolar disorder.

DSM-5 differs from earlier editions in that, if substance use precipitates a manic or hypomanic episode, but the episode lasts longer than anyone would expect from the substance alone, bipolar disorder is still the appropriate diagnosis. So, if you took an antidepressant and then started rapid cycling for several months, the position taken by DSM-5 is that the antidepressant may have triggered a vulnerability to bipolar mood swings, but was not the core cause of the syndrome. I will say more about what we mean by a vulnerability to bipolar disorder in Chapter 5.

● ● ● ● ● ● ● ● ● ● ● ● ● ●

I hope you can see now how important it is to obtain a proper diagnosis and to rule out competitive diagnoses. Knowing the diagnostic criteria for bipolar disorder and understanding how these symptoms manifest themselves, both in you and in others, is empowering. As you'll see later, awareness of the symptoms that you typically experience during mood episodes will go a long way in helping you prevent these episodes from spiraling out of control.

In the next chapter, I'll discuss the problems people have in adjusting to or coping with the diagnosis of bipolar disorder. Some deny the reality of the disorder and believe that their symptoms are just exaggerations of their personality. Some overcommit to the diagnosis and unnecessarily try to limit their career and personal aspirations, and others reluctantly agree to the diagnosis but continue living their lives as if they were illness free. No one likes to believe that he or she has a psychiatric disorder that requires long-term treatment. Coming to accept the diagnosis is a difficult emotional process.

CHAPTER 4

"Is It an Illness or Is It Me?"
Coping with the Diagnosis

In Chapter 3 we discussed the rather dry (though useful) DSM-5 diagnostic criteria. What these criteria do not address or convey is the emotional impact of learning you have bipolar disorder and acknowledging its reality. Most of my patients go through painful struggles in coming to terms with this diagnosis. Initially, they experience anger, fear, sadness, guilt, disappointment, and hopelessness. These are not manic–depressive cycles but rather a healthy process of forming a sense of self that incorporates having biological dysregulations and mood disturbances. It may sound like I'm talking about people who have had only one or two manic or depressed episodes and are surprised by the diagnosis, but I've also seen these reactions in people who have been hospitalized for the disorder numerous times.

Why is the process of acceptance so painful? Coming to terms with having the disorder may mean admitting to a new role for yourself in your family, in the workforce, or in your personal relationships. It may require you to make decisions about restructuring your life and priorities, which may mean viewing yourself differently. For example, Luiz, age 25, gave up his apartment and returned to live with his parents after his hospitalization. He then had to deal with their hypervigilance and increased attempts to control his behavior, which made him feel like he was a child again. Rob, age 38, had been quite successful in his work as a civil engineer. After his bipolar I diagnosis was revealed, he found that people at work seemed afraid of him. He attributed losing his job to the disclosure of his illness. Nancy, age 44, noted that after she learned of her bipolar II diagnosis and told many of her friends about it, at least one "dumped me because I was too 'high maintenance.'"

You can imagine the pain and confusion you might feel when there are such costs to acknowledging the disorder.

What's Unique about Bipolar Disorder?

People who have to live with medical diagnoses such as diabetes or heart disease go through similar emotions in coping with their diagnoses. Nobody likes to believe he or she has a long-term illness that requires treatment. But it's a lot easier to attribute your abnormally high blood pressure to an inherited biological condition than to do the same for your mood changes. As I mentioned in Chapter 2, bipolar disorder can be difficult to distinguish from the normal ups and downs of human life. You may have always been moody or temperamental and believe that your high or low periods are just exaggerations of your natural moodiness. How do you know what is really your illness and what is your "self" or personality (your habits, attitudes, and styles of relating to others—the way you are most of the time)? How do you train yourself to know the difference between you when you're well and you when you're ill and not fool yourself into thinking that changes in mood, energy, or activity are just "how I've always been"?

On a practical level, the ability to recognize differences between personality traits and disorder symptoms is important so that you and others know when emergency procedures need to be undertaken. On an emotional level, understanding these distinctions can contribute to a more stable sense of who you are. Maureen, for example, knew she had always been extraverted but realized she needed to visit her doctor when she began staying up late to call people—all over the country—to whom she hadn't spoken in years. Having to increase her dosage of lithium did not interfere with her appreciation of others.

The reaction of many of my clients upon learning of the diagnosis is disbelief or denial, which is only natural. After all, they have to revise their image of themselves, which is painful and difficult to do. Others, especially those who were diagnosed some time ago, come to believe they have the disorder but continue to lead their lives as if they did not. You can imagine why people would react this way; in fact, you may even recognize these reactions in yourself. Nevertheless, these styles of coping can cause trouble for you, especially if you refuse to take medications that would help you, or regularly engage in high-risk activities (for example, staying up all night, getting drunk or high frequently) that can worsen your illness.

Antonio, age 35, behaved in self-destructive ways to cope with his confusion and pain. He went off his medications to try to prove to others that he wasn't sick, but then relapsed and ended up back in his psychiatrist's office, with more medication being recommended. Rosa, who had received her diagnosis years ago, often turned to alcohol when she experienced the shame, social stigma, and hopelessness she felt the diagnosis conferred on her.

After they have lived with the disorder for a while, some people begin thinking of themselves as if they were nothing more than a diagnostic label or a broken brain or a set of dysfunctional molecules. They start automatically attributing all of their personal problems to the illness, even those problems that people without bipolar disorder routinely experience. They usually accept the need for medications but unnecessarily limit themselves and avoid taking advantage of opportunities that they actually could handle.

By the end of this chapter you will have a greater sense of the various emotional reactions people have upon learning of the diagnosis. You'll feel empowered knowing that your own emotional reactions are shared by others and that admitting to the diagnosis doesn't mean giving up your hopes and aspirations. The chapter ends with suggestions for coping with the difficult process of coming to terms with the illness.

The Emotional Fallout of the Diagnosis

Most of the people who consult me have been told by someone at some time that they have bipolar disorder, even if they don't believe it themselves. When we actually sit down and begin discussing the disorder, they experience a wide range of emotions, including bewilderment, anxiety, and anger. Some people feel relief: learning that you have a psychiatric disorder that has a name, and that explains a great deal of what has happened to you, can help alleviate your feelings of guilt or self-blame. More often, however, the diagnosis raises more questions than it answers—most of which concern what the future holds for you and those close to you.

When you first learned that you had the disorder, you may have asked yourself questions like the following:

"Why me?"
"Why is this happening now?"
"Am I 'only bipolar' now, or do I still have a separate identity?"
"Where does my identity stop and the disorder begin?"
"Were my prior periods of high energy, creativity, and accomplishment nothing more than signs of an illness?"
"How much mood variability am I 'allowed' before people think I'm getting sick again?"
"How responsible am I for my own behavior?"
"How do I become more convinced that this is what I have?"
"Will I have a normal life and achieve my goals?"

> **Effective prevention:** *Bipolar disorder is something that you have, but it is not who you are.* Knowing this difference can keep you from rejecting the diagnosis or, at the other extreme, giving your life over to the illness.

Even if you've had numerous episodes of bipolar disorder, you may ask yourself these questions. It's natural to do so, and healthy—to the extent that struggling with these questions helps you clarify your feelings, goals, and sense of self. Unfortunately, ambivalence about the diagnosis and perceived discrimination from others can make you want to reject all treatments. Some people do this to prove to others that they don't need treatment and can function independently. These choices can lead to recurrences of their illness and a decreased quality of life.

If any close family members (for example, your spouse or parents) learned of your diagnosis at the same time as you did, they probably had questions of their own. They may not have voiced these questions to you directly because they understood that hearing their worries might be painful for you or because they didn't wish to cause family conflict. For example, Kyana's parents worried that she would always be tagged as mentally ill and never have a normal life. They worried that they would have to take care of her for the rest of their lives and that their hopes and dreams for her had been dashed. Greg's wife wondered if she had married the wrong man and whether she should leave the relationship. None of these family members raised their worries until they began talking openly about the disorder with Kyana or Greg. On the positive side, learning more about the disorder was comforting to Kyana, Greg, and their families, because they learned together that the prognosis was not as poor as they had feared.

"It's No Big Deal": Rejecting or Underidentifying with the Diagnosis

"I want to go back to the place where I used to live in Miami, back before all this mess started. Who knows? Maybe the apartment I lived in is still available. People liked me there. I had so many friends. I sometimes think if I go back there, I'll find the old me sunning herself under some big old palm tree."

—A 26-year-old woman who had just been hospitalized for her second manic episode

Perhaps you remember the first time someone told you that you had bipolar disorder. Did any of the "common reactions" in the box on page 77 describe how you felt then or now?

Consider the first reaction of rejecting the diagnosis outright. Did you then (or do you now) believe that the diagnosis was all just a misunderstanding of your behavior? Did you think others were just trying to rein you in and weren't interested in your private experiences? Did you get confused about whether your medication was meant to treat your mood swings or whether it caused them in the first place? Were you convinced that the diagnosis was wrong and that alternative treatments (for example, acupuncture) were the answer?

Carter, age 49, rejected the diagnosis, refused to see his doctor, and refused to take medications despite having had manic, mixed, and depressive episodes (with hospitalizations) for almost 15 years. His obstinate stand usually surfaced when he was manic, but he also dug in his heels when he had few or no mood symptoms at all. The longer he stayed well, the more he doubted that he had any kind of mood disorder. He believed that whatever problems arose could be controlled by diet (particularly by limiting his sugar intake) and Chinese medicines. He argued that his behavior—no matter how dangerous or bizarre it had been—was just being misunderstood and misinterpreted. He blamed his aggressive actions on people he thought had provoked him—typically, family members, employers, or romantic partners. During the few intervals in which he did agree to take medications, he mistakenly concluded that they had caused his illness ("My moods were fine until they gave me Depakote, and after that they swung all over the place").

As I discussed in Chapter 3, you will certainly want to explore with your doctor why he or she thinks the diagnosis applies to you and why other possible diagnoses are being ruled out. Second opinions are often helpful, and there is no substitute for learning as much as you can about the symptoms of the disorder, the purposes of various medications, and effective self-management strategies. But rejecting the diagnosis outright is a dangerous stance to take, because, as in Carter's case, it can lead to the rejection of treatments that may be lifesaving. People who take this

---

Common Reactions to Being Told You Have Bipolar Disorder

Rejecting the diagnosis:

- "The diagnosis is wrong; it's just a way for other people to explain away my experiences."

Underidentifying with the diagnosis:

- "I'm just a moody person."
- "They just want to straitjacket me with drugs to stop me from having experiences that no one else understands."

Overidentifying with the diagnosis:

- "My illness and my moods are everything that I am, and I have no control over them."
- "I want to go to parties, travel, and work but I'm afraid I'll set off another episode, so I rarely leave my house."

stance often go through several episodes and hospitalizations before they admit that anything is wrong, and even then distrust the diagnosis, the doctors, and the medications.

Now consider the second reaction, what I call underidentifying with the diagnosis. Underidentification is a common reaction style, and, for many people, a stage in coming to terms with having the illness. It is similar to being in denial, which is not quite the same thing as rejecting the diagnosis. *Denial* or *thought suppression* refers to the process of avoiding emotionally painful problems by pushing them out of conscious awareness. Being told that you have an illness that will recur and that requires rethinking your life goals is extraordinarily painful. Who wouldn't want to push away this emotional reaction and try to keep living as if the diagnosis were not right?

People who learn that they have other medical diagnoses also react by underidentifying. For example, people who have had heart attacks may acknowledge to others that they need to make lifestyle adaptations yet go on smoking, exercising little or not at all, taking on too many work assignments, or sleeping irregularly. People with diabetes or hypertension sometimes superficially acknowledge their diagnoses but go on eating sugary or salty foods.

Ellen Frank, a professor of psychiatry at the University of Pittsburgh, has termed the emotional issues underlying the denial of bipolar disorder "grieving the lost healthy self" (Frank, 2007). Many people with bipolar disorder were very energetic, popular, bright, and creative before they became ill. Then, once their illness is diagnosed and family members or friends start treating them like a "mental patient," they become resentful and start yearning for who they used to be. They may think that if they go on acting as if nothing has changed, their old self will come back, like a long-lost friend—the way the woman quoted earlier dreamed of finding her old self back in Miami. Underlying these reactions are deep feelings of loss over the dramatic life changes the illness has brought. For some, even the label "bipolar" can bring to mind painful memories of lost hopes, disappointments, and dashed expectations. Understandably, these painful memories make people prone to deny the illness when faced with evidence of it.

In my experience, people with bipolar disorder have strong feelings about the importance of personal achievement and independence. The disorder has a way of derailing achievements, making the person feel like a failure, and bringing negative self-appraisals to the surface. When I was on sabbatical at Oxford University (2006–2007), we conducted an experiment in which we asked adults with bipolar disorder, major depression, or no psychiatric history to unscramble six-word strings (example: "am ruining I life my improving") to produce five-word sentences (Miklowitz, Alatiq, Geddes, Goodwin, & Williams, 2010). The task required that they leave out one word. The sentences could be completed in a negative way ("I am ruining my life") or a positive way ("I am improving my life"). In one condition of the experiment, in which participants heard a reward bell for every four sentences they completed, the participants with bipolar disorder completed more sentences in the negative direction than participants with major depression or with no psychiatric history. We interpreted these findings to mean that, for people with bipolar disorder, reward brings to mind memories of failure in achievement situations and feelings of low self-worth.

Isn't Denial Healthy?

Denial of the illness can be a way of coping with fears of failure or pessimistic views of the future. Unfortunately, it only works in the short term, because negative self-evaluations have a way of reemerging during the next life challenge.

If you're just now being diagnosed for the first time, it's normal to be in a certain amount of denial. But even if you have had the diagnosis for some time and feel you've accepted its reality, you may be able to recall times when you were in denial about it. When you were last hypomanic or manic, did you:

- Doubt that the illness was real or believe that it had been a mistake all along?
- "Test" the diagnosis by staying out all night, drinking a lot of alcohol, or taking street drugs?
- Forget to take your lithium, Depakote, Seroquel, or other mood medications?
- Believe you could take your medications without any supervision (that is, regular doctor's appointments to discuss your side effects and measure your blood levels)?

Inconsistency with medications is a big problem for people with bipolar disorder. People miss between 20 and 40% of their prescribed medication doses (Levin, Krivenko, Howland, Schlachet, & Sajatovic, 2016). Many factors affect an individual's willingness to take medications as prescribed (for example, the supportiveness of the physician), but denial of the illness is one such factor. I devote a full chapter of this book (Chapter 7) to issues surrounding medication nonadherence.

"If I'm Bipolar, So Is Everybody Else"

"My mother really gets on my case about my medications, about my visits to my doctor, about the men I'm going out with, my job, my sleep—you name it. She's always asking me if I've been drinking. She goes behind my back to try to find out. She's always been critical and disapproving of me. I think she's the one who's bipolar."
            —A 29-year-old woman with bipolar II disorder and alcoholism

Sometimes people who deny they have the disorder say it's because they're confused about where normal mood variation ends and bipolar illness begins. Recall the discussion in the introductory chapter about the continuum of bipolar symptom severity, from mild ups and downs to severe manic and depressive episodes requiring hospitalization. Perhaps you've wondered at times whether your emotional reactions to events or situations are really any different from other people's. Have you found yourself thinking or saying, "People around me have it, but they just don't know it yet"? You are most likely to think this way when your relatives or friends become angry or overcontrolling, or accuse you of being sick even when you feel you are doing well and having fairly ordinary ups and downs. These different perceptions are most common in bipolar II disorder, in which hypomania/depression cycles can be quite subtle: people may not believe their moods have changed as much as others seem to think.

You may be right that others around you are moody. We do know that bipolar disorder runs in families (see Chapter 5) and that people with the disorder tend to find mates who themselves have mood disorders (also called *assortative mating*; Smoller & Finn, 2003). So it's not impossible that others in your family have the disorder or a mild form of it. Of course, if you or I asked them why they're so moody, they might say they're only reacting to your behavior. In turn, you may think that your behavior occurs in reaction to their moods.

Being aware of the moodiness of your close relatives or friends is not necessarily a bad thing. You can learn to avoid doing the things that provoke them and, even better, help them find appropriate sources of help (for example, a support group). Their mood fluctuations may occur because of matters that have nothing to do with you. Chapter 13, which discusses communicating with family members, should help you address some of these issues.

Simply having moods that shift doesn't make one bipolar (recall the role of symptom and impairment thresholds in making the diagnosis, discussed in Chapter 3). But if you find yourself seeing bipolar disorder in everyone else, the reason may be that you don't want to feel alone or isolated. Admitting that you're ill and different from others is stigmatizing and painful. However, as we'll see later, acknowledging the disorder can also be empowering. It doesn't mean that life as you know it has to stop.

The Personality-versus-Disorder Problem

"I feel like everything I do is now somehow connected to my being sick. If I'm happy, it's because I'm manic; if I'm sad, it's because I'm depressed. I don't want to think that every time I have an emotion, every time I get angry at somebody, it's because I'm ill. Some of my feelings are justified. People say I'm a different person every day, but that's me! I've never been a stable person."

—A 25-year-old woman who had a severe manic episode
with psychosis, followed by a 6-month depression

Having a sense of how your personality, habits, and attitudes differ from your symptoms is an important part of learning to accept the disorder. Understandably, most people want to feel that they have a "self" that is separate from their symptoms and biological vulnerabilities. They especially feel this way if they've been led to believe, by their doctors or by anyone else, that their illness is a "life sentence." Defining yourself in terms of a set of stable personality traits that have been with you through most of your life may make you feel less vulnerable to the kinds of conflicts the young woman just quoted is experiencing.

Another reason to distinguish between your personality and your disorder is that it will help you determine when you are truly beginning a new episode rather than just going through a rough time. For example, if you are extraverted by nature, socializing a great deal in one weekend may be less significant in determining whether you are developing a manic or hypomanic episode than changes in your sleep patterns, increases in irritability, or fluctuations in your energy levels. In contrast, if you are habitually an introverted person, a sudden increase in your socializing may be quite useful as a sign of a developing episode.

Bipolar Disorder and Temperament

You may believe—and others who interact with you may believe—that your symptoms of mania are just your exuberant, optimistic, high-energy self; that your depression is just your tendency to slide into pessimism or overreact to disappointments; or that your mixed episodes or rapid cycling reflect your natural moodiness or dark temperament. In fact, there is evidence that people with bipolar disorder have mood swings or *temperamental disturbances* that date back to childhood. A questionnaire given to members of the Depression and Bipolar Support Alliance (DBSA) revealed that many people with bipolar disorder had depressive and hypomanic periods even when they were children, well before anyone diagnosed them (Lish, Dime-Meenan, Whybrow, Price, & Hirschfeld, 1994).

One of the more creative thinkers in our field, Hagop Akiskal, has an interesting slant on the whole question. He believes that, for many people with bipolar disorder, the behaviors, habits, and attitudes that sound like ongoing personality attributes are really mild or "subthreshold" forms of mood disorder, or bipolar disorder in its early stages of development. He describes four temperamental disturbances that he believes predispose people to bipolar disorder (see the box on page 82) and presents evidence that people with these temperaments, even if they have never had a major depressive, hypomanic, mixed, or manic episode, often have a family history of bipolar disorder and are vulnerable to developing the illness (Akiskal et al., 2006).

Why is it important for you to examine whether one of these temperaments applies to you? Because if you have one of them, you're at risk for a worsening of your disorder if you are not getting proper treatment. For example, if you had dys-

---

Akiskal's Four Temperamental Disturbances

- *Hyperthymic:* chronically cheerful, overly optimistic, exuberant, extraverted, stimulus seeking, overconfident, meddlesome

- *Cyclothymic:* frequent mood shifts from unexplained tearfulness to giddiness, with variable sleeping patterns and changing levels of self-esteem

- *Dysthymic:* chronically sad, tearful, joyless, lacking in energy

- *Depressive mixed:* simultaneously anxious, speedy, irritable, restless, and sad, with fatigue and insomnia

---

thymia or cyclothymia in adolescence, you are at risk for developing bipolar depressive episodes earlier rather than later (Hillegers et al., 2005; Lewinsohn, Seeley, & Klein, 2003; Van Meter et al., 2017). Lithium can be used to treat cyclothymia as well as bipolar disorder. If you had dysthymia or hyperthymia as a child or adolescent, you are at risk for developing hypomanic episodes, especially if you take an antidepressant medication and are not simultaneously taking a mood stabilizer such as lithium (Van Meter & Youngstrom, 2012). If you have any of the four temperaments, you may still experience mood variability even once you return to your baseline after a manic or depressive episode. The notion is that these temperaments are relatively constant and reflect a biologically based vulnerability to your disorder. They come before the onset of the disorder and remain present even after the worst of the symptoms have ceased.

So, in one sense, when people with bipolar disorder say that they have always been moody, they're right. But the key point is that your moodiness may reflect changes in the brain related to bipolar disorder rather than your character or personality. This is not to say that you don't also have a distinct personality consisting of traits like sociability or extraversion, openness to new experiences, reliability, or conscientiousness. But what may look like personality traits can really be subthreshold mood symptoms that require more aggressive treatment.

Comparing Personality Traits with Symptoms: A Checklist

It may be impossible to fully distinguish your personality and your disorder, particularly if you've had a number of episodes and have become accustomed to the wide mood swings and the changes in energy and behavior that go with them. Nonetheless, thinking through the differences between your personality traits and the symptoms you have had during manic and depressive episodes can be illuminating.

In the following checklist, under "personality traits," try to think of the way you are most of the time, not just when you're having mood cycles. Does your personality consist of a group of traits that "hang together" (for example, sociable, optimistic, affectionate, open)? See if you can distinguish the cluster of traits that have described you throughout your life from those that typify the way you feel, think, or behave when you are manic, hypomanic, or depressed. How do you usually relate to other people, and does this change when you get into high or low mood states? When you're racing and charged up, are you really "affectionate and open" or just physical with many different people and talkative across the board?

What's Me and What's My Illness?

Check as many of the following as apply.

Your personality traits	Your manic or depressive symptoms
_____ Reliable	_____ Euphoric
_____ Conscientious	_____ Grandiose
_____ Dependable	_____ Depressed
_____ Indecisive	_____ Loss of interest
_____ Assertive	_____ Sleeping too much
_____ Open	_____ Sleeping too little
_____ Optimistic	_____ Racing thoughts
_____ Sociable	_____ Full of energy
_____ Withdrawn	_____ Doing too many things
_____ Ambitious	_____ Highly distractible
_____ Aloof	_____ Feeling suicidal
_____ Critical	_____ More easily fatigued
_____ Intellectual	_____ Unable to concentrate
_____ Affectionate	_____ Irritable
_____ Spirited	_____ Feeling worthless
_____ Passive	_____ Taking big or unusual risks
_____ Talkative	_____ Wired
_____ Seeking novelty	_____ Highly anxious

Would people describe you as boisterous, assertive, or energetic even when you're not in a manic episode? Are you pessimistic and withdrawn when you're not feeling depressed?

If you're not sure about whether you have certain personality traits, check with others to see if they would describe you with these trait terms. Frequently, those close to you will have different ideas than you do about what your personality is like and how it differs from your mood symptoms. Of course, you may feel uncomfortable approaching certain close relatives with these questions, especially if you feel these family members have an agenda, such as getting you to take more medication. For now, try to select someone you think is not invested in the outcome of the discussion (that is, whether you conclude that certain behaviors are your illness rather than your personality, or vice versa). A close and trusted friend is the best choice. Perhaps frame the question like this: "I'm trying to figure out why I've had so many mood changes. I want to know whether I've really changed or whether I've always been like this. Can you help me with a simple exercise?"

"Won't Bipolar Disorder Change My Personality?"

The flip side of this "personality versus disorder" question is whether one or more episodes of mania or depression can actually change your personality or character. This is a very complicated question. Many people, particularly those who have had many mood episodes, feel that the disorder and the experiences of hospitalization, medications, psychotherapy, and painful life events have fundamentally changed who they are. People who have just been diagnosed may not worry so much that their personality will be changed by the diagnosis. They may worry instead that people will relate to them differently because of it—and then start acting differently as a result.

Certainly, a long-standing mood disorder—especially if it has not been treated—can profoundly affect your attitudes, habits, and styles of relating to others. It can also require lifestyle changes that are a lot like changes in personality. But if you were really free of your mood disorder symptoms for a long period of time, would you go back to being the way you were before the illness began?

We really don't know whether there are fundamental changes in a person's character as a result of long-term bipolar illness. It is possible that what look like changes in personality (for example, becoming less sociable, acting more aggressively) are really just *subthreshold symptoms* that never fully disappeared after the last major episode. But no one doubts that the experience of bipolar mood swings is very profound and can change the way you view yourself and those around you.

"I Am My Disorder": Overidentifying as a Coping Style

"I've become very worried about having another episode. I keep thinking that even the smallest thing will push me over the edge—a glass of wine, traveling, eating a rich dessert, even just going to the store. I'm terrified about even small changes in my sleep. My husband wants me to do more, like go with him to restaurants or shows, but I'm afraid going out will make me manic. I'm now leading a pretty sheltered life, I guess."

—A 58-year-old woman in a depressed phase of bipolar I disorder

"I was depressed most of my life, and then I found out I had bipolar II, and everything changed. It explained so much, like why I hadn't gotten better on antidepressants, why cognitive therapy seemed like a bust, why I was always rapid cycling. It explains why I haven't been able to hold a job and why relationships haven't worked out. Now that I know my right diagnosis, I know I shouldn't do anything that might trigger my highs, including new relationships! When I think through my goals, I have to accept that depression is going to be a major part of my life."

—A 38-year-old woman with bipolar II disorder

Some people deal with the emotional pain of the disorder by giving themselves over to it. They *overidentify* with the illness, viewing all of their problems, emotional reactions, viewpoints, attitudes, and habits as part of their disorder. If your last period of illness was quite traumatic for you (for example, your life was threatened, you experienced public shame or humiliation, you lost a number of friends, or you lost a great deal of money or status), you may have become fearful of the disorder's power over you and placed severe restrictions on your life as a way of warding off future damage. If this coping style does not describe you now, perhaps you can recall periods of time when it did.

There are many reasons that people overidentify with the illness. First, you may have received inaccurate information from your doctors or other mental health sources. You may have been told that your illness is quite grave, that you shouldn't have children, that you can't expect a satisfying career, that you may end up spending a considerable amount of time in hospitals, that your marital problems will worsen, and that there is little you can do to control your raging biochemical imbalances. If you've been given this kind of information, it's not surprising that you would give up control to this affliction that destroys everything—or so you've been told.

Being given this kind of "sentence" by your doctor may make you start reinterpreting your life in the context of the label. You may start thinking back on normal developmental experiences you had (for example, being upset about breaking up with your high school boyfriend or girlfriend) and labeling them as your first depressive episode. You may start to think that you can accomplish little in your life, believing "All I am is bipolar, and I can't change. It's all a brain disease, and I can't expect much from myself." This way of thinking may make you avoid going back to work, withdraw from social relationships, and rely more and more on the caregiving of your family members.

In case it isn't obvious, I disagree with this way of characterizing bipolar disorder. Many—in fact, most—of my patients are productive people who have successful interpersonal relationships. They have adjusted to the necessity of taking medications, but they don't feel controlled by their illness or its treatments. They have developed strategies for managing their stress levels but don't completely avoid challenging situations either. I have been amazed by how many of my most severely ill clients call me years later to tell me they've gotten married, had kids, and/or started an exciting new job or even a company. But without knowing the future, some people overarm themselves and go too far in trying to protect themselves from the world.

You may find that you're more likely to underidentify with the disorder when in the manic pole of the illness, whereas you may overidentify with it when experiencing the depressive pole. This is, in part, because depression dampens your motivation to initiate certain activities, like work, socializing, or sexual intimacy. You may have subtle problems with memory or concentration as well, rendering the world a confusing, blurry place that demands too much. The illness can seem like an incredible burden that erases any hopes for the future. When you feel this way, you may, understandably, begin to merge the illness with your sense of who you are and who you will become.

If you have symptoms of depression, it's important not to take on more than you can handle and to stick to your guns about what you do and don't feel able to do (even when others want you to do more). But remember also that your depression is likely to go away, with the proper combination of medications, psychotherapy, family and friendship support, physical exercise, and time. So, it's a good idea to set some limited goals for what you can accomplish even while you're depressed, to help you become more energized. Maintaining a certain level of *behavioral activation* can protect you against a worsening mood state (see Chapter 10).

"What Is the Best Way for Me to Think about the Diagnosis?"

Getting into debates with yourself or others about whether your behavior stems from your personality or your disorder can be quite discouraging. You may disagree intensely with your family members about whether you really have changed or whether you're just being yourself and reacting to circumstances. Alternatively, you may disagree with others who expect you to be "up and rolling" when you feel like you're not back to full capacity. But if underidentifying and overidentifying are both problematic, what is a helpful view? Is there an accurate *and* empowering way to think about the disorder? Keep in mind several "mantras" about the diagnosis.

1. *Bipolar disorder is not a life sentence.* As I've discussed, underidentifying and overidentifying are based on painful experiences from the past and understandable fears and uncertainties about the future. But having bipolar illness doesn't mean you have to give up your identity, hopes, and aspirations. Try to think of bipolar disorder in the same way you might think of another chronic medical illness that requires you to take medication regularly (for example, high blood pressure or asthma). Taking medication over the long term markedly reduces the chances that your illness will interfere with your life. There are also certain lifestyle adaptations you will need to make (such as visiting regularly with a psychiatrist or therapist, arranging blood tests, keeping your sleep–wake cycles regulated, moderating your exposure to stress, choosing work that helps you maintain a stable routine). None of these changes, however, requires that you give up your life goals, including having a successful career, maintaining good friendships and family relationships, being physically healthy, having romance, or getting married and having children.

2. *Many creative, productive people have lived with this illness.* Bipolar disorder is one of a very small set of illnesses that may have an upside to it: people who have it are often highly productive and creative. This is because, in part, when you're not actively cycling in and out of episodes of the disorder, your innate mental capabilities, imagination, artistic talents, and personality strengths come to the fore. In her book *Touched with Fire,* Kay Jamison (1993) discusses the link between bipolar disorder and artistic creativity. In reading her work, you will discover that you are not alone in your struggles. Some of the most influential people in art, literature, business, and politics have had the disorder and have produced work that has had lasting effects on our society. A recently documented example is the poet Robert Lowell, whose life and struggle with bipolar disorder are described in Jamison's (2017) book *Setting the River on Fire.*

3. *Try to maintain a healthy sense of who you are and think about how your personality strengths can be drawn on in dealing with the illness.* As you reflect on who you were before you were diagnosed, and once you have completed the trait checklist on page 83, you will probably recall many of your personality strengths. Perhaps you are assertive, sociable, or intellectual. How can you be appropriately assertive in getting proper medical treatment? Can you use your natural sociability to call on your friends, family, and neighbors to help you through rough times? Can you use your natural intellectual inclinations to read up on and learn as much as you can about your illness? Doing so may generate a feeling of continuity between who you used to be and who you are now.

4. *The way you feel right now is not necessarily the way you will feel in 3 months, 6 months, or a year.* You may be feeling bad about your diagnosis and unable to function at the level that you know you're capable of. This rough period may make you feel like you have to give up control to your family, your doctors, and, worst of all, your illness—a prospect that feels highly distasteful. But in all likelihood, with proper treatment, you will return to a state that is close to where you used to be or that at least is more manageable. In the same way that someone who has had a bad viral flu has to stay in bed for another few days after the worst symptoms have cleared, you may need a period of *convalescence* before you can get back to your ordinary routines and functioning.

5. *There are things you can do in addition to taking medications to control the cycling of your mood states.* Coming to terms with the diagnosis of bipolar disorder also means learning certain strategies for mood regulation. Later chapters (8–11) describe these strategies in detail. Acquiring these practical self-management skills will keep you from feeling victimized by the disorder.

• • • • • • • • • • • • • • •

I hope the last chapters have given you a sense of the challenges the disorder can bring to your view of yourself, and how, when you're challenged in this way, it is natural to want to reinterpret the events that have occurred in ways that feel more acceptable. Your reactions to the illness label are shared by others with the disorder. You may be able to make even more sense of bipolar disorder when you think about changes within the brain's neural circuitry that are associated with different extreme mood states and how certain stressful circumstances in your life can trigger these changes. Becoming familiar with the causes of bipolar disorder will help ensure that you ask for, and get, the right treatments.

PART II

Laying the Foundation for Effective Treatment

CHAPTER 5

Where Bipolar Disorder Comes From

Genetics, Biology, and Stress

Stacy, 38, had two young daughters and worked part time for an accounting firm. She had been diagnosed with bipolar I disorder more than 15 years ago and took valproate (Depakote) and a thyroid supplement on a regular basis. Although she agreed that she'd had severe mood swings, her interpretations of their causes tended toward the psychological rather than the biological. She often doubted that she had bipolar disorder: she was scientifically trained and felt that the absence of a definitive biological test meant the diagnosis should remain in doubt. Her psychiatrist frequently reminded her of her family history: her uncle had been diagnosed with bipolar illness and alcoholism, and her mother suffered from periods of major depression. But she remained unconvinced and continued to wonder whether she really needed medication. After all, she had been feeling fine for more than a year. She toyed with the idea of discontinuing her valproate but was talked out of it, time and time again, by her psychiatrist. Over the course of a year, Stacy went through a series of life changes, including divorcing her husband. Other than some mild depression, she made it through the initial marital separation reasonably well. It wasn't until she and her children had to undergo a child custody evaluation that she began to show symptoms of mania. As the evaluation proceeded, she found that calls from her lawyer made her spring into action: She would rush off to the library and copy every legal precedent that was even remotely pertinent to her case, call friends all over the country to ask them to speak to lawyers they knew, and fax numerous documents to her lawyer's and doctor's offices. She often called her estranged husband and screamed threats into the phone. Her lawyer assured her that the divorce and custody agreement would be comfortable for her and her children, but his assurances did little to stop her from working harder and harder and sleeping less and less.

When her psychiatrist suggested to her that she was getting manic, she shrugged and said "probably," adding that she needed to spend every minute preparing for her upcoming court date. As her mania escalated, her doctor convinced her to add risperidone (Risperdal), an SGA. She reluctantly agreed to these modifications but still insisted her problems were stress related.

The divorce and custody arrangement were eventually settled out of court (and in Stacy's favor). Perhaps due to the additional medication and the removal of this life stressor, her mania gradually stopped and a major crisis was averted.

Two major questions plague virtually everyone diagnosed with bipolar disorder: "How did I get this?" and "What triggers an episode of mania or depression?" Some people put it more simply: "What's wrong with my brain?"

As you read this chapter, you'll make distinctions between factors that cause the onset of the disorder and factors that affect the course of the disorder once it is manifest. These factors are not necessarily the same. Specifically, the initial cause of the disorder is strongly influenced by genetic factors (having a family history of bipolar disorder or at least depressive illness) and a history of childhood adversity, which usually means physical, sexual, or emotional abuse. In contrast, new episodes that develop after the first one (also called recurrences) appear to be more heavily influenced by life or family stressors, sleep disruption, alcohol and substance abuse, inconsistency with medications, and other genetic, biological, or environmental factors.

If you have been learning about the disorder for quite some time, you may have read that mood swings have a strong biological or neural basis, often called a "chemical imbalance." (Although there is some validity to this idea, we now know that what is happening in the brain involves much more than a chemical imbalance; more on this later in the chapter.) You may also be aware that bipolar disorder runs in families, and that relatives in your family tree had it or had versions of it. You may have also learned that the cycling of the disorder is influenced by disruptions of *regulatory mechanisms* in the brain and that medications are designed to correct these disruptions or dysregulations. Knowledge of the genetic and biological origins of the disorder will help you accept the illness and educate others close to you about what you are going through (see also Chapter 13). Also, knowing about the biological bases of your disorder will probably make taking medications feel more reasonable to you when you have doubts.

Of course, genetics and biology are not the whole story. As Stacy's case reflects, a major life stressor, such as going through a divorce, can serve as a catalyst for the cycling of mood states. Everybody gets mad, sad, or happy depending on the nature of the things that happen to them. People with bipolar disorder, because of their inherited biological dysregulations, can develop extreme moods in reaction to events in their environment. We don't think that external stress alone can cause people to have bipolar disorder in the first place, but we're fairly certain that it makes the course of the illness worse in people who already have it.

Vulnerability and Stress

We needn't think of bipolar disorder as "only a brain disease" or "only a psychological problem." It can be both of these things, and each can influence the other. Most professionals think of the cycling of bipolar disorder—and, for that matter, the waxing and waning of most illnesses—as reflecting a complex interplay among:

- *Genetic vulnerabilities*—inheriting a propensity toward the disorder from one or more blood relatives
- *Neurocognitive processes*—abnormal functioning of brain circuits and neurotransmitters such as dopamine or serotonin
- *Psychological processes*—your personality, beliefs, or expectations about your ability to control things or make good things happen
- *Stress agents*—either events that bring about positive or negative changes (for example, transitions in your job or living situation, financial problems, or a new romantic relationship), or the worsening of chronic problems (such as ongoing and severe conflicts with your family members; living in close, cramped quarters; or taking care of someone who is severely ill)

Think of it this way: You have underlying genetic vulnerabilities with which you were born. Essentially, the strength of the signals transmitted through the spaces between the nerve cells in your brain (synapses) is different from that of people without bipolar disorder. This dysregulation is called *abnormal synaptic plasticity* (Schloesser, Huang, Klein, & Manji, 2008), and it can show up in different ways:

- Your brain may be over- or underproducing certain neurotransmitters, such as dopamine, serotonin, norepinephrine, or GABA (gamma-aminobutyric acid).
- You might undergo changes in the structure or function of your nerve cell receptors.
- You might also have changes in the functioning or volume of certain brain structures, such as the subgenual prefrontal cortex or the amygdala. These changes are only detectable in brain scans.

If these disturbances seem alarming, know that most of the time they are dormant and have little effect on your day-to-day functioning, although they still make you more susceptible to experiencing manic or depressive episodes. When stressors reach a certain level, biological vulnerabilities or predispositions get expressed as the symptoms you're already familiar with—irritable or elevated mood, racing thoughts, paralyzing sadness, and sleep disturbance. In other words, your biological predispositions affect your psychological and emotional reactions to events (and in all likelihood, vice versa). Likewise, when the stress agent is removed (for example, you end a relationship that was causing you grief), your biological dysregulations may become dormant again (as happened for Stacy).

Some psychiatrists and psychologists use a vulnerability–stress model to explain a person's bipolar symptoms. This model requires thinking about the interactions among several levels:

- *Molecular factors*—genes that make you susceptible to bipolar disorder or, alternatively, genes that protect you from getting severe mood swings
- *Cellular events*—such as how quickly cells grow or die
- *Brain systems*—the circuits or nerve pathways involved in mood regulation
- *Behavior*—how you react emotionally and what you do when you encounter stressful situations
- *Environmental stressors*—life events, particularly those that cause sleep deprivation; excessive goal striving (for example, taking on too many work assignments), family conflicts, poverty, or adverse living conditions (Schloesser et al., 2008)

Look at the graph on page 95. If you were born with a great deal of genetic or biological vulnerability—for example, the disorder is present in multiple past generations of your family—a relatively minor stressor, such as a change in your working hours and the resulting loss of sleep, could be enough to elicit mood symptoms. Less genetic vulnerability (only one extended relative, like an uncle, had bipolar disorder, or a few relatives had depression, but no one was bipolar) could mean that mood symptoms will be triggered only by relatively severe stressors, such as the death of a parent or a major car accident or trauma.

To make matters more complex, certain genes can predispose you to favor certain environments. Someone who inherited a strong physique, for example, might choose work that builds muscles, like building construction. A person who is socially withdrawn might choose activities that don't require interacting much with others—forestry, for example. Likewise, as a person with a genetic vulnerability to bipolar disorder, you may be drawn to highly stimulating, creative, and spontaneous or unpredictable activities, like writing, painting, and performing music or, for some, stock trading. You may have the energy to perform well in these endeav-

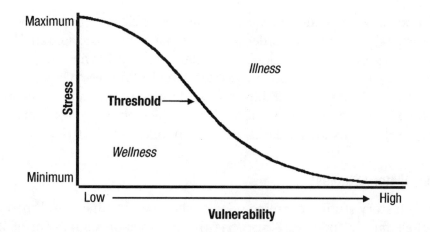

A vulnerability–stress model for understanding periods of illness and wellness. Adapted by permission from Zubin and Spring (1977). Copyright © 1977 by the American Psychological Association.

ors most of the time but then become emotionally dysregulated by the constant stress and changes in stimulation associated with these activities. You may become depressed when you experience a letdown related to these activities (for example, the stock market has a "correction") and find it impossible to do them anymore.

This chapter provides examples of what is meant by genetic and biological vulnerability and ways to determine whether your family tree puts you at greater or lesser risk. You'll also learn more about the kinds of stressors that have been shown in research to trigger mood cycling. Recognizing that you may be biologically and genetically vulnerable to mood swings and that certain factors are particularly stressful for you is empowering: these are the first steps in learning to manage your disorder. By the chapter's end you should have a general idea of how genetics and biology answer the question "How did I get this?" and how these factors combine with stress to bring about new episodes of bipolar disorder. Later chapters provide practical suggestions for minimizing the impact of stressful events or interpersonal circumstances.

"How Did I Get This?": The Role of Genetics

We have known for many years that mood disorders are genetically heritable and run in families. Genetic studies of persons with bipolar disorder (reviewed in the next section) have consistently supported this position, although no one thinks that genetics provide all the answers.

As I said in Chapter 3, your family history should be a part of your initial diagnostic evaluation. Stacy, as it turned out, had a mother and an uncle who showed signs of mood disorders, although it was only her uncle who had bipolar disorder. It is not unusual for bipolar disorder to *co-segregate* or be associated in family trees with other kinds of mood disorders, particularly various forms of depression.

How do we know that bipolar disorder runs in families? Geneticists usually establish that an illness is heritable through family, twin, and molecular genetic studies. If you want to know more about these topics, there are some great reviews you can consult (for example, Ikeda, Saito, Kondo, & Iwata, 2017).

Family History Studies

Family history studies examine people who have an illness and then find out who in their family "pedigree" also has the disorder or some form of it (recall from earlier chapters that bipolar disorder can look quite different among different people). We know that when one person has the disorder, often a brother, sister, parent, or aunt or uncle will also have it. We also know that some relatives of people with bipolar disorder will have other mood disorders, such as major depressive disorder or dysthymic disorder. They may be affected by alcoholism, drug abuse, panic or other anxiety symptoms, or an eating disorder (for example, obesity with binge eating), which, while not mood disorders themselves, are problems that co-occur with and sometimes mask underlying depressive or manic symptoms. The diagram at the bottom of this page depicts Stacy's family pedigree. The circles represent women, and the squares represent men. Notice that some of her relatives had mood disorders and some did not.

The average rate of mood disorders (major depression, dysthymia, or bipolar disorder) among first-degree relatives of bipolar persons is about 25%. That is, one of every four siblings, parents, and children of a person with bipolar disorder will have some kind of mood disorder. On average, about 9% of a person's first-degree

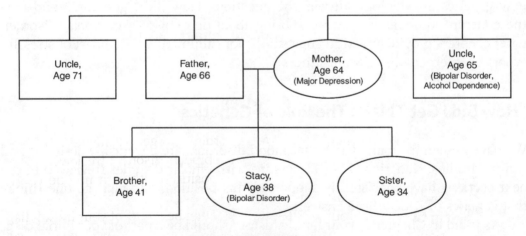

Stacy's family pedigree.

relatives have bipolar I or II disorder (compared to about 1–2% of the general population), and about 14% have strictly defined major depressive disorder (without mania or hypomania). These numbers are averages: some people have many more relatives who have mood disorders, and some have fewer. Nonetheless, if you have bipolar disorder, the chances that one of your first-degree relatives has it are 9–10 times the general population rate. On the other hand, the same statistic means that if you have bipolar disorder, your child's chances of developing it during his or her lifetime is only about 10%.

Twin Studies

Another way to establish heritability is to ask this traditional question: When one identical twin has the disorder, what is the probability (percentage) that the other identical twin also has it? Identical twins, as you probably know, came from the same egg and share 100% of their genes. Fraternal twins (from two different eggs) share only about 50% of their genes (on average), just like brothers and sisters. If we think a disorder is heritable, we would expect the identical twin pairs to have higher *concordance* or agreement rates—when one twin is bipolar, the other should be also—than fraternal twin pairs.

The most recent twin studies find that concordance rates for bipolar disorder among identical twins average 48% and between fraternal twins 6% (Barnett & Smoller, 2009; Ikeda et al., 2017). Stated another way, when one identical twin has bipolar disorder, there is about a 1 in 2 chance that the other identical twin does too. When a fraternal twin has bipolar disorder, there is only about a 1 in 16 chance that his or her twin has it. This means that bipolar disorder has a strong genetic component, but if the illness were entirely genetic, the identical twin rate would be 100%. We know there must be nongenetic environmental causes as well, and these are discussed later in this chapter.

Genes are powerful determinants of the likelihood that a person will develop bipolar disorder; in fact, bipolar disorder is one of the most heritable of psychiatric conditions. Knowing these facts may or may not make you feel better about your condition. Some people feel absolved of self-blame upon learning the disorder is inherited, especially if they previously believed or were told that their symptoms of depression or mania were expressions of a character weakness. Other people feel "defective" or fearful that they will pass on bad genes to their children. I will talk about these issues more below, but first let's consider what it is that is actually passed on from generation to generation.

What Exactly Is Inherited?

We know that inheriting bipolar disorder can't be as simple as inheriting brown hair or blue eyes. Too many people with the disorder do not have any relatives with mood disorders, or have not had mood disorders occur in their family for several generations. This means that the way the disorder is passed on is more complicated than, for example, hair color. It may be that the tendency to become *emotionally dysregulated*—extremely moody—runs in families. It may be that people inherit a mild form of bipolar disorder, or perhaps just a moody temperament, but develop the full bipolar condition only in the presence of other predisposing conditions, like these:

- Inheriting genes for bipolar disorder from both sides of the family
- Being "in utero" when the mother contracted a virus and undergoing a difficult, complicated birth
- Taking street drugs when growing up
- Sustaining a head injury
- Surviving highly adverse childhood circumstances

Some people with bipolar disorder experienced highly traumatic sexual, physical, or emotional abuse as children, not necessarily from their parents but often from other relatives, family associates, babysitters, or strangers. Traumatic experiences in childhood strongly contribute to difficulties in regulating one's emotions in adulthood, although we don't think that abuse alone can cause bipolar disorder. Street drugs like methamphetamine can trigger a manic episode that is then followed by one or more depressive episodes. However, when this pattern occurs it is usually in a person with a family history of bipolar disorder.

Is there direct evidence for the hypothesis that a person's genetic inheritance or biological vulnerabilities interact with specific environmental conditions to produce bipolar disorder? The data on this question are just beginning to come in. For example, a group of researchers at the University of Pittsburgh School of Medicine found that children of parents with bipolar disorder were more likely to develop the disorder than children whose parents were not bipolar, but the risk for bipolar disorder was highest when (1) the parent had a young onset of illness (under age 18) and (2) the child showed evidence of depression, anxiety, or mood instability throughout childhood (Hafeman et al., 2016). Longitudinal studies that show the separate effects of environmental factors (such as childhood adversity) and their interaction with genetic factors will be of considerable value in understanding these complex relationships.

Molecular Genetic Studies

Recent advances in *molecular genetics* allow researchers to examine regions of the chromosomes in an attempt to locate genes for bipolar disorder. These studies require huge numbers of participants to avoid spurious findings. Although a number of genes have been found to be associated with bipolar disorder, no single gene provides an adequate explanation. Rather, researchers suspect that many genes—each with a quite small effect—contribute to a genetic vulnerability to the illness. Examples of these "candidate genes" include:

- Genes for brain-derived neurotrophic factor (BDNF), which encourages the development of new brain cells, the connections between cells, and synaptic plasticity; it is also believed to have a role in the stress response

- The SLC6A4 gene, which encodes the serotonin transporter (SERT), a protein that transports the neurotransmitter serotonin from the synaptic cleft to the presynaptic neuron

- The gene for the NMDA (*N*-methyl-D-aspartate) glutamate receptor

- Genes that contain instructions for building calcium channels (CACNA1C), promoting neural connectivity (TENM4), or cortical thickness (NCAN)

- The gene for monoamine oxidase A (MAOA), which breaks down serotonin into metabolites

- "Clock genes" that drive our circadian rhythms (see the pullout to the right; Barnett & Smoller, 2009)

> **New research:** Recent research suggests that genes that control our circadian rhythms (for example, "clock genes") are involved in the risk for bipolar disorder and its recurrences. For example, laboratory mice with mutations in clock genes behave in ways that resemble the behavior of people with mania (for example, increases in activity, decreased sleep, reward-seeking behavior). These changes are reversed when the mice are given lithium (Roybal et al., 2007).

Quantitative Trait Studies

A new method of studying genetics is to determine what changes in thinking, behavior, or the brain get inherited alongside bipolar disorder. An innovative study was conducted in the pedigrees of people who lived in isolated regions of Costa Rica and Colombia, where families with high rates of bipolar disorder have lived for many generations. Investigators found a number of cognitive, temperamental, and neuroanatomical attributes that were influenced by genes being passed through family members and that were also associated with bipolar disorder, such as decreased thickness of the prefrontal and temporal cortices (Fears et al., 2014). In other words, a person who inherits bipolar disorder is more likely to also inherit brain changes that may be important in regulating emotions.

One particularly interesting finding in these families was that measures of creativity were significantly higher in individuals who had bipolar disorder and in their family members than among individuals in the same communities who did not have bipolar disorder (Fears et al., 2014). In other words, not all genes that contribute to bipolar disorder are "bad" or undesirable. However, in the wrong combination, genes that influence positive traits like creativity may combine with genes that influence less desirable attributes of the illness, such as extreme difficulty in regulating one's emotions or becoming overly goal driven. Possibly, combinations like these can lead to excessive workaholism, sleep disruption, or grandiose thinking.

• • • • • • • • • • • • • • •

What can we conclude from all of this? At this stage, we can say with confidence that bipolar disorder is highly heritable, but there is a lot we don't know about how it is inherited, what genes are involved, and what these genes do. Once the genes are located (and there will probably be many), more accurate diagnoses and better treatments are likely to follow. The long-term goal of this research is to *personalize our treatment choices,* which means predicting what medications or therapies are best suited to people with genetically distinct forms of bipolar disorder.

"Do I Have a Genetic Vulnerability?": Examining Your Own Pedigree

Before we get into the issue of what the genetic data might mean for your own life, take a look at whether bipolar disorder runs in your family. Are you genetically predisposed to the disorder? To begin this exercise, fill out the form on page 101 to the best of your knowledge. Confine yourself to your own children, your siblings (note in the table if the person is a full sibling or a half sibling), your parents, grandparents, aunts, and uncles. Leave out cousins, nephews, and nieces unless you know them very well—the information people have on these relatives tends to be unreliable. Consult your parents or siblings if you want more information. I have filled in the first four lines for Stacy's family as examples.

Next, place a star next to anyone you think may have had (or still has):

1. Full bipolar I or bipolar II disorder or even a milder form of bipolar disorder, such as cyclothymia or unspecified bipolar disorder
2. Major depressive episodes or long-term periods of mild to moderate depression (dysthymia)
3. Any other psychiatric problem that may be masking mood disturbances (for example, drinking or drug problems, panic attacks, or eating disorders)

Collecting Information to Draw Your Pedigree

Name of relative	Relationship to you	Age now (or at death)	How did he/she die?
1. Robert	Father	66	Heart attack
2. Isabelle*	Mother	64	(Still alive)
3. Mark	Brother	41	(Still alive)
4. Valerie	Sister	34	(Still alive)
5. _____	_____	___	_____
6. _____	_____	___	_____
7. _____	_____	___	_____
8. _____	_____	___	_____
9. _____	_____	___	_____
10. _____	_____	___	_____

* = major depression.

Answers to the following questions will give you clues as to your relative's health or illness:

- How did the relative die (if deceased)? Was it an accident, suicide, or an illness?
- Was the person ever unable to work for a period of time, or did she constantly switch jobs?
- Did he have multiple marriages or a succession of relationships that did not last?
- Are there family stories about the person being drunk, hurting himself or others, or having a "nervous breakdown"?
- Was this relative a recluse, shutting herself away in a room for days at a time?
- Did he ever take psychiatric medications? What kind?
- Was he ever in a psychiatric hospital?

Now assemble your information into a pedigree. Again, circles refer to female relatives and squares to males. Fill in the circle or square of any relative you think may have had bipolar disorder. Fill in only half of the circle or square if the person had major depression, dysthymia, cyclothymia, or any of the other problems we have discussed that can mask a mood disorder. Put an *S* above anyone who committed suicide. Put a question mark in the circles or squares of any relatives you don't know about.

Next, examine the pedigree (paying particular attention to the solid and half-solid circles or squares) and ask yourself the following: How many of your relatives probably had bipolar disorder? If none, are there relatives in your family tree who are or were depressed or addicted to alcohol or drugs? If so, consider whether these relatives may have had a hidden depressive or bipolar condition. For example, if a person had bursts of rage even when not drunk and became withdrawn for periods of time even when "on the wagon," he or she may have had an underlying mood disorder as well as alcoholism.

Disorders like alcoholism or drug abuse tend to affect males more than females, whereas major depressive episodes and eating disorders affect more females than males. Does this pattern help you determine whether specific relatives in your family tree had psychiatric conditions? Did any relative spend time in a psychiatric hospital or take psychiatric medications for a long period of time? Did anyone commit suicide? Suicide attempts or completions are more common among people with bipolar disorder than among people with major depression, especially when they also have an alcohol or substance dependence disorder.

If you have children, you may know whether one or more of them has a psychiatric disorder and can fill in those circles or squares. Of course, your children may not yet have reached an age when a disorder is recognizable—bipolar disorder

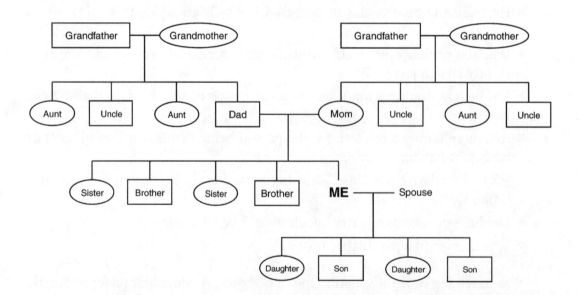

Locating relatives with mood disorders in your family pedigree.

can be diagnosed at any age, but the majority of people develop it in their middle to late teens (see Chapter 14). Be sure to fill in any psychiatric information relevant to your children's other parent and draw in "tree branches" to any affected or unaffected relatives in his or her family of origin. As you know, it is possible that your children inherited mood disorders from the other side of the family or from both sides.

"What Does the Genetic Evidence Mean for Me?"

Practical Implications of Genetics

One's degree of vulnerability to bipolar disorder is usually described in general terms like *low, medium,* or *high.* One way of assessing your family tree is to ask whether the number of late-teenage or adult first-degree relatives in your pedigree who have had mood disorders exceeds the average rate of 25% among people with bipolar disorder. If your family tree is dotted with people who have had bipolar disorder or some other mood disorder—if more people are affected than unaffected—your vulnerability is high. Likewise, if bipolar disorder or other mood disorders are present in several generations (for example, in your siblings, parents, and grandparents), then your genetic vulnerability is higher than that of a person with bipolar disorder in only one generation. If only one of your first-degree relatives had a mild dysthymic depression and no one had bipolar disorder, your genetic vulnerability is probably on the low end of the continuum.

Now, what do you do with the information if you have concluded that bipolar disorder, or at least depression, runs in your family? Genetic evidence has practical implications for your life. First, the fact that the disorder runs in your family

---

PERSONALIZED CARE TIP:
Making sense of gene–environment interactions

There is an important distinction to be made between the original causes of bipolar disorder and the triggers of new episodes (recurrences) or the factors that affect functioning or quality of life once you have the illness. As discussed in this chapter, environmental factors play a key role in recurrences. While it is empowering to understand the role of both genetic and environmental factors in your individual pattern of recurrences, keep in mind that we don't have full control over what environmental triggers come our way. Like the genes we're born with, environmental stressors can occur independently of our actions. In later chapters, you'll learn some strategies for reducing the effects of life events on your mood stability.

should make you feel less ashamed of having the illness. None of us can control the genes with which we come into this world. We also don't know how to engineer the environment to prevent the original onset of the disorder. As you'll see in later chapters, there are things you can do to control the cycling of your illness. But getting the disorder in the first place is heavily influenced by your genetic makeup. *In other words, it isn't your fault—a fact that your family members may also need to hear* (see Chapter 13). As the father of one young man with bipolar disorder told me, "For a long time we thought he was just a screw-up. He seemed able to screw up everything. But eventually we realized there was an illness and that there was something really wrong with his brain. He had a real problem that had a chemical basis, and it was probably something he got from me or from my side of the family. He wasn't doing all that stuff to hurt us. That's when we came to some understandings as a family."

Having a family history of bipolar disorder may also help confirm your diagnosis if you still have doubts (see also Chapter 3). If bipolar disorder clearly runs in your family, this fact should sway you and your doctor toward the validity of your own bipolar diagnosis more than, say, ADHD or schizophrenia.

A family history of bipolar disorder is not a conclusive piece of evidence; it provides only one piece of the diagnostic puzzle. Even if bipolar disorder runs in your family, you probably feel that your mood swings are a product of more than just your clock genes or circuits in your brain that have gone haywire. Stacy certainly felt this way. That's why it's very important to think of genetics as providing only a background for problems you may have in regulating your emotions, thinking, or activity levels. It's the same way with cardiovascular (heart disease) risk: it certainly runs in families, but not everyone in a genetically susceptible family ends up with high blood pressure, and certainly not everyone with a family history of heart disease ends up dying of a heart attack. What people eat, whether they smoke, their weight, how much they exercise, their levels of stress, and a whole host of other factors come into play.

"What If I Don't Have a Family History of the Disorder?"

"My grandpa, he's another story. I doubt he was ever depressed, 'cause he was too busy torturing his wife, his kids, and his farmhands. He just disappeared on a horse one day. Probably somebody shot him."
　　　　—60-year-old woman with bipolar II disorder reviewing her family tree

You may examine your family pedigree and see no evidence of any mood disorders or other mental illness. This is unusual, but it does happen. The thing to ask yourself is whether you know enough about the people in your pedigree to say that they had no illness. Could the "exhaustion" that your mother describes in her own mother have been depression? If your grandfather is described as "dominating," "angry," or "aggressive," could he have also been manic? Could bipolar illness have occurred in someone several generations back?

Usually, your older relatives will know more about your family pedigree than you do, in which case you can enlist their help in filling out your pedigree chart. Your parents, if they are alive, will almost certainly know more about the lives of their parents, siblings, and other relatives. Sometimes, doctors will conduct thorough family history interviews with your relatives as part of your initial evaluation (see Chapter 3), but in my experience this is rare.

Even with high-quality information, you may not be able to identify any relatives in your pedigree who had a mood disorder. There are probably forms of bipolar disorder that are triggered by environmental or at least nongenetic factors. For example, it's possible that prolonged drug abuse can bring on bipolar disorder in some people. An injury to the head or a neurological illness such as encephalitis or multiple sclerosis can bring on mood swings that look just like those of bipolar disorder. Perhaps we will find that in some people the onset of bipolar disorder can be attributed to complications that occurred during their birth or to viruses their mothers contracted during pregnancy, as has been found for schizophrenia. As I said above, adverse childhood experiences such as physical or sexual abuse may also contribute to the onset of bipolar disorder.

Even if your disorder doesn't have an obvious genetic basis, you may respond to the medications that are used to treat bipolar disorder (see Chapter 6), just as a headache caused by environmental stress can be alleviated by aspirin. An increasing number of studies indicate that if you have people in your family tree who had bipolar disorder and responded well to lithium, you will respond well to lithium yourself (Duffy et al., 2014; Grof, Duffy, Alda, & Hajek, 2009). But family history evidence is still not strong enough to guide our choice of treatments, given how little most of us know about what drugs our relatives did well on. To make drug treatment recommendations your physician will probably place greater emphasis on

New research: The pathways from genes to environment to the occurrence of manic symptoms are quite complex. In an epidemiological study of 811 people with a lifetime history of mania, childhood adversity (physical and sexual maltreatment) was associated with a higher risk for both onset of manic symptoms and recurrent manic episodes in adulthood. Stressful events that occurred in the year before the study, such as financial problems, were more closely associated with onsets or recurrences of mania among individuals who had both a family history of bipolar disorder *and* childhood adversity, compared to those without childhood adversity. In other words, childhood adversity may potentiate the effects of later stressful events in provoking mania, especially in people who are genetically susceptible to the disorder (Gilman et al., 2015).

your current and past symptoms and pattern of mood cycling than on your family history.

"What about Having Children?"

As indicated above, if you have bipolar disorder, your chances of passing it on to your kids average about 9%, with an additional 14% chance that they will develop major depression. These probabilities are comparable to those for other psychiatric disorders—the rate of schizophrenia in the children of mothers with schizophrenia is about 13%. So, the odds are in your favor: in most cases, your children won't develop anything. See Chapter 14 for more information on children.

Of course, the question of whether to have children goes well beyond statistics. Whether you are a woman or a man, your answer to this question should be based on considerations such as whether you want children, are clinically stable enough to take care of a child, whether you are physically healthy in other ways, and, where applicable, whether you are satisfied with your relationship with your partner or with your ability to take care of a child on your own. I'll talk more about these concerns in Chapters 12 and 13.

Genes Are Not Destiny

Despite the relatively small chance that bipolar disorder will be passed genetically from parent to child, many people feel doomed by the evidence that they may have susceptibility genes. They assume that having the associated genes means they and their children have nothing to look forward to but a lot of mood cycling, doctors, medications, and hospitals. Being genetically prone or vulnerable to a disorder means that, due to your biology, you are more likely to get an illness than someone without the same genetic susceptibility. But being genetically vulnerable does *not* mean that you will necessarily get ill within a certain stretch of time; it does not predict the probability or the timing of your recurrences. It also does *not* mean that there is nothing you can do to control your cycling. High blood pressure, high cholesterol, and diabetes are all heritable, but exercise, diet,

Effective prevention: If you're worried that your children might develop bipolar disorder, be alert for these early warning signs (see Chapter 14 for more details):

- Irritability that occurs in episodes
- Highly reactive moods, rapid mood shifts
- Aggressiveness
- Sleep disturbance
- Anxiety
- Suicidal or morbid thinking
- School problems
- Inappropriate sexuality
- Drug or alcohol abuse
- Sadness
- Lethargy and withdrawal

and appropriate medications go a long way in controlling these diseases. Likewise, lifestyle management and medications are critical to controlling episodes of bipolar illness (see Chapters 6–10).

Genetics are not destiny for your first-degree relatives either. Illnesses skip generations or can be transmitted in a milder form. Even if you see signs of disturbance that suggest the beginnings of bipolar disorder, there are steps you can take to get your child treatment—see Chapter 14 and the strategies I have written about in *The Bipolar Teen* (Miklowitz & George, 2007). Start by getting a thorough diagnostic evaluation from a psychiatrist or psychologist who specializes in pediatric mood disorders. Talk to your child's teachers about what accommodations can be made in your child's educational plans (see *www.jbrf.org*).

What Is a Biological Dysregulation?

Stacy had been told that her illness was "probably chemical." She understood that having a biological dysregulation meant that her illness was not fully under her control, but she was not sure what "chemical" meant. Unfortunately, "chemical imbalance" is, we now know, inadequate to describe the nature of dysregulations that occur in the brains of those with bipolar disorder. As mentioned earlier, biological dysregulation affects more than neurochemicals. Stacy wanted to know more:

- Was this dysregulation something that could be measured?
- Why was there no blood test or brain scan for detecting it?
- Were the relevant changes in her brain occurring only when she was manic or depressed?
- What were the medications doing for the dysregulation?
- Were the medications creating a different kind of dysregulation?
- Could these vulnerabilities be corrected by diet?

Stacy became frustrated that her doctor didn't give clear answers to these questions, even though he seemed quite knowledgeable otherwise. She felt that she was being asked to accept a lot of things on faith, and her scientific background made her feel doubtful.

Biological Vulnerabilities: Neural Circuits and Second Messenger Systems

Given that genetic background so strongly influences the onset of bipolar disorder, surely anatomical and/or physiological factors play a role as well. As I discussed in the preceding sections, a biological vulnerability can be dormant and then become activated by a trigger, such as environmental stress or drug abuse. Defining the nature of this biological vulnerability is much trickier, however. If you have been told that you have a "biochemical imbalance in the brain," you may feel that this explanation raises as many questions as it answers, as it did for Stacy.

You may find you're more willing to adopt a medication regimen if you understand what your doctors mean by a biological vulnerability or dysregulation. They are usually referring to something that is part of you even when you're not having any symptoms. To use the blood pressure analogy, people with hypertension always have a vulnerability to an attack of high blood pressure, even when they're doing fine. Their system is such that their blood pressure is above normal even when they are relatively stress free and eating well, and stress causes their blood pressure to rise even higher. Likewise, we think that in bipolar disorder, biological dysregulations are present even when you are feeling well.

In bipolar disorder, biological vulnerabilities may be evoked by stress agents (for example, a sudden change such as loss of a job), alcohol or street drugs, or, for some people, antidepressants (see Chapter 6). When a stressor brings biological vulnerabilities to the foreground, the symptoms of bipolar disorder are more likely to appear.

For a long time, scientists talked about bipolar disorder in terms of the amount of certain neurotransmitters: people with the disorder had too little serotonin, too little norepinephrine, or too much dopamine. A major figure in our field, Husseini Manji, encourages us to think instead about the disorder as an "impairment of synaptic and cellular plasticity" (Manji, 2009, p. 2). This means that people with bipolar disorder have genetically influenced problems with information processing in synapses (the spaces between nerve cells) and circuits (the neuronal connections between one brain structure and others), rather than too much or too little of a certain chemical.

To get technical for a moment, we suspect that people with bipolar disorder have disturbances in *intracellular signaling cascades*, which regulate the neurotransmitter, neuropeptide, and hormonal systems that are central to the limbic system. The limbic system, which includes the amygdala and the hippocampus, regulates emotional states, sleep, and arousal, all of which are strongly affected in bipolar disorder. Additionally, when people with bipolar disorder and major depression are under stress, their adrenal glands may overproduce certain hormones (for example, glucocorticoids). Long-term stress and glucocorticoid overproduction may damage or destroy cells in the hippocampus, a brain structure that is centrally involved in memory and conditioned fear reactions (Manji, 2009; Schloesser et al., 2008).

New research involving persons with bipolar disorder has also found problems in their *second messenger systems* (also known as *signal transducers*), which are molecules inside brain nerve cells. When one nerve cell fires, it sends neurotransmitters (the "first messengers") to the next nerve cell. Then a second messenger system informs the second nerve cell that the first nerve cell has fired. In other words, second messengers help to determine whether a cell communicates messages to other parts of the same cell and to nearby cells. For example, lithium and valproate slow down activity of the *protein kinase C signaling cascade,* an important mediator of signals within the cells when their receptors are stimulated by neurotransmitters (Harrison, Geddes, & Tunbridge, 2018; Newberg, Catapano, Zarate, & Manji, 2008). This exciting research suggests that changes in second messenger systems may constitute one form of biological vulnerability to bipolar disorder—one that may be partially correctable by medications.

An Alternative Theory: Immune Dysregulation

A novel area of investigation concerns the role of immune functioning in people with bipolar disorder (B. I. Goldstein et al., 2015). When the body is under biological or psychological stress, such as when it is being attacked by an infectious agent, it produces molecules called *inflammatory cytokines* that bring about a flu-like state: changes in sleep, loss of pleasure from everyday activities, and low energy. Just as neurons communicate with one another using signaling molecules (neurotransmitters), immune cells communicate using cytokines as signaling molecules. These symptoms are a lot like those of depression, and in fact depression and physical illness states co-occur in many people. There has been increasing interest in the relevance of neuroinflammation to depression: people with major depression have higher levels of proinflammatory cytokines than healthy volunteers (Miller, Maletic, & Raison, 2009).

Might people with bipolar disorder also have irregularities in immunological processes? A meta-analysis of 30 studies concluded that adults with bipolar disorder could be distinguished from healthy adults on concentrations of several cytokines, with names like IL (interleukin)-2, IL-4, or IL-6 (Modabbernia, Taslimi, Brietzke, & Ashrafi, 2013). Levels of these markers are highest during mood episodes, whether manic or depressed, and may also remain elevated when people are free of symptoms. We think there is a subgroup of people with bipolar disorder or major depression who have high levels of proinflammatory cytokines even when they're between episodes and feeling well.

Although psychiatric medications are thought to act by modifying neurotransmitters, lithium, antipsychotics, and antidepressants are also known to reduce inflammation in patients (Boufidou, Nikkolaou, Alevizios, Liappas, & Christodoulou, 2004). In addition, several studies have shown that even over-the-counter anti-inflammatories like aspirin and ibuprofen can help reduce depression symptoms in some people. We don't yet know whether immune-suppressing drugs will be effective for bipolar disorder, a topic we're likely to have an answer to in the next decade.

The Lack of a Definitive Test

"I've been told for years that there's something wrong with my brain. I just wish there was a blood test or a brain scan or something that I could look at and see my illness. Then I'd be more convinced that I need medications. What if I'm taking all these drugs to treat some chemical deficiency that I don't even have?"

—A 57-year-old man with bipolar I disorder

Despite this promising research, there is no definitive biological or genetic test for the impairments of synaptic and cellular plasticity or the inflammatory abnormalities characteristic of bipolar disorder. Most professionals, patients, and families wish there were, because that would make diagnosis and treatment planning much easier.

The absence of a definitive test makes it easy to forget that you have a biological dysregulation and even easier to believe that you never had one in the first place. Stacy, who had been free of symptoms for quite some time, started to wonder whether she really had a biological predisposition. Asking this question is certainly understandable. Could your manic or depressive episodes have been one-time occurrences that were set off by unpleasant life circumstances? Many people start to think, "I had this illness once, but now it's under my control," especially when they've been well for a while. But bipolar symptoms have a way of recurring when you least expect them. We believe this is because genetic and biological vulnerabilities are still present, even when your symptoms are controlled by medications and psychotherapy.

Despite the limitations of our current technologies, I believe we will see some real advances in diagnostic tests for the illness in the next decade. The neural circuits most associated with mood symptoms are being mapped through brain-imaging techniques such as functional or structural magnetic resonance imaging (MRI). Many studies find that the amygdala—a structure that is central to identifying and responding to environmental threats (real or imagined)—is both more active and larger in volume in people with bipolar disorder. Areas of the prefrontal cortex, the "executive center" in the brain that inhibits lower brain areas like the amygdala, may be correspondingly less active and smaller in volume in bipolar disorder (Phillips & Swartz, 2014).

These are not the only brain structures or circuits involved in the disorder, nor are we able to diagnose bipolar disorder from brain scans alone. Be skeptical of showmen who claim they can do so. It is possible that diagnosis by neuroimaging will be available in the future, but we have a lot of work to do first.

What Turns a Biological Vulnerability into an Episode?

Learning that you may have certain inherited biological dysregulations, although perhaps distressing, should help to arm you against recurrences of your illness.

Like the person with diabetes who knows he or she must avoid ice cream, or the person with high blood pressure who must avoid high-salt foods, you can exert a degree of control over bipolar disorder by learning to avoid triggers that influence the expression of your biological vulnerabilities. When people who do not have biological dysregulations experience these triggers (for example, they take drugs or alcohol or intentionally subject themselves to high levels of stress), they may experience changes in mood, but not to the degree that characterizes a person with bipolar disorder.

Some triggers may directly impinge on a person's biological vulnerabilities and set them off, kind of like lighting a fuse connecting a string of firecrackers. For example, bipolar disorder is believed to be related to diminished functioning of the serotonin system. LSD stimulates the action of serotonin receptors in the brain, which produces other biochemical events that can increase your risk of developing a manic episode. Another example: bipolar disorder has been related to increased sensitivity of the dopamine receptors and changes in the regulation of dopamine-rich "reward pathways" of the brain. Studies of laboratory animals as well as humans find that amphetamine (speed) stimulates the release and prolongs the activity of dopamine in the brain, which can cause a state of high arousal, paranoid thinking, irritability, and increases in energy or motor activity.

Alcohol inhibits the activity of your central nervous system (for example, it increases the effects of the inhibitory neurotransmitter GABA on its receptors) and, like caffeine and other substances, interferes with your sleep–wake rhythms. When you stop drinking, your brain circuits become more excitable, much like they do in mania.

Environmental stress can aggravate your biological vulnerabilities also, but the mechanisms by which this happens are not well understood by scientists. Stress cannot be avoided in the same way that alcohol or drugs can be avoided, but knowing what kinds of environmental changes are particularly troublesome for you (for example, the onset of daylight saving time or the beginning of the school year) will help you plan preventively to avoid recurrences (for example, changing your nightly routines). Let's take a closer look at how stress affects mood episodes.

Stress and Bipolar Episodes

Can bipolar disorder be caused by environmental factors, such as a high-conflict marriage, problems with parents, life changes, a difficult job, or a history of abuse as a child? These are extremely important questions. Indeed, people with bipolar disorder are 2.6 times as likely to have been in an abusive environment as children than healthy people, with emotional abuse being the most common form (being severely criticized or humiliated or threatened with a loss of basic securities) (Palmier-Claus, Berry, Bucci, Mansell, & Varese, 2016). Most scientists in the field doubt that a traumatic event or an emotionally abusive family alone can *cause* bipolar disorder without the contributing influences of genetics and biology. However, we are reasonably certain that stress and trauma increase the chances that you will have a recurrence of mania or depression. It may also affect the timing of your first episodes (for example, whether the illness starts in childhood). Your level and type of stress may also affect how long it takes you to recover from an episode or your risk of having another episode within a certain time frame. Clinicians are interested in knowing about the role of stress in your life because it can help them in treatment planning, such as deciding what type of therapy to recommend to you.

What kinds of environmental stressors are particularly influential in recurrences of the illness? Encountering a major life change—whether positive or negative—increases your likelihood of having a manic or depressive recurrence. Stacy's divorce had relatively little immediate effect on her mood state, but the child custody evaluation played a major role in her manic episode. Other kinds of stress include sleep–wake cycle disruptions and conflicts with significant others. I'll be talking about each of these and giving examples. I'll also talk about some of the current thinking about mechanisms by which biological vulnerabilities might be affected by stress.

Life Changes

Changes are a part of life, and sometimes they are quite welcome. Examples of positive life changes include getting married, having a child, buying a new house, making a large sum of money from an investment, or getting a job promotion. Negative life changes include the death of a loved one, the loss of a relationship, the loss of a job, a car accident, or the development of a medical illness in yourself or a family member. Stress can come in the form of conflicts or unpleasant interactions with people you know well, particularly your family.

Manic and depressive episodes often follow major life changes, both positive and negative. Sheri Johnson, a psychology professor at the University of California, Berkeley, has written extensively about the role of life events in bipolar disorder. She points out that it is not always clear whether life events are a cause or an effect of mood episodes. Patrick, age 36, provides an illustration. When he was cycling into mania, he would become overconfident and frequently tell off his employers. He often lost jobs as a result. When discussing his history, he would argue that his pattern was to lose jobs and *then* become manic—when the reality was probably the other way around. But even when considering only events that couldn't have been brought about by the illness itself (for example, the death of a parent, losing one's job at a plant that closed down, or a significant event at the national level), researchers still find that life events play a role in the onset of manic and depressive episodes.

All of us are emotionally affected by stress, but not everyone has the severe mood swings that people with bipolar disorder have when under stress. Are these people somehow more sensitive to life events? Johnson and her colleagues (2008) point out that the kinds of events that precede manic episodes are often goal or achievement oriented. Examples of these kinds of events include job promotions, new romantic relationships, financial investments, and athletic successes. Johnson et al. have supported this hypothesis in research showing that, among people with bipolar I disorder, manic episodes are often preceded by events that stimulate goal-directedness.

Johnson and her colleagues postulate that goal attainment events activate a circuit in the brain known as the *behavioral activation system,* which regulates the activity of the brain when stimuli indicating reward are present (for example, investments that signal the possibility of great financial gain). One theory is that the prefrontal cortex, which is important in foresight, planning, and control over emotions and impulses, becomes underactive and fails to "dampen down" the activity of the amygdala, the ventral striatum, the nucleus accumbens, and other brain structures when these structures become activated by a reward opportunity, resulting in manic mood and behavior (Nusslock et al., 2012; Townsend & Altshuler, 2012).

In contrast, other kinds of events cause people to shut down and withdraw, as they do when they get depressed. These events, which usually involve loss, grief, or rejection, may activate a different set of neural circuits, called the *behavioral inhibition system.* This system motivates the person to avoid circumstances that, to the individual, signal punishment. For example, the loss of a relationship may make a person withdraw from others as a way of avoiding further rejection.

Stressful Events: Examining Your History

Have stressful events played a role in your previous episodes? If you have had more than one clear-cut episode, you may find the following exercise useful. In the form on page 114, fill out the dates of three or more of your previous manic/hypomanic or depressive episodes and see if you can determine whether life events occurred before (or during) any or all of them. If your previous episodes have been mainly mixed, indicate this in the second column of the table so that you can keep them separate when evaluating the exercise. Currently, we don't know whether mixed episodes have different environmental triggers than manic or depressive episodes.

Include major events (for example, a move to a new state, new romantic relationships or relationship breakups, car accidents, job changes, unexpected financial problems, deaths or illnesses in the family) as well as events that, by comparison, are less severe or disruptive (for example, getting a new pet, having the flu, taking a vacation, changing your job hours). Include both positive and negative life events.

What Role Has Stress Played in Your Illness?

Approximate date of episode (or your age at the time)	Type of episode (manic, hypomanic, depressed, mixed, other)	Stressful events (describe)
_____	_____	_____
_____	_____	_____
_____	_____	_____
_____	_____	_____

Try to take a somewhat removed stance when examining the role of life stress in your own illness. Are particular types of events consistently related to your episodes? Has an event involving loss or grief ever preceded one or more of your depressive episodes? How many of your prior manic or mixed episodes were related to romantic relationships, even if the event was positive (such as finding a new partner)? Do events that signify achievement (for example, an award or public recognition of your work) often precede manic or hypomanic episodes? How many of these events might have resulted in changes in when or how much you slept? More generally, do these events occur independently of your mood disorder? Or does your manic or depressive behavior play a significant role in bringing about these events?

Don't be disappointed if you have difficulty answering these questions. Many people with bipolar disorder have trouble recalling when their episodes started and ended and when certain stressful events occurred, and it can be especially hard to tell whether your episodes caused them. If you are having trouble, try consulting a family member or a doctor who has seen you through several episodes. Go through the exercise together and see if he or she can help jog your memory about when certain events occurred, whether these events came before or after an episode, and what type of mood episode you had.

The time relationship between a life event and a resulting mood state can be quite complicated. For example, 27-year-old Annie became mildly depressed after she broke up with her live-in girlfriend, but she did not develop a full bipolar depression. However, when her physician started her on an antidepressant, she developed a mixed episode. In this case, the environmental stressor (the relationship ending) was related to the outcome (the mixed episode) only because she started a new medication.

As I said earlier, discovering a linkage between life events and your mood disorder episodes does not mean that you are somehow at fault for causing your own illness. Many life events are unavoidable. Some events are more likely to occur when you get manic or depressed, but that still doesn't mean you are fully in control of their occurrence. For example, you may have lost certain jobs once your mood cycled into irritability or depression, but that doesn't mean you should have been able to control these mood states or their effects on others, particularly without having any tools to do so.

The Role of the Sleep–Wake Cycle

We've already talked about one set of mechanisms by which stress can affect bipolar symptoms—the behavioral activation and inhibition systems. Another mechanism concerns circadian rhythms, notably sleep. If you remember back to your first episode or any subsequent episodes, you will probably agree that sleep played some role in all of them. Perhaps it is simply that when you were manic you slept less, and when you were depressed you slept more. But changes in sleeping and waking are important in another way. Researchers believe that people with bipolar disorder are very sensitive to even minor changes in sleep–wake rhythms, such as when they go to bed, when they actually fall asleep, and when they wake up (Frank, 2007). If so, events that change your sleep–wake cycle will also affect your mood.

Stacy became quite manic when she began the child custody proceedings, possibly because the preparations were stressful and forced her to stay up later at night. Darryl, age 24, became manic shortly after his graduate school finals, during which he had stayed up later and later. Losing even a single night's sleep can precipitate a manic episode in people with bipolar disorder who have otherwise been stable (Malkoff-Schwartz et al., 2000). In parallel, sleep deprivation can improve the mood of a person with depression, although only briefly (Harvey, 2011).

What Affects Our Sleep–Wake Regularity?: Social Zeitgebers and Zeitstorers

Unless you speak German, you've probably never heard these terms before—nor had I until I started reading about the *social rhythm stability hypothesis* of Cindy Ehlers and her associates at the University of Pittsburgh (Ehlers, Kupfer, Frank, & Monk, 1993). This theory helps us understand why life events might affect the mood cycles of people with bipolar disorder.

Ehlers's theory states that the core problem in bipolar disorder is one of instability. Usually, people maintain regular patterns of daily activity and social stimulation, such as when they go to bed, when they get up, when they eat, how many people they ordinarily interact with, or where they go after work. These *social rhythms* are important in maintaining our *circadian rhythms*, which are the more biologically driven cycles such as when you actually fall asleep, the production of hormones like melatonin (which occurs when you are approaching sleep), or your pattern of rapid-eye-movement activity during sleep.

Social rhythms stay stable, in part, because of *social zeitgebers,* which are persons or events that function as an external time clock to regulate your habits. Your dog can be a social zeitgeber if he or she needs to be walked at a certain time of the morning. Your spouse or partner, if you have one, almost certainly plays a role in organizing your eating and sleeping schedules and probably affects how much stimulation you have from other people during the day. Breaking up, or even having your partner go away on a business trip for a period of time, would disrupt your daily and nightly routines. Your job also keeps you on a regular routine.

In contrast, a *social zeitstorer* (time disturber) is a person or a social demand that throws everything off balance. When you start a new relationship, your patterns of sleeping, waking, and socializing change. The same thing will happen if you have a baby. In these cases, the new romantic partner or your baby is a zeitstorer. If you take on employment that has constantly shifting work hours or requires that you travel across different time zones, your social and circadian rhythms will be disrupted considerably.

What does all of this mean for a person with bipolar disorder? Events that bring about changes in social rhythms, either by introducing zeitstorers or removing zeitgebers, alter circadian rhythms. You are particularly vulnerable to a manic episode after you have experienced a social-rhythm-disrupting life event (Malkoff-Schwartz et al., 2000). Let me give you some examples.

Debra, a 36-year-old woman with bipolar II disorder, lived with her husband, Barry. During a therapy session with the couple, Debra complained that Barry had changed the schedule for feeding their two cats. He had begun feeding them both in the morning instead of the evening, and as a result one or both of the cats were coming into the couple's room in the middle of the night, crying for food. Debra wanted to feed the cats before she and Barry went to bed, but he refused, saying it would make the cats overweight. After three consecutive nights of poor sleep, she became irritable, experienced mental confusion at work, and developed racing thoughts. This was the first time I had heard of a hypomanic episode being induced by a crying cat.

Barry finally agreed to the new evening feeding schedule, which alleviated the problem with the cats. As Debra got back on a regular sleep–wake cycle and experienced several nights of restorative sleep, her hypomania started to settle down. In Debra's case, a major episode was averted by reestablishing routines that had been disrupted by a relatively minor event.

Miriam, a 47-year-old woman with bipolar I disorder, developed hypomanic symptoms the day after drinking alcohol, even if she drank only small quantities. It wasn't entirely clear to me why a small amount of alcohol would make her hypomanic until I considered her sleep cycle: alcohol was acting as a disruptive zeitstorer. She had much more difficulty falling asleep after drinking. Once she stopped drinking (or limited herself to one beer, usually consumed early in the evening), she had less trouble sleeping and fewer shifts in her moods.

In Chapter 8, "Tips to Help You Manage Moods," I'll tell you about a method for keeping your social routines regulated even when events conspire to change them (the social rhythm stability method). This self-monitoring technique can help you keep your mood and sleep–wake cycles stable.

Conflicts with Significant Others

"I started writing a blog about my moods and what was going on with me. Each night, I described what I felt like and what had happened that day. It wasn't of much interest to anyone but me, but I was surprised to find that each 'up and down' went along with something involving my family. I always knew this to be true on some level, but it was so obvious once I kept track of it.

"Sometimes my mood would drop because of something stupid, like an annoying phone call from my mother about forgetting someone's birthday. Other times it was more serious, like when my brother's wife said she didn't want me to babysit my nieces anymore because she didn't trust me not to be crazy. A criticism that felt like a shock to the system. And then if something good happened—like my stepmom complimenting my cooking or my dad telling me he liked my writing—I could feel my mood escalating. Every time I had some interaction with my family, anything involving emotion, I would get stressed out and my mood would change."

—A 32-year-old woman with bipolar II disorder

So far, we've talked about single life events and changes in your routine. The other major type of stress has to do with your ongoing relationships. Chapter 13 discusses dealing with family members, so I'll give it only brief mention here. There is no evidence that disturbances in family relationships (for example, being parented poorly as a child) are a primary cause of bipolar disorder, but high-intensity, high-conflict family or marital situations can increase your likelihood of having a recurrence of bipolar disorder once you have it.

In the middle to late 1980s, I conducted my dissertation research on this topic with colleagues at UCLA (Miklowitz, Goldstein, Nuechterlein, Snyder, & Mintz, 1988). We worked with young adults who were hospitalized, usually for their first manic episode, and who were planning to live with their parents after hospital discharge. We examined the level of tension, conflict, and criticism between these patients and their parents while the patients were in the hospital and once they got out. Not surprisingly, those who returned to high-conflict, high-intensity families were more likely to have manic and depressive recurrences within 9 months after their discharge than those who returned to low-conflict families. Other researchers have found similar associations between family relationships and outcomes for patients with bipolar disorder, whether or not they had been hospitalized at the outset (for a review, see Miklowitz & Chung, 2016).

We don't know exactly why conflict-ridden family environments make bipolar people more recurrence prone, but we do know that family environments characterized by conflict and criticism affect the course of many other psychiatric disorders, including schizophrenia, depression, alcoholism, and eating disorders. We also suspect that it is not only conflicts with family members or a spouse that can affect the cycling of your disorder but also conflicts with other significant people in your life, such as your employer, coworkers, or close friends. In Stacy's case, conflicts with her ex-husband may have played a role in her escalating mania. Had she been able to work things out with him in a civil manner, her chances of keeping a stable mood might have been better. But she really didn't have that option.

For now, let's simply recognize that family and interpersonal conflicts can be risk factors in the course of your illness. Begin thinking about what role family or marital conflict has played in your disorder. Do your episodes typically coincide with significant family or marital arguments? Do these conflicts come before the episode, after the episode has begun, or is it impossible to tell? Many of my cli-

---

New research: *"Is that my mother I hear?"*

Expressed emotion (EE) refers to the degree to which parents, a spouse, or other close relatives express critical comments, hostile statements, or emotionally overinvolved or overprotective attitudes when discussing you with a neutral third party. It has long been known that people with mood or psychotic disorders who hail from "high-EE" families have a rougher course of illness over time than those from low-EE families (with relatives who are less critical or overprotective). Jill Hooley, a professor of psychology at Harvard University, has an innovative way of studying this phenomenon. In a study by Hooley, Siegle, and Gruber (2012), people with and without a history of depression were asked to fill out a simple measure of how critical they thought their mothers were, using a 1–10 scale of "perceived criticism." Then they lay in an MRI tube while hearing recorded messages from their mothers expressing critical comments, praise, or neutral statements toward them (for example, "I really don't like the hours you keep"). Sound like a nightmare? Hooley and colleagues found that when hearing maternal criticisms, formerly depressed people who rated their mothers as high in perceived criticism showed increased activity in the amygdala and decreased activity in the prefrontal cortical regions of the brain compared to healthy volunteers. They did not show similar activation of these brain regions when hearing praise. These regions are part of the neural circuit that drives emotional reactivity and regulation, processes that become destabilized in depression and bipolar disorder.

unts say that the family conflicts came before their episodes; others say that the conflicts arise once they've become manic, mixed, or depressed—but that these conflicts also make it harder to get better. Some report that family conflicts that have been there all along get worse when they become ill or that buried issues come out in their dealings with family members. When you are becoming ill, it can be difficult to edit the things you want to say to your family members, and these family members may have similar difficulties in editing what to say to you (see Chapter 13).

When thinking through these issues, try to avoid blaming members of your family or significant others for their role in your illness cycling—in most cases they are trying their best to be helpful and often don't know what to do or say. As you'll see in Chapter 13, there are good and bad ways to deal with your family members regarding your disorder. Managing your family relationships is an important element of maintaining wellness.

• • • • • • • • • • • • • • •

Bipolar disorder does not have clear-cut causes, but we know enough to say that it involves biological dysregulations that are partly under genetic control. These biological vulnerabilities can be set off by various kinds of stressors, conflicts, or life changes, both positive or negative. Stacy's experiences with life stress, family conflict, and sleep–wake disturbances may mirror some of your own.

Medications prescribed for bipolar disorder are designed to correct the underlying biological vulnerabilities of people with the disorder. The next chapter describes the available medications, what we think they do, their side effects, and the role of psychotherapy as an adjunctive treatment. Later chapters describe lifestyle management techniques. Usually these techniques are recommended alongside medications as a way of improving your ability to cope with stress. As you read on, try to think of biology and environment as interacting with each other—you'll have an easier time making choices about treatments if you can keep these multiple causes of bipolar disorder in mind.

CHAPTER 6

What Medications and Psychotherapy Can Do for You

We have known for a long time that medication is the first-line treatment for bipolar disorder. We know that people with bipolar disorder get better faster and remain well longer if they take medication regularly. But we also know that medication requires careful monitoring by you and your physician and often demands that you deal with unpleasant side effects. Fortunately, research continues to produce treatments that are both effective and more easily tolerated.

People have strong feelings about taking mood-stabilizing medications and sometimes don't take them even when they would clearly benefit—often because they lack accurate information about the medications and their side effects. This chapter's overview of the medications used to treat bipolar disorder will allow you to take on a much more powerful role in dealing with your disorder. Knowing about the track record of these medications, which side effects are common and which are rare, and how you can deal with side effects will help you plan your medication regimen with your doctor and manage it over time.

The different medications in your regimen will make more sense if you think of each of them as belonging to a certain class of drugs (for example, antidepressants, mood stabilizers, antipsychotics) and having a specific purpose (such as improving sleep or anxiety). Because it is so important to take medications consistently, I've devoted Chapter 7 to exploring the factors that can stand in the way of your sticking with a medication regimen even when it could prove beneficial to you.

I strongly believe that people with bipolar disorder do best when they are taking medications and simultaneously working with a therapist. In study after study, we find that people who take medications and get therapy for their bipolar disorder do better than those who only take medications (Miklowitz & Chung, 2016). Although psychotherapy is not a substitute for medications, there are things you can accomplish in therapy that won't be accomplished by medications. There are also things that medications can do for you that therapy won't. In this chapter I discuss what we do and don't know about psychotherapy as an adjunct to medications.

What Will You Gain from the Latest Research Findings about Treatment?

Knowing the facts about your medications and psychotherapy—including what the latest studies say about their effectiveness and side effects—is a crucial foundation for staying with a treatment regimen. You'll feel more confident about the medications you take and the psychotherapy sessions you attend if you know about the research that has been conducted on these strategies.

Medications have to be validated through *randomized controlled trials* (RCTs) before they can obtain a U.S. Food and Drug Administration (FDA) indication for use in bipolar or other conditions. In most RCTs, a coin is flipped and people receive the medication or a placebo (an inert tablet like a sugar pill), and neither they nor their doctor knows which they have received. To receive an FDA indication, the medication has to either (1) work better in alleviating depressive or manic symptoms than a placebo, or (2) work better than placebo in preventing recurrences of mania or depression. Additionally, the medication cannot cause significant side effects that overwhelm its benefits. These effects have to be observed in multiple studies conducted by different groups of investigators. Sometimes medications are tested as singular treatments for mania or depression (*monotherapy studies*) and sometimes as adjuncts to other drugs in *combination therapy* studies.

In the sections that follow, I'll be referring to various RCTs on medication effectiveness. I won't spend much time on the specifics of how these studies were conducted (although, if you are of a scientific bent, I'd encourage you to look over some of the articles referenced so that you can draw your own conclusions). Instead, I refer to *meta-analyses* whenever possible. These are methods of aggregating many studies together to draw overall conclusions concerning whether a certain drug works better than a placebo for outcomes like "recovery" (how long it takes to stabilize from an acute episode of depression or mania) or "recurrence" (whether a new episode of mania or depression occurs while in treatment or afterward).

Psychotherapies can also be evaluated in RCTs, such as when we compare the illness outcomes of people who are assigned randomly to receive cognitive therapy and medication or medication alone. Psychotherapies do not undergo the same FDA certification process that drugs do, although some clinical psychologists think they should. I agree with their position. Currently evidence that one psychotherapy is more effective than another for a specific type of bipolar disorder is lacking.

What Medications Can Do for You

You'll recall from earlier chapters that bipolar disorder follows a relapse/remission course. When people with bipolar disorder are treated with mood stabilizers, their chances of having a recurrence average 37–49% in 1 year and up to 73% over 5 years (Gignac, McGirr, Lam, & Yatham, 2015). The polarity of these episodes is not consistent: depressive recurrences are about three times as common as manic or hypomanic recurrences (Perlis et al., 2006; Judd et al., 2002). The good news is that taking medication cuts recurrences substantially. For example, lithium reduces the likelihood of manic episodes in people with bipolar disorder by about 50% over intervals of 1–2 years (Severus et al., 2014). Of course, not everyone responds to lithium; you and your doctor may decide that another mood stabilizer (for example, valproate, lamotrigine) or one of the second-generation antipsychotic (SGA) medications is more appropriate for you.

Effective prevention: Lithium decreases the chances that a person with bipolar disorder will commit suicide or make suicide attempts (Cipriani, Hawton, Stockton, & Geddes, 2013). But it is not only the drug that makes the difference; it is also the regular contact and collaboration with a caring professional.

One only has to read autobiographical accounts of people with bipolar or depressive disorders to know the positive impact that medication has had on their lives, including the reduction in suicidal thoughts, impulses, and attempts (for example, Jamison, 2000a; Solomon, 2002). Sadly, many people who commit suicide had little or no access to psychiatric treatment. They did not receive the appropriate medications or therapy, or their illnesses were not even detected by mental health professionals in the first place. Not surprisingly, regular contact with a caring mental health professional who *collaborates* with you on your health care (for example, asks you what side effects are tolerable for you or helps you find payment options if your insurance doesn't cover your medications) will increase your feelings of hopefulness (Morris et al., 2005).

Acute versus Preventive Treatment

Think of your disorder as having an *acute treatment phase* (during which the goal of medication is to treat an existing manic, mixed, or depressive episode) and a *maintenance treatment phase* (during which the goals are to keep you stable and prevent future episodes). The medications you take during the two phases may be different. Your daily regimen during the acute phase is likely to involve more medications at higher dosages than your regimen during the maintenance phase. For example, it is common for people to be treated with an SGA like risperidone as well as a mood stabilizer like lithium when they are manic. As they recover, they may be able to taper and then discontinue the SGA and get along with a lower dose of lithium.

The acute phase involves bringing you down from a severe manic high or up from a depressive low. Acute-phase treatment is usually done on an intensive out-patient basis through regular psychiatry appointments or in some cases through inpatient or partial hospitalization. On average, the acute phase lasts up to 3 months, although nowadays in the United States less than a week of this (if any) is spent in the hospital. The length of the acute phase may be shorter or longer, depending on your response to specific medications in your regimen and the degree to which the environment facilitates your recovery.

In contrast, the maintenance phase involves preventing more severe symptoms. The maintenance phase does not have a prescribed length, although some doctors say that, following an acute episode, at least 6 months of being clinically stable on medications is necessary to prevent the same mood episode from coming back. As you'll see in Chapter 7, many people take their medications during the acute phase but mistakenly want to stop them during the maintenance phase, thinking they no longer need them. Often the result is that they have rapid recurrences of the disorder, even though they were better at the point when they discontinued their medications.

The two graphs on page 124 show how acute and maintenance treatment works. Two patterns are described in each: one in which a person with bipolar disorder takes medications (solid line) and one in which he does not (dotted line). In the first figure, Albert, a 32-year-old with bipolar I disorder, began developing a severe manic episode. Just before the mania would have crested, he began taking two medications, lithium and quetiapine (Seroquel), an SGA. The dotted line shows what would likely have happened if he hadn't taken medications at that point.

The second graph shows what the longer-term course of Albert's illness looked like with medications (lithium and quetiapine) and what it would have looked like without them. Notice that medications do not eliminate Albert's mood cycling, but they do slow it down and help prevent full recurrences. The periods of wellness are longer, his mood episodes are shorter and less severe, and his symptoms between episodes are milder.

When your symptoms are well controlled, as was the case for Albert, you can expect to be more in control of your life and have an easier time pursuing your goals. Having a sense of personal control will decrease your anxiety about the future and increase the chances that you'll be able to function better at work and in your family and social life.

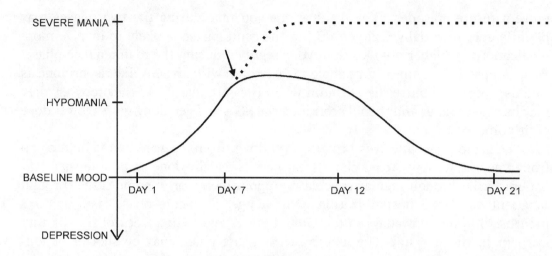

The effects of medications on Albert's acute manic episode. The arrow indicates the point at which Albert began taking lithium and Seroquel. The dotted line indicates what might have happened to his mood had he not taken these medications.

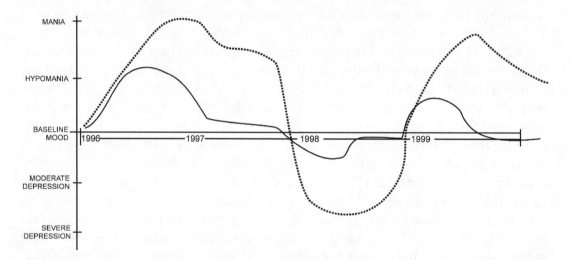

Albert's longer-term mood cycling as it would appear on appropriate medications (solid line) and off medications (dotted line).

"Do I Have to Take Medication Forever?"

This is an understandable and very important question, but one we really don't know how to answer. As you know from Chapter 5, bipolar disorder is related to underlying biological vulnerabilities involving the activity of nerve cells, neurotransmitters, and intracellular signaling systems. These vulnerabilities are inherited in many cases. We also believe that medications help correct disruptions in neurotransmitter or intracellular systems in some of the ways described below. For

> # A Medication Regimen Should Do Three Things for You:
>
> 1. Control and help resolve an episode that has already developed
>
> 2. Delay future episodes and minimize the severity of those that do occur
>
> 3. Reduce the severity of the symptoms you experience between episodes

this reason, most people with bipolar disorder must take medications indefinitely, especially if the diagnosis is certain and they have had multiple depressive and manic or hypomanic recurrences. In this way, bipolar disorder is like other medical illnesses that require long-term medication, such as high blood pressure or asthma.

There are exceptions to this rule, such as if a woman wants to become pregnant: certain mood stabilizers can increase the risk to the fetus of central nervous system or cardiac defects. I'll be talking about pregnancy in some detail in Chapter 12. You may also have to stop your medications if you develop a medical condition that prevents you from taking mood stabilizers (for example, certain diseases of the liver or kidney). Fortunately, your mood-stabilizing medications are not addictive or habit forming: you will not crave them when they are withdrawn.

If you have had only one manic or mixed episode, your doctor may recommend that you take medicines for 1 year and then reassess your need for them. But that recommendation will vary from doctor to doctor and will depend on how stable your mood remains over the year.

Needless to say, accepting a long-term medication regimen is a very significant personal decision. For now, let's focus on the mechanics of medications: which ones you are likely to be prescribed, in what dosages, their effectiveness (as shown in research studies), their likely side effects, and how long they take to work. I'll say more about the emotional significance of taking medications in Chapter 7.

What Is a Mood Stabilizer?

To be defined as a mood stabilizer, a medication has to effectively (1) treat manic/hypomanic, mixed, and/or depressive episodes of bipolar disorder without causing mood cycling (rapid switching from one mood polarity to another—for example, from depression to mania or hypomania), (2) prevent future mood episodes from occurring, and (3) not worsen the illness (Rybakowski, 2014). As you'll soon see, antidepressants such as fluoxetine (Prozac) are not considered mood stabilizers, because they impact only depression, not mania, and because they can cause rapid cycling if given alone.

PERSONALIZED CARE TIP:
Combining two or more medications

If you are taking one mood stabilizer and still experiencing symptoms of depression or mania, your doctor may recommend that you combine this medication with another mood stabilizer or an SGA. Taking more than one medication doesn't mean that you are sicker than the next person with bipolar disorder or that you're getting worse—it just may mean that your unique physiology doesn't respond as well as that person's to an individual compound. Many people with bipolar disorder do better when taking more than one mood stabilizer; in fact, over 80% of individuals with bipolar disorder take more than one medication. Agents like lithium and valproate have different but complementary effects on brain mechanisms, such as the protein kinase C signaling pathway (Schloesser et al., 2008; see Chapter 5). Additionally, people vary in their response to medications because of their individual pattern of symptoms, such as whether they have pure manic highs versus mixed episodes, rapid cycling versus infrequent and distinctive episodes, or long periods of depression with occasional periods of hypomania. People also respond differently to medications as they age. Lastly, your regimen can be affected by your consistency in taking the medications as prescribed—many people end up on multiple drugs because they take their medications irregularly (see Chapter 7).

Medications have at least two names: a generic name (which I'll give first) that reflects their chemistry, followed by a specific brand name created by the pharmaceutical company for commercial use (given in parentheses). Doctors and pharmacies usually refer to drugs by their brand name, but this is not consistent from place to place. The main mood stabilizers in use today are *lithium carbonate* (Eskalith, Lithobid, or *lithium citrate* if taken in liquid form) and the *anticonvulsants,* typically *valproate* (Depakote, Depakene) and *lamotrigine* (Lamictal). Certain SGAs, such as *quetiapine* (Seroquel), *aripiprazole* (Abilify), and *olanzapine* (Zyprexa), also qualify as mood stabilizers.

Types of Mood Stabilizers

Lithium

The most well-known mood stabilizer is lithium, which is dispensed under brand names like Eskalith, Lithobid, Lithonate, and Cibalith-S. Lithium was the first medication proven to stabilize mood in bipolar disorder and also to prevent manic or depressive episodes from returning. The discovery of lithium treatment is usually attributed to John Cade (1949) (see the box on page 127). Lithium is considered a first-line agent in treating manic episodes, often in combination with an SGA. The supporting evidence for lithium in preventing recurrences (maintenance treatment) is more conclusive than for any other medication (Leucht et al., 2013).

Lithium is given in 300- or 450-milligram (mg) tablets. Typically, people with bipolar disorder have starting doses of 600 mg, with final doses of 900–1,800 mg or higher.

How well does lithium work? In a meta-analysis of lithium maintenance trials, which included 1,580 participants followed for up to 2 years, researchers concluded that lithium was 50% more effective than placebo in preventing manic relapses and about 22% better than placebo in preventing depressive relapses (Severus et al., 2014). The same meta-analysis indicated that lithium was more effective than anticonvulsants like valproate or lamotrigine in preventing manic episodes.

Despite its less than impressive effectiveness in treating bipolar depression, lithium is the only medication that has been found to reduce the risk of suicide or suicidal behaviors. In a study of 21,000 patients by Dr. Frederick Goodwin and colleagues (2003) at George Washington University, people with bipolar disorder who were taking lithium were less likely to attempt or complete suicide, and less likely to require hospitalization for suicide attempts than people taking either valproate or carbamazepine (both mood stabilizers). A meta-analysis of 48 RCTs indicated that lithium reduced suicides by 87% compared to placebo (Cipriani et al., 2013). So, on balance, lithium is still the first choice for the long-term treatment of bipolar disorder and may even be life-saving in some people.

The Discovery of Lithium

Lithium has been known to have mood-calming properties since at least 200 A.D., when a Greek doctor named Galen used it in baths for people with mental illness. Various lithium bromide compounds were marketed to the public in the 1800s but were found to be highly toxic. If you bought a 7UP soft drink prior to 1948, it would have had lithium in it.

John Cade, an Australian physician, happened upon lithium by accident (Cade, 1949). His experiment involved injecting uric acid mixed with lithium into the bloodstream of guinea pigs. Injection with lithium calmed the animals down and made them less active. Dr. Cade then thought to try lithium with a human guinea pig, one of his most severely ill manic patients, a 51-year-old man. The patient responded very well and for the first time was able to function outside of a hospital. This story of scientific serendipity is tempered by the fact that this patient took himself off the medication 6 months later, against medical advice, perhaps foreshadowing the wide-ranging problem of nonadherence among people taking lithium. Nonetheless, lithium came into general use in the 1960s and has been used regularly in the United States since 1970, to the great benefit of many people.

> ## PERSONALIZED CARE TIP:
> # Lithium dosing
>
> Some people take their lithium in divided doses, several times a day, and some only once. This is one of the decisions you and your doctor can make when trying to figure out how best to control your side effects. For example, there is an extended-release form of lithium that can be substituted if you have severe nausea.
>
> A correct dosage is one that brings your blood level into a *therapeutic range.* The therapeutic range your doctor targets for you during treatment of your acute episode (usually between 0.8 and 1.2 milligrams per milliliter (mg/ml), a chemical measure of lithium concentration in the blood) may be higher than the one targeted during your maintenance treatment (commonly, 0.6–1.0 mg/ml), when your dosage may be correspondingly lower. Children with bipolar disorder often need higher doses of lithium than adults to get a therapeutic blood level, whereas persons over the age of 65, who may be more sensitive to the side effects of lithium, are given lower dosages.

How Do You Know Whether You'll Respond to Lithium?

A lot of studies have tried to predict who will respond to lithium, but the results have been inconclusive. The box on page 130 lists some of the factors that are correlated with a good response to lithium. Knowing about these factors may help you understand why your doctor is recommending lithium versus an anticonvulsant or an SGA.

How Lithium Works

Lithium appears to affect pathways that determine whether chemical messages are sent successfully from the brain to other parts of the body or from one part of the brain to another. Additionally, by increasing some proteins and enzymes and inhibiting others, lithium slows down or even stops the process of cell destruction in various brain structures, including the prefrontal cortex, which is central to emotional processing and higher-order control over lower parts of the brain

Effective treatment: Don't give up on lithium if you don't feel its benefits right away. It will probably take at least a week and often a few weeks before you start seeing improvement in your manic or depressive symptoms. When you take lithium for the first time, you might feel a slight elevation in your mood for the first week or so. If you have no response after 3 weeks, your doctor will probably adjust the dosage upward or recommend another medication.

PERSONALIZED CARE TIP:
Will you respond to lithium?

The more your illness reflects the textbook description of bipolar disorder (euphoric, grandiose highs followed by deep depressions and periods of mood stability in between), the more likely you are to respond to lithium (Grof, 2010). Having family members who were treated successfully with lithium also increases your chances of a positive response. If your disorder is less typical (for example, you have rapid or continuous cycling, or mainly mixed episodes), some doctors will recommend you start with an anticonvulsant instead of (or in addition to) lithium.

There are probably many genes for lithium response (as well as for antipsychotic or antidepressant response) that interact with each other in highly complex ways. Nonetheless, we have some promising candidates for genes that predict lithium response. For example, good responses to lithium in people with bipolar disorder are correlated with a polymorphism in the BDNF gene (Dmitrzak-Weglarz et al., 2008). BDNF is involved in neural processes such as cell proliferation and synaptic plasticity and cognitive functions, including memory (Rybakowski, 2014). In the not-too-distant future, a blood or saliva test may help determine the drugs to which you will respond best (and that hopefully will yield the fewest side effects)—a key goal of personalized medicine.

(for example, the amygdala). Lithium may improve the structural stability of cells and even cause new cells to grow or proliferate (Machado-Vieira, Manji, & Zarate, 2009).

People with bipolar disorder who take lithium have been found to have larger gray matter volumes in the brain than people with bipolar disorder who are not taking lithium (Sun et al., 2018). The gray matter is rich in neuronal cell bodies, axons, and dendrites, all parts of the nerve cells that are essential for communicating chemical messages. So lithium does not cause long-term brain damage, as many people fear. Instead, it may actually reverse some of the damage caused by the illness.

Side Effects of Lithium

When you take any medication, it's important to know the possible side effects so that changes in your body will not come as a surprise to you and you'll know to discuss them with your doctor. All mood-stabilizing agents have some side effects. Be skeptical of "natural" or "homeopathic" mood remedies that presumably have no adverse effects. No substance is both free of side effects and effective as a mood stabilizer or antidepressant. For example, Hypericum perforatum (St. John's wort) can cause high blood pressure and headaches; omega-3 fatty acids (fish oil) can cause stomach upset, nausea, and diarrhea.

Your doctor should include any side effects you report as an important source of information in planning your treatment. Side effects can often be controlled in some of the ways described in the box on page 131. In Chapter 7 you'll find a side-effect recording sheet that will help you communicate with your doctor about complications associated with your medications.

Individuals have some predictable side effects with lithium, but their severity will vary a great deal from person to person. Common side effects of lithium include thirst, nausea, water retention, frequent urination, hand tremors, fatigue,

---

Predictors of Lithium Response

Predictors of a good response to lithium:

- Pure euphoric or elevated manic highs
- Mood cycling marked by manias followed by depressions
- A good response to lithium previously
- Later age at onset of illness (later than adolescence)
- Relatively symptom-free intervals between episodes
- Few or no comorbid disorders
- Relatives in the family tree have been treated effectively with lithium
- Having a "hyperthymic" personality (cheerful, overly optimistic, exuberant even between episodes)

Predictors of a poor response to lithium:

- Irritability, hostility, and dysphoria during manic episodes (mixed features)
- Psychotic symptoms occurring outside of mood episodes
- A pattern of continuous cycling or frequent hospitalizations
- Depressive episodes usually come before manic episodes
- No family history of mania or hypomania
- Co-occurring substance or alcohol abuse
- Mania symptoms that occur after a neurological illness or brain injury

Sources: Grof (2010); Rybakowski (2014).

> ## PERSONALIZED CARE TIPS:
> ## Reducing lithium's side effects
>
> ■ Frequent urination can be reduced by taking lithium once instead of several times a day; talk to your doctor about this option.
> ■ Thirst can be controlled by drinking more water, chewing on ice chips, or using sugarless cough drops.
> ■ Stomach irritation can be helped by taking lithium after a full meal or even switching to an extended-release formulation to reduce gastrointestinal symptoms.
> ■ Adding thyroid supplements (for example, levothyroxine [Synthroid]) or beta-blockers for hand tremors (for example, propranolol [Inderal]) can reduce the impact of these side effects.

diarrhea, or a metallic taste in the mouth. More troublesome side effects include weight gain, mental sluggishness or problems with memory, development or flare-up of skin conditions (such as acne or psoriasis); or stomach discomfort, nausea, or diarrhea. Some people also develop hypothyroidism, a condition in which the thyroid gland does not produce enough hormone. Kidney functioning (the ability of the kidney to concentrate urine) can also be affected if lithium is taken over a long period of time. Make sure your doctor is monitoring your creatinine levels, a measure of kidney functioning.

Before taking lithium, you should have certain blood tests to make sure you do not have kidney or thyroid disease. If you show evidence of renal insufficiency or failure, lithium is not recommended. Thyroid abnormalities—those present before lithium treatment—do not necessarily rule out lithium but it may be necessary to treat them (for example, using a thyroid supplement) first. Depending on where you're seen, your doctor may also recommend a serum calcium measure, an electrocardiogram (if you're over 40), and, if you're female, a pregnancy test.

The side effects of lithium can be related to the dosage you take. Many doctors adopt the "start low, go slow" approach, in which you start taking the medicine at a low dosage and gradually increase it in small steps to a therapeutic dosage as a way of keeping your side effects in check. If you are already taking a certain dosage of lithium but have unpleasant side effects, your doctor may recommend you reduce your dosage, although doing so may make the medication less effective for you.

Lithium Blood Tests and Toxicity

People who take lithium must have their blood drawn regularly to make sure they are getting the proper dosage. If you are starting lithium for the first time and are being stabilized from a manic or depressive episode, you will probably have to

---

PERSONALIZED CARE TIP:

Will lithium affect your mental sharpness or creativity?

A less well-known side effect of lithium is "cognitive dulling," where people feel like they have lost their usual mental sharpness or edge or that emotions are blunted. This is especially a problem for those in the arts. If you are a person who writes music or poetry, paints, or has other artistic abilities, you may feel that your creativity is diminished when taking lithium. You may yearn for your hypomanic days, when ideas, images, or solutions to problems seemed to flow more readily. The best solution to the problem of cognitive dulling is to talk to your doctor about getting a lower dose of lithium or a different dosing plan. If you are in the maintenance phase, your dosage should already be lower than it was during acute treatment, but your doctor may recommend that you adjust downward even further until you find the "sweet spot" that allows you full artistic expression while still protecting you against significant mood swings. Alternatively, you may decide to try another mood-stabilizing agent (for example, valproate or lamotrigine) that may be less likely to cause this side effect.

---

get your blood tested every 2–3 weeks for the first 1–2 months of treatment and then every month for the next 3 months. If all has gone well up to that point, your doctor will probably recommend you get it tested every 3 months or so. The purpose is to make sure you have a therapeutic level of lithium in your bloodstream. Generally, your physician will check your blood level 10–14 hours after your last lithium dosage.

Effective prevention: *Should hypomania be treated as aggressively as mania?*

Hypomania, by definition, does not cause the level of impairment that mania causes. But it does herald the development of more severe depressive episodes. It can also be the first in a series of rapidly cycling mood states or, for people with bipolar I disorder, the first stage of a full-blown manic episode. So treating hypomania can be an important preventive maneuver. The medication options usually involve increasing your mood stabilizer dosage or adding a low-dose SGA to your regimen. If you have bipolar II disorder and have never been fully manic, you may decide instead that "watchful waiting" is the best option. If you have bipolar II hypomanic episodes and are not taking medications, it is especially important to monitor your moods with a self-rated mood chart (see Chapter 8) and pay particular attention to the regularity of your sleep and wake times.

It is helpful to become familiar with the blood-level scale so that you can become an active participant in your lithium treatment. As stated earlier, the target range during an acute episode is 0.8–1.2 mg/ml and during maintenance treatment 0.6–1.0 mg/ml. Ask your doctor which blood level he or she is targeting for you so that you'll know when your levels are getting too low or too high. If you decide to see another doctor, that doctor will want to know what therapeutic blood levels you are currently maintaining and what levels have been problematic for you in the past.

Having your blood tested regularly also helps prevent *lithium toxicity*, in which your body accumulates lithium at very high levels. The signs of toxicity include problems with balance and coordination, severe diarrhea, abdominal discomfort, blurry vision, slurring of speech, extreme shakiness of the hands, severe nausea or vomiting, and mental confusion or disorientation. These signs are most likely to occur when you have changed your diet, become dehydrated due to an illness or excessive exercise, or are taking diuretic drugs (for example, for blood pressure) or anti-inflammatory drugs like ibuprofen (for pain or fever). *Because this toxic state is extremely dangerous and even potentially deadly, it is important to know the signs (and acquaint your close relatives with them as well) so that you can get in to see your doctor as soon as possible, have your blood level checked, and, in most cases, have your lithium adjusted or stopped.*

You may find blood testing difficult: no one likes to be stuck with a needle, and it can remind you of being ill. But blood tests are a very important component of your care. If you find it particularly unpleasant, discuss it with your doctor, who may suggest a different mood stabilizer that requires less frequent blood testing. Whether to go that route is, of course, up to you.

PERSONALIZED CARE TIP:
Adjusting lithium dosages to minimize side effects

Treatment with lithium can be a balancing act in which you and your doctor collaborate to find the blood level that best stabilizes your mood but also allows you to function with the fewest annoying side effects (for example, not having to deal with slowed-down thinking). Your levels can be too high (putting you at risk for toxicity) or too low (and nontherapeutic). There are considerable differences between people in lithium dosing depending on their age, weight, and other factors. If you have been unable to find an acceptable lithium level, discuss with your physician the relative advantages and disadvantages of the other mood stabilizer and SGA options so that you can find a more workable treatment plan.

Valproate (Depakote)

Valproate, also called valproic acid or divalproex sodium, is an anticonvulsant that has been used for decades to treat epilepsy and other seizure disorders. Many anticonvulsant drugs have mood-stabilizing properties. Valproate is a fatty acid similar to compounds found in animal fats and vegetable oils. It works in several ways, including reducing activity of the protein kinase C pathway and enhancing the action of the inhibitory neurotransmitter GABA (Manji et al., 2003).

Valproate, marketed under the names Depakote and Depakote ER (extended release), is in wide use as both an acute and a long-term preventive agent. Like lithium, valproate appears to be effective as a treatment for manic episodes. A meta-analysis of randomized trials found that valproate had a 151% advantage over placebo in terms of improvement from mania; lithium had a 189% advantage (Smith, Cornelius, Warnock, Tacchi, & Taylor, 2007). Valproate also can help alleviate depression, although, like lithium, its antimanic effects are more impressive (Reinares et al., 2013). Some studies indicate that valproate has greater antimanic effects than lithium in people with mixed episodes or rapid cycling states (Rosa, Fountoulakis, Siamouli, Gonda, & Vieta, 2011). It is not as effective as lithium in treating or preventing suicidal thinking or actions.

PERSONALIZED CARE TIP:
Lithium or valproate?

Evidence from the Oxford BALANCE trial suggests that, given a choice of lithium or valproate, you may be better off (on average) choosing lithium, especially if you have some of the features that predict a good lithium response (see the box on page 130). If you are already taking valproate, you may benefit from adding lithium to it. Valproate may also be effective when combined with an SGA.

If you have not responded to lithium in terms of symptom reduction, you may respond better to valproate (and vice versa). Valproate is more sedating than lithium, so if you are struggling with agitation and sleeplessness, valproate may be recommended. It works a bit more quickly than lithium, even within as few as 3–5 days after the onset of a major manic episode. In contrast to lithium, your dosage of valproate can usually be raised rapidly without severe side effects. These advantages must be weighed against the greater abundance of supportive research on lithium, particularly as a preventative agent for manic episodes and in the treatment of people who are suicidal.

It is not clear whether valproate can *prevent* episodes of either depression or mania. In the large cross-national BALANCE trial, Oxford University researchers John Geddes, Guy Goodwin, and others randomly assigned 330 patients with bipolar I disorder to lithium, valproate, or a combination of both in maintenance treatment (BALANCE investigators et al., 2010). In a 2-year follow-up, they found that the combination of lithium and valproate *or* lithium alone prevented mood disorder recurrences for longer than valproate alone. By itself, valproate was no more effective than placebo in preventing recurrences. The combination of lithium and valproate was not substantially more effective than lithium alone.

People usually take valproate in 250- to 500-mg tablets, with daily doses of 1,500–3,000 mg. It is usually given once a day, at night. As with lithium, regular blood tests can tell you and your doctor whether you are getting the proper dosage of valproate, although not all doctors order them. If your doctor thinks that valproate levels are informative, he or she will probably recommend a therapeutic serum level between 94 and 125 micrograms per milliliter (mcg/ml; the measure used to indicate valproate concentration in the blood). You should have liver function tests and a complete blood count before you start taking valproate.

Side Effects of Valproate

Because valproate is broken down by the liver, you can develop an elevation in liver enzymes, which in rare instances can lead to liver inflammation. Valproate can also affect the production of blood platelets. Your doctor should conduct liver enzyme tests and blood platelet counts at regular intervals. When you start taking valproate, you may feel nauseous, sleepy, sedated, or have indigestion. As with lithium, you may have a hand tremor. These side effects usually disappear relatively quickly. Some people also develop hair loss or hair thinning. More worrisome is significant weight gain, which can contribute to other medical problems (for example, cardiovascular disease or diabetes). Women of childbearing age are not usually given valproate as a maintenance treatment because of its association with polycystic ovarian syndrome (see Chapter 12).

As with lithium, your doctor will treat side effects by changing your dosing schedule or dropping the dosage (for example, to make you feel less sedated). Different formulations of valproate help people who are very sensitive to the side effects of the 500-mg tablets. Depakote 125-mg "sprinkles"—a popular alternative for many adults and children—can be put on food to reduce stomach irritation. There is also an extended-release

Effective solution: Your doctor may recommend certain drugs as adjuncts to valproate to resolve side effects: ranitidine (Zantac) for nausea, metformin (Glucophage) for weight gain, or vitamins containing selenium and zinc for hair loss.

500-mg tablet (Depakote ER) that may be less likely to cause stomach distress or significant weight gain.

It's always a good idea to give your doctor a list of other medications you take regularly, even if they are unrelated to your mood disorder. Anticonvulsants like valproate and carbamazepine often interact with other medications, meaning that side effects or medical complications can occur when these drugs are used together with other drugs.

Lamotrigine (Lamictal)

"My partner, Beth, swears by Lamictal. She gets really down and can't get back up again, and it's the only thing that helps her. But it didn't help me, so I stopped taking it. My depressions are more like these periods of being mopey and all "poor me" and stuff, but I still go to work, feed the cats, and once in a while drag myself to the gym. I think I do better when I stay active."

—A 29-year-old woman with bipolar II disorder

Lamotrigine (Lamictal), another anticonvulsant used in the treatment of epilepsy, is being used more and more for people with bipolar depression. Its popularity reflects its mild side-effect profile and ability to treat depressive episodes without causing a switch into mania or hypomania. A meta-analysis of five randomized clinical trials found that lamotrigine has modest effectiveness in the treatment of bipolar depression (Geddes, Calabrese, & Goodwin, 2009). As illustrated by the young woman quoted above, it is most effective for people who have more severe bipolar depression when they start treatment (for example, intensely sad mood that rarely lifts, nightly sleep disturbance, severe inertia) and less effective with people whose depressions are milder (for example, feeling tearful and sad but able to function with extra effort). Lamotrigine is somewhat better than lithium in protecting people against depressive recurrences, but not as good as lithium in preventing manic relapses (Goodwin et al., 2004). As a result, it is often recommended as an adjunct to lithium.

Lamotrigine is easier to take than lithium or valproate because it is less likely to cause serious weight gain, tremors, or other unpleasant side effects. Typically, the side effects are temporary and include problems with physical coordination, dizziness, vision problems, nausea, vomiting, and headaches (Malhi, Adams, & Berk, 2009). Nonetheless, there are concerns about lamotrigine because 5–10% of people who use it develop a skin rash within 2–8 weeks of beginning treatment. In rare instances (about 1 in 1,000), people who take lamotrigine develop Stevens–Johnson syndrome, a potentially life-threatening condition involving a whole-body rash, a blistering or burning of the skin tissue or lining of the mucous membranes, and a fever. Doctors are usually conservative and stop prescribing lamotrigine at the first indication of a rash.

Your doctor can try to prevent rashes by increasing your dosage very slowly. Generally, doctors recommend starting at 25 mg per day and then gradually increasing the dosage for the first 4–6 weeks until you are getting mood benefits, with 200 mg being a typical daily dose. Rashes are more likely when doctors increase the dosage of lamotrigine too quickly, or when they combine it with valproate, which has the unintended effect of increasing lamotrigine blood levels.

Carbamazepine (Tegretol) and Oxcarbazepine (Trileptal)

Carbamazepine (Tegretol, Carbatrol, or Atretol), an anticonvulsant, was quite popular as a treatment in the 1980s, especially when used in combination with lithium. It appears to be just as effective as lithium in controlling mania, but there is less evidence for its role in treating depression (Shim, Woo, Kim, & Bahk, 2017). It can be challenging to find the appropriate dose with carbamazepine because of its difficult side-effect profile; as a result, doses must be increased slowly, and it is being recommended less and less.

Typical dosages of carbamazepine are between 400 mg and 1,600 mg per day. The most common side effects are sedation, nausea, and mild memory impairment. Some people experience blurry vision, constipation, or loss of muscle coordination. There is less of a problem with weight gain on carbamazepine, which is why some people prefer it. People taking carbamazepine can also develop a mild elevation in liver enzymes. Your doctor will probably discontinue carbamazepine if you develop signs of hepatitis, such as feeling sluggish and experiencing stomach pain or other gastrointestinal problems. From 10 to 15% of people develop skin rashes. As with lamotrigine, rashes should be reported to your doctor immediately. A small percentage of people taking carbamazepine develop Stevens–Johnson syndrome (see page 136).

The most serious side effect of carbamazepine—although quite rare (affecting about 1 in 100,000 people)—is a bone marrow reaction called *agranulocytosis,* which involves a dramatic drop in white blood cells. Fever, infection, sore throat, sores in your mouth, and easy bruising or bleeding are signs of this condition. If

---

PERSONALIZED CARE TIP:
Why carbamazepine?

Your doctor may prescribe carbamazepine (alone or with other drugs) if you have had a difficult time with the side effects of other anticonvulsants or if you haven't responded to lithium or valproate. Like valproate, carbamazepine seems to work best in people with mixed episodes, rapid cycling, or manias with psychosis (delusions or hallucinations).

you are taking carbamazepine, your doctor will probably monitor your white blood count, although doing so will not necessarily prevent agranulocytosis from occurring.

A medication that is chemically similar to carbamazepine, *oxcarbazepine* (Trileptal), came on the scene about 20 years ago but has fallen out of favor. It does not appear to work as well as other anticonvulsants (for example, valproate) in treating mood episodes (Rosa et al., 2011). Its side effects include fatigue and a possible decrease in sodium levels, but it is easier to take than carbamazepine and does not carry the same risk of liver or blood dysfunction.

Other Mood Stabilizers

Other drugs are used for bipolar depression and sometimes for mania, although they are not meant to be used as solo treatments. *Topiramate* (Topamax), an anticonvulsant, has not been shown to be any better than placebo in treating mania and has virtually no record in treating depression (Pigott et al., 2016; Reinares et al., 2013). Why, then, do psychiatrists prescribe it? Unlike most other mood stabilizers, it can cause weight loss rather than weight gain. For this reason, many people want to substitute it for lithium or valproate, even though the research does not justify this substitution. This drug has side effects, such as concentration or memory problems (for example, trouble finding words), tingling feelings in the hands or face, fatigue, feeling slowed down, tremors, nausea, dizziness, and in some, a vulnerability to kidney stones.

Gabapentin (Neurontin) is an anticonvulsant that was once thought to be a mood stabilizer but failed to beat placebo in a large-scale trial (Cipriani et al., 2011). Because it is sedating, its main use in bipolar disorder is to treat comorbid anxiety when antidepressants or benzodiazepines are not recommended.

A class of drugs known as *calcium channel blockers,* although used mainly for the treatment of heart disease and blood pressure, may have mood-stabilizing properties. These drugs include verapamil (Calan, Isoptin), nimodipine (Nimotop), and other agents. They are sometimes recommended for treatment-resistant mania, but only rarely, given their questionable efficacy.

Right now, topiramate and calcium channel blockers are recommended only as add-ons to traditional mood stabilizers or as alternatives for people who can't tolerate the side effects of any of the first-line choices. The table on page 139 summarizes some of the information you've just read. You may want to refer to it from time to time to see if your side effects for any given medication are consistent with those listed and if your dosages or blood levels are within the expected range.

Common Mood-Stabilizing Medications

Drug	Dosage	Blood level	Common side effects
Lithium	300–2,400 mg per day	0.8–1.2 mEq/L	• Weight gain • Fatigue, sedation • Stomach irritation, diarrhea • Thirst and frequent urination • Metallic taste in mouth • Hand tremor • Thyroid dysfunction • Acne or psoriasis • Mental sluggishness, memory problems • Kidney clearance problems
Valproate (Depakote)	1,500–3,000 mg per day	45–125 mcg/ml	• Nausea, stomach pain • Fatigue, sedation • Hand tremor • Hair loss, curlier hair • Dizziness • Headaches • Weight gain • Elevated liver enzymes • Drop in platelet count
Lamotrigine (Lamictal)	200–400 mg per day	—	• Skin rashes • Dry mouth • Nausea, vomiting • Dizziness • Headaches • Sleepiness or insomnia • Stevens–Johnson syndrome (low risk)
Carbamazepine (Tegretol)	400–1,600 mg per day	4–12 mcg/ml	• Fatigue, sedation • Nausea, stomach pain • Mild memory impairment • Constipation • Dizziness, lightheadedness • Blurred vision • Skin rashes • Problems with physical coordination, unsteadiness • Elevated liver enzymes • Drop in white blood cell count • Stevens–Johnson syndrome (low risk)

Note. mEq/L: milliequivalents per liter; mcg/ml: micrograms per milliliter.

Second-Generation Antipsychotics

"What a great medication. There's no question that it improved my mood. Too bad it made me blow up like a balloon."
> —A 44-year-old woman with bipolar II disorder, upon discontinuing the antipsychotic olanzapine (Zyprexa)

Increasingly people are being treated with SGAs (also called atypical antipsychotics) instead of or in addition to mood stabilizers. The notion of taking an antipsychotic medication is scary to many people because they equate these drugs with having severe delusions, hallucinations, or even schizophrenia. The fact that doctors refer to them as "major tranquilizers" doesn't help much. Antipsychotic medications are not to be taken lightly, but they have broader applicability than just the treatment of psychosis. In fact, several of the SGAs have strong mood-stabilizing properties. The medications in this category include *olanzapine* (Zyprexa), *quetiapine* (Seroquel), *risperidone* (Risperdal), *aripiprazole* (Abilify), *ziprasidone* (Zeldox, Geodon), *lurasidone* (Latuda), *asenapine* (Saphris, Sycrest), *clozapine* (Clozaril), *cariprazine* (Vraylar), and *paliperidone* (Invega).

What Is "Atypical" about Atypical Antipsychotics?

Twenty years ago, doctors were recommending a traditional line of "typical" antipsychotics that you may have heard about: chlorpromazine (Thorazine), fluphenazine (Prolixin), haloperidol (Haldol), and others. These drugs have severe long-term side effects, including abnormal facial or finger movements that can progress into an irreversible syndrome called *tardive dyskinesia*. Overall, SGAs or "atypicals" have less severe side effects and are substantially less likely to cause tardive dyskinesia than the typical antipsychotics, but they carry risk for another category of problems: metabolic disturbances, which I'll say more about momentarily.

SGAs are used in bipolar disorder for several purposes. First, some people with the disorder do have severe disturbances in thinking and perception (psychosis) that are not fully controlled by traditional mood stabilizers. During the period in which they are escalating into mania or during the manic episode itself, they may hear their name being called or music being played (even though no one else is around), see movement out of the corner of their eyes (even though nothing is there), or believe they are being followed or that someone is reading their thoughts. These symptoms can be alleviated by antipsychotic medicines.

Second, SGAs have antimanic and sometimes antidepressive properties when given alone or in combination with lithium or anticonvulsants. In fact, several of the SGAs qualify as mood stabilizers—they control acute episodes, decrease the vulnerability to future episodes, and do not worsen the course of the illness. A meta-analysis of 24 studies found that SGAs were significantly better than placebo in treating mania and just as effective as mood stabilizers like lithium, valproate, or carbamazepine (Scherk, Pajonk, & Leucht, 2007). The most effective treatment for mania was found to be the combination of an SGA and a mood stabilizer (for example, olanzapine or quetiapine plus valproate or lithium).

SGAs are sometimes substituted for mood stabilizers when people haven't done well on the latter. They work more rapidly in stabilizing acute manic or mixed episodes than either lithium or valproate and are often recommended for rapid cycling, severe anxiety, or sleep problems. The Food and Drug Administration also recommends certain SGAs (currently olanzapine, aripiprazole, and risperidone) as solo agents in maintenance treatment for preventing relapses. The role of these SGAs in treating depression is less clear.

Unfortunately, most of the SGAs cause some degree of weight gain. They also can cause metabolic disturbances, such as increased cholesterol, triglycerides, and blood sugar. These side effects put you at risk for cardiovascular disease or diabetes. Less severe side effects include shakiness or stiffness, daytime sleepiness, and sedation (Tohen & Vieta, 2009). Fortunately, some of the SGAs have less burdensome side effects than others, and the effects can sometimes be minimized with dosage adjustments.

If SGAs are recommended to you, it doesn't necessarily mean that your illness is getting worse or that you are psychotic. In fact, your doctor may recommend that you take an antipsychotic medication during an acute episode and then discontinue it gradually once you have begun to stabilize.

> **Effective prevention:** To head off the side effects of an SGA, your doctor should regularly monitor you for weight gain and metabolic disturbances (glucose, triglycerides, lipid levels), especially if you have had these problems before. Also, tell your doctor if you think you might be developing any unusual physical movements, such as twitching, tics, stiffness, or smacking your lips. These movement problems may be more easily detected by those around you.

Which SGA Should You Take?

Each medication has a different side-effect profile (see the table on page 143). The most well studied is olanzapine (Zyprexa), which has particularly strong effects on mania, mixed states, and rapid cycling. Its efficacy in preventing manic or mixed-episode recurrences appears to be comparable to or even better than that of lithium or valproate; it can also strengthen the effects of mood stabilizers when given in combination (Tohen et al., 2005). Unfortunately, olanzapine causes more weight gain and metabolic side effects than the other SGAs.

Many doctors prefer quetiapine (Seroquel) over olanzapine because it appears to have a milder side-effect profile and may work better in treating depressive episodes. It has a strong evidence base for treating depression and mania as well as preventing episode recurrences (Cipriani et al., 2011; Thase, 2010). Moreover, quetiapine is effective among patients with rapid cycling or comorbid anxiety disorders and does not appear to cause a switch into mania. Nonetheless, quetiapine is associated with a moderate degree of weight gain, sedation, dizziness, and high blood cholesterol and triglycerides.

Two other SGAs—risperidone and aripiprazole—have antimanic as well as antipsychotic properties and are usually prescribed either as solo treatments or as adjuncts to mood stabilizers. Both appear to have antidepressant properties, although aripiprazole has greater efficacy when added to lithium or valproate for depression than when given by itself. Both SGAs can cause side effects including motor tremors, restlessness or jitteriness, or rigidity of the muscles. Risperidone can also elevate your levels of the hormone prolactin, which is a particularly important issue for women (discussed in full in Chapter 12). Aripiprazole has a lower risk of weight gain than other SGAs.

> **Effective solution:** About 50% of people gain significant weight within the first 6–8 weeks of taking an SGA. If you opt to stay on an SGA, there are a number of things you can do to maintain your health, in consultation with your physician: (1) implement "healthy lifestyle" interventions (for example, exercise, keep regular sleep hours), recognizing that your health goals will be much harder to achieve when you are depressed (see Chapter 10), (2) take an adjunctive weight-loss drug that alters triglyceride, lipid, or glucose levels (for example, metformin), and (3) consult with a dietician regarding your eating habits (Correll, Sikich, Reeves, & Riddle, 2013).

Some doctors recommend ziprasidone, usually as an add-on agent rather than as a primary treatment for mania or mixed episodes. Its evidence base in bipolar disorder is weak, although it works better than placebo in alleviating manic symptoms. Side effects of ziprasidone include motor coordination problems, sleepiness, dizziness, and agitation, but it is much less likely to cause weight gain than olanzapine or quetiapine (Leucht et al., 2013). Finally, your doctor may recommend a newer SGA called asenapine (Saphris) for manic symptoms, although it tends to be sedating, and people complain about its bitter aftertaste.

A newer SGA option is lurasidone (Latuda), which has been shown to be effective alone or in combination with a mood stabilizer in treating bipolar depression (Loebel et al., 2014). Its supporting evidence from clinical trials is limited, but it has gone into wide use due to an intensive marketing campaign. It does not appear to cause mania or hypomania even though it works well for depression. Its side effects are considered relatively mild and include nausea, restlessness, and problems with motor movements.

The other SGAs in use, such as zonisamide (Zonegran), paliperidone (Invega), and cariprazine (Vraylar), do not have enough randomized trial data to determine whether they will be more or less effective or tolerable than the other SGAs listed in the table on page 143. The good news is that we have far more options for treating manic and depressive episodes and for preventing recurrences than ever before.

Second-Generation Antipsychotics Used During Maintenance Treatment

Drug	Starting dosage (mg)	Maintenance dose range (mg)	Common side effects
Olanzapine (Zyprexa)	5	10–15	Sedation, weight gain
Aripiprazole (Abilify)	5	10–30	Restlessness/anxiety, sedation
Quetiapine (Seroquel)	25–50	200–800	Sedation, weight gain, dizziness upon standing
Ziprasidone (Geodon)	40	80–160	Sedation, restlessness
Risperidone (Risperdal) (oral preparation)	1–2	2–6	Sedation, weight gain, restlessness/anxiety
Asenapine (Saphris)	10	10–20	Sleeping too much, dizziness, restlessness, mild weight gain, bitter taste
Lurasidone (Latuda)	20	20–120	Nausea, restlessness, sedation

Adapted from Miklowitz and Gitlin (2014a, p. 119).

Antidepressants

"When I'm depressed, anything bad that happens, no matter how minor, can really destroy me. On antidepressants, it's like putting on a suit of armor or something. It's not that I don't care, or that I'm walking around like "I'm happy now." I'm just not as bothered by things that happen. I feel like I can handle them."

—A 23-year-old woman with bipolar II disorder

Because mood stabilizers and SGAs are generally more effective in preventing the manic pole than the depressive pole of the illness, your doctor may discuss with you the option of combining your mood stabilizer with an antidepressant medicine. *In bipolar I disorder, antidepressants are usually recommended only in combination with mood stabilizers or SGAs, not by themselves.* These agents can be effective in alleviating the often incapacitating symptoms of depression, particularly insomnia, fatigue, and the painful inability to experience pleasure.

In recent years there has been considerable controversy about whether antidepressants should be used at all in bipolar disorder because of questions concerning their efficacy and the possibility that they will provoke a switch into mania or hypomania (El-Mallakh et al., 2015). Nonetheless, given the suffering and impairment caused by bipolar depression, most clinicians believe they should be kept as an option, especially for people whose depression has not responded to mood stabilizers or SGAs.

There is a seemingly endless list of available antidepressants; some are more effective than others, and some have more easily tolerated side effects. You have probably heard a lot about the *selective serotonin reuptake inhibitors* (SSRIs). These include *fluoxetine* (Prozac), *sertraline* (Zoloft), *paroxetine* (Paxil), *fluvoxamine* (Luvox), *citalopram* (Celexa), and *escitalopram* (Lexapro). There are also *novel antidepressants,* including *bupropion* (Wellbutrin), *trazodone* (Desyrel), and *mirtazapine* (Remeron); and *dual-action (serotonin–norepinephrine)* agents, including *duloxetine* (Cymbalta), *venlafaxine* (Effexor), and *desvenlafaxine* (Pristiq).

Concerns about Antidepressants

There has been some alarmism, particularly in the United States, about the use of antidepressants for individuals with bipolar depression. One concern is that they cause people to become suicidal (see "Effective Prevention" on this page). Another concern is that antidepressants can bring on hypomanic or manic switches or a speeding up of mood cycles, especially in those who have a rapid cycling history. My read of the literature is that antidepressants can indeed cause mania or worsen rapid cycling, but mainly in bipolar I patients and primarily when given alone, without an accompanying mood stabilizer or SGA. There is not much evidence that these drugs make people with bipolar I worse if given in combination with traditional mood stabilizers or SGAs. Antidepressant-induced mania usually occurs when people are misdiagnosed as having depression (without mania) and then learn that they have bipolar disorder when an antidepressant— taken alone—causes their first manic episode. DSM-5 still classifies this as a bipolar I manic episode if the symptoms continue after the antidepressant has been stopped.

The bigger question (in my view) is whether antidepressants really add anything. The research is not entirely consistent in answering this question. One large-scale randomized trial study found that people with bipolar depression recovered just as quickly on the combination of mood stabilizers and placebo as on the combination of mood stabilizers and antidepressants (paroxetine or bupropion; Sachs et al.,

> **Effective prevention:** Do antidepressants make people suicidal? The FDA has mandated that a "black box" warning be put on the package inserts of antidepressants concerning the increased risk of suicidal thinking and behavior among children during the first few weeks of treatment. The risks are not large (4% of children develop suicidal thoughts, threaten suicide, or attempt self-injury, compared to 2% on placebo) and are not limited to children with bipolar disorder. Although the risk seems confined largely to children and young adults, you should be aware of feelings of restlessness, irritability, anxiety, pessimistic thinking, hopelessness, or aggressive impulses when you start taking an antidepressant. You may need to stop taking it if these feelings persist.

PERSONALIZED CARE TIP:
Making your history work for you

If you are considering taking an antidepressant but have a history of becoming highly activated by antidepressants, or have a history of rapid cycling, tell your doctor about this history—he or she will probably recommend that you combine the antidepressant with a mood stabilizer or SGA background, or try lamotrigine before trying an antidepressant. This information may not have been discussed during your initial diagnostic workup.

2007). A smaller study, but one that followed people longer, found that those who recovered from their bipolar depression with the combination of a mood stabilizer and an antidepressant—and who had not become manic on antidepressants—were better off staying with this regimen than stopping the antidepressant, in terms of preventing later relapses of depression (Altshuler et al., 2003).

The biggest change in our views about antidepressants has come from studies of bipolar II depression. Jay Amsterdam and his colleagues (2010) at the University of Pennsylvania found that venlafaxine (Effexor) was helpful in alleviating depression in people with bipolar II disorder but did not cause switches into the hypomanic or manic state even when given alone. Most recently, the late Lori Altshuler of the UCLA Semel Institute and her colleagues in the Stanley Research Consortium (Altshuler et al., 2017) conducted a 16-week randomized trial of 142 patients with acute bipolar II depression who were assigned to lithium by itself, sertraline (Zoloft, an SSRI) by itself, or the combination of lithium and sertraline. A total of 63% of the patients showed a significant reduction in depression symptoms over 16 weeks, but it did not matter which of the three treatments they received. The three groups did not differ on the likelihood of switching to a manic or hypomanic or mixed state during the trial. So, at least for people with bipolar II depression, antidepressants may be a safer alternative than we once believed.

If your doctor has recommended combining an antidepressant with an SGA, ask about the single-capsule formulation called OFC (*olanzapine–fluoxetine combination*), marketed under the trade name *Symbyax*. The FDA has approved OFC for the treatment of bipolar I depression, and it is reasonably effective in bipolar mixed states (Benazzi et al., 2009). Few doctors use this medication because they prefer to adjust the two medications individually (in separate prescriptions) rather than rely on a combination pill with fixed dosages of each agent.

Will You Do Well on an Antidepressant?

Given the potential risks of taking antidepressants, what guidelines can we offer to determine whether an antidepressant is right for you? University of Pennsylvania psychiatrist Michael Thase (2010), who has been studying antidepressants for years, recommends taking adjunctive antidepressants if the conditions in the tip at the bottom of this page are met.

Which Antidepressant Should You Take?

Some antidepressants appear safer than others in terms of provoking manic or hypomanic states. A meta-analysis of 57 studies of people in either unipolar or bipolar depressive states found that the highest rates of manic/hypomanic switch occurred with dual-action antidepressants (for example, venlafaxine [Effexor]) and the older line of tricyclics (for example, imipramine, desipramine). Lower rates of manic switch were found for bupropion (Wellbutrin) and the SSRIs (Allain et al., 2017). SSRIs (for example, escitalopram or sertraline) are the most frequently recommended of the antidepressants, especially if you have comorbid anxiety symptoms.

If you have not responded well to SSRIs or these other commonly used antidepressants or have had bad side effects, your doctor may recommend a monoamine oxidase inhibitor (MAOI), usually tranylcypromine (Parnate) or phenelzine (Nardil). Many people do quite well on MAOIs, but they are more difficult to take because they require you to avoid foods that are high in the amino acid tyramine, such as aged cheeses, sausage, or chianti wines.

About one in three people develops sexual side effects on SSRIs or MAOIs. These can include a lower sex drive and delayed orgasm. If these side effects become significant, your doctor may recommend a different antidepressant or advise you to take breaks from the medication. For some people, sexual side effects are reason enough to stop taking an antidepressant, but as with any side effect, you should discuss this with your physician before discontinuing the drug. Going off an antidepressant quickly has been known to increase a person's risk of developing mania or rapid cycling. Other side effects of antidepressants can include weight gain, insomnia, headaches, and daytime sedation.

PERSONALIZED CARE TIP:

Should you take an antidepressant over the long term?

Consider long-term adjunctive treatment with an antidepressant (that is, in combination with a mood stabilizer or an SGA) if you (1) are currently depressed and your illness has been dominated by depression, (2) have done reasonably well on antidepressants before, and (3) have no history of becoming manic or hypomanic or less stable when taking antidepressants. If you have been keeping a mood chart (see Chapter 8), it will be easier to determine if your periods of mood instability co-occur with taking an antidepressant. If you opt to try an antidepressant, reexamine its effectiveness and side effects with your physician biweekly or monthly at first and then at 3- to 6-month intervals.

Treatment-Resistant Bipolar Depression

Some people with bipolar disorder have *treatment-resistant depression* (TRD), meaning they have not done well on at least two mood stabilizers or at least two antidepressants, and psychotherapy has not been particularly helpful either. For some, this means that their depression never gets better beyond a certain level, which is unacceptable; or there are sudden episodes of "breakthrough depression" in a person who has been stable on mood stabilizers or SGAs. TRD has been described in both unipolar depression and bipolar disorder, and many of the studies lump those two together.

Not everyone likes the term "treatment-resistant," because it can imply that you have some sort of built-in resistance to treatments to which you should have responded, or that you are not accepting what is being given to you. I'm not a big fan of the term either but recognize that it is meant as shorthand for the idea that the biological vulnerabilities associated with depression are resistant to medical modification, not that you are a resistant person.

People with TRD may do well with two antidepressants taken together, especially if they have different mechanisms of action (for example, an SSRI and bupropion, which augments both norepinephrine and dopamine). Alternatively, your doctor may recommend two mood stabilizers/SGAs together, such as lithium with lamotrigine or lurasidone. But not everyone with TRD responds to these approaches.

One welcome advance of the past few years has been the availability of new, adjunctive medications to supplement traditional mood stabilizers, SGAs, or antidepressants for bipolar depression. None of the newer medications has the track record of the standard mood stabilizers, but you may want to discuss them with your doctor if your existing medications are either causing unpleasant side effects (for example, memory problems, significant weight gain) or not improving your mood or energy sufficiently.

Thyroid Supplements

It's not unusual for doctors to recommend thyroid medications to supplement drugs like lithium for depression (and particularly rapid cycling depression). Thyroid supplements are usually marketed under the name levothyroxine (Synthroid, Levoxyl, Levothroid) or liothyronine (Cytomel or T3). People with bipolar disorder often have comorbid hypothyroidism, a condition of hormonal insufficiency in which people feel inertia, low mood, slowness, and sleep disturbances. Certain mood stabilizers, such as lithium, can have the unintended effect of suppressing thyroid hormones. This is useful to know if you're feeling fatigued or slowed down on lithium: a thyroid supplement may help bring you back to a normal energy level. Additionally, having a normal thyroid level may increase the chances that you'll respond to an antidepressant.

You may benefit from thyroid supplements even if you have a normal thyroid test result but are not responding to mood stabilizers alone. However, be aware of some of the issues regarding treatment of women with hypothyroidism (see Chapter 12).

Ketamine

There has been quite a lot of excitement in the popular press about the drug ketamine for depression. A sedative used during surgical procedures for anesthesia, ketamine produces rapid antidepressant effects in people with TRD (both the unipolar and bipolar types), with improvements in mood occurring between 4 and 72 hours after its infusion (Katalinic et al., 2013; Zarate et al., 2012). Ketamine inhibits glutamatergic signaling in the brain, which is thought to be dysregulated in depression. It also increases levels of BDNF, which we have already discussed as enhancing the strength of cells and synaptic plasticity (see Chapter 5).

One meta-analysis found that ketamine reduced suicidal ideation in depressed people within 1 day following a single intravenous dose, with the effects on suicidal ideation lasting up to a week (Wilkinson et al., 2018). Its effects are most rapid and consistent in alleviating anhedonia—the loss of pleasure in activities. Ketamine has only been studied as a treatment for bipolar depression when added to a mood stabilizer. Nonetheless, several randomized trials have shown that it improves depression and suicidal ideation in bipolar depression in as little as 40 minutes, with few side effects (Zarate et al., 2012). It has beneficial effects on regulation of circadian rhythms, which, as you learned in Chapter 5, are central to the physiology of bipolar disorder (Duncan, Ballard, & Zarate, 2017).

One of the main concerns about ketamine has been its mode of delivery through an intravenous tube, limiting its acceptability to many recipients. There are now nasal sprays that deliver "esketamine" directly to the brain, but we don't know yet whether this form of administration will prove equally powerful. Second, although as many as 70% of people with depression show rapid improvement with ketamine, the effects appear to be short-lived (a week to 10 days), with depressive relapses common after that. Third, there are some dose-related side effects, such as perceptual distortions, temporary elevations in blood pressure and heart rate, and short-lived cognitive problems (Abbasi, 2017). Finally, there is a question of whether it is addictive: ketamine is a schedule III controlled substance because it is hallucinogenic and sold as a street drug (where it is called "special K"). Currently, we don't know how long people can be treated with ketamine.

Research is being conducted to find effective alternatives to ketamine that have fewer side effects and do not have its perceptual or hallucinogenic properties. For now, if you have bipolar depressions that have not responded to antidepressants, ketamine is certainly an option to consider. There is an advocacy network for locating ketamine providers (*www.ketamineadvocacynetwork.org/provider-directory*).

Omega-3 Fatty Acids (Fish Oil)

One popular alternative for treatment-resistant depression is the *omega-3 plan*. You can get omega-3—or "long-chain fatty acids" as they're sometimes called—in a health food store, with dosages of 1,000–2,000 mg/day. The most effective kind of omega-3 contains ethyl-eicosapentaenoate (EPA) acid, which is also used to reduce levels of triglycerides (the main component of body fat). Interest in omega-3 as an antidepressant began with the observation that societies in which fish is a major part of the daily diet have lower prevalence rates for depression (Hibbeln, 1998). Because it is a "natural" over-the-counter substance, some people feel better about taking it than a pharmaceutical, but it is meant as an adjunct, not a substitute for lithium, valproate, or SGAs. Its side effects are considered minimal and include a "fishy" aftertaste, upset stomach, diarrhea, or nausea.

The jury is still out in determining whether omega-3 is a good treatment for bipolar depression, because relatively few studies have been done. A meta-analysis of 10 studies involving 329 people with major depression found that omega-3 was significantly better than placebo in reducing depressive symptoms, but only two of these studies concerned bipolar disorder (Lin & Su, 2007). A recent trial found positive effects of omega-3 in children ages 7–14 with depression (many of whom could be presumed to be at risk for later onset of bipolar disorder) (Fristad et al., 2016).

On the whole, omega-3 probably has weak antidepressant effects and may be good for one's general health. It will not be adequate as a solo agent for treatment-resistant bipolar depression. If your child is depressed or has significant mood swings, adding omega-3 may be a way of augmenting the effectiveness of mood stabilizers or SGAs without increasing their side effects, but always discuss this option with your child's doctor before proceeding.

Medications for Comorbid Conditions

Benzodiazepines for Anxiety

Many people with bipolar disorder also take one of the benzodiazepines, a class of drugs that may calm you down, help manage your anxiety or panic symptoms, and help with sleep. Remember Valium? Drugs like diazepam (Valium) and alprazolam (Xanax) were prescribed quite readily in the 1970s as a way of managing stress and tension. Other drugs in this class include clonazepam (Klonopin) and lorazepam (Ativan). These drugs need to be taken with caution, because unlike the other drugs discussed so far, the benzodiazepines are addictive. People may need higher and higher dosages over time to get the same effects and can have withdrawal symptoms when stopping them—including seizures. But if you're having considerable problems getting to sleep or staying asleep at night, or if you feel chronically anxious during the day, these medications may help you. Your doctor may also recommend a benzodiazepine instead of an SGA to help quell your manic or mixed symptoms, although they do not appear to be as effective toward that end.

Neuroenhancers for Cognitive Functioning

Neuroenhancers are drugs used to enhance brain function, either in people with neurological illnesses or in healthy people who are looking for a boost, such as help staying awake or increasing their ability to focus. *Pramipexole* is a neuroenhancing drug that increases the availability of dopamine in the synapses of cells; it is used regularly in Parkinson's disease. It may improve cognitive functioning and mood in some people with bipolar disorder. In one small trial, pramipexole, when combined with mood stabilizers, alleviated depressive symptoms among people who had not done well on other antidepressants (Goldberg, Burdick, & Endick, 2004). Another small-scale trial showed that adjunctive pramipexole was more effective than a placebo add-on in treating depression in bipolar II disorders (Zarate et al., 2004). It appears to have a mild side-effect profile, although any drug that increases dopamine can increase the risk of mania or psychosis.

Modafinil and *armodafanil* (Provigil and Nuvigil), also neuroenhancers, are used in the treatment of daytime sleepiness or narcolepsy. They have the effect of making you feel mentally sharper or more focused, with improved recall or verbal fluency. They have been found to treat bipolar depression without an increased risk of manic switch (Grunze, 2014). Neuroenhancers have less of an effect on blood pressure than dopamine stimulants such as Adderall.

Electroconvulsive Therapy: What Is and Isn't True about It?

Josh, a 35-year-old man with bipolar I disorder, was hospitalized for a manic episode and then returned home on a combination of lithium and risperidone. Shortly after his discharge he swung into a severe depression, which was characterized by sleeping most of the day, suicidal thoughts, low energy, mental slowness, and loss of interest in his family and work. He began to have unusual thoughts, such as fearing that his body was rotting. His physician was unwilling to give him an antidepressant because he'd had several bad reactions to antidepressants before, including periods of rapid cycling and mixed symptoms. Increasing his dosage of lithium did not help his depression and gave him more side effects—and "more to be depressed about" (his words).

Josh eventually asked to be admitted to the hospital again. Although he had been quite frightened of electroconvulsive therapy (ECT) the first time he had it, this time he asked for it, thinking it was the only option that would help. He was started on a course of ECT three times a week. He responded to this treatment within 3 weeks and was discharged from the hospital, his depression largely lifted. He felt brighter, mentally sharper, and more able to engage with his wife and children. His suicidal thoughts had diminished.

ECT, or what is often disparagingly called "shock treatment," is one of the more powerful treatment options available for people with bipolar depression and other severe (and often treatment-resistant) forms of depression. ECT works quickly and efficiently. It is one of the most effective methods we have for pulling someone out of a severe depressive or mixed episode. ECT can also be used to bring a person down from a manic high, although it is rarely used for that purpose.

What Happens During ECT?

Typically you stop taking your mood-stabilizing or antidepressant medications, although you can continue taking SGAs. Once these drugs are washed out of your system, which can take a week or two, an appointment is scheduled. During this session, you are given a general anesthetic (for example, sodium pentathol) and another medication (succinylcholine) to help relax your muscles and prevent a full-body seizure. These drugs will make you unconscious while you are undergoing the treatment. The doctor then administers an electrical pulse that creates a mild seizure in your brain. The theory behind ECT is that this pulse and the resulting seizure "jump-start" the brain's production of neurotransmitters.

Usually between 4 and 12 treatments are needed, or up to three times a week for about 1 month. Because ECT is generally not considered a maintenance (preventive) treatment, you will usually restart your mood stabilizer, antidepressant, or antipsychotic regimen after the course of ECT is over.

Because of the difficult and turbulent history of ECT—it was once used as a punishment in psychiatric hospitals—people with bipolar disorder and their family members often don't want to consider it even in the most dire of circumstances. This is unfortunate, because ECT can be lifesaving. It can pull people out of serious depressions that might otherwise have resulted in suicide. Nowadays, ECT is a safe and effective outpatient treatment that is fairly routine in its administration. Because of its side effects and high economic cost, it is typically considered only when a person has not responded adequately to mood stabilizers or antidepressants and is incapacitated by depression, psychosis, or suicidality. Although this may be surprising, it is considered one of the safest options for women who are pregnant and severely depressed or manic. Most mood stabilizers and antidepressants carry some risk of harm to the unborn baby, but ECT does not when administered under standard medical conditions (see Chapter 12).

ECT will not be done against your wishes. Like any psychiatric treatment, ECT is based on a joint decision between you and your doctor.

"Won't ECT Destroy My Memory?"

Some physicians recommend ECT reluctantly because one of its side effects is a loss of memory. The memory loss is usually most noticeable for events that occurred during the months after the treatments are given (Fraser, O'Carroll, & Ebmeier, 2008). But some people also forget events that occurred prior to the ECT procedures. This probably occurs because ECT can affect the transfer of information usually held in short-term memory (the kind of memory that encodes and briefly holds information in your mind, such as when you first hear people's names and phone numbers) to long-term memory storage. A recent study found that patients who had received ECT did not perform as well on verbal learning and memory tests as those who had never received ECT, but it was not clear whether these effects were permanent (MacQueen, Parkin, Marriott, Bégin, & Hasey, 2007).

The memories do not appear to be lost for good. In fact, some memories of events that occurred before the ECT come back several months after the treatment. It appears that about two-thirds of people who receive ECT experience problems in memory functioning, but the problems seem to be temporary and disappear with time.

New Electrical Stimulation Techniques

Rapid transcranial magnetic stimulation (rTMS) has been proposed as a simpler and less invasive way to stimulate parts of the cerebral cortex than ECT. In this method, pulses of electrical stimulation produced by a stimulator coil (placed over the scalp) are used to enhance neuronal activity in the dorsolateral prefrontal cortex, a major site for executive functioning, cognitive flexibility, inhibition, planning, and mood regulation. RTMS may improve cognitive functioning as well as mood. Studies have shown that rTMS can stabilize depressive symptoms in unipolar depression and, if treatment is continued during the maintenance phase, prevent depressive relapses (Oldani, Altamura, Abdelghani, & Young, 2016; Rachid, 2017a). It has not been studied extensively in people with bipolar disorder.

Some transient side effects occur with rTMS, like headaches, neck pain, or toothaches. The treatment has to be administered in conjunction with a mood stabilizer because, like antidepressants, it carries a risk of inducing mania or hypomania (Rachid, 2017b). It does not appear to be as effective as ECT for people with TRD (Oldani et al., 2016). A bigger problem is that rTMS is very expensive, and many insurance companies will not cover it for use in bipolar depression; its FDA approval is for major depressive disorder.

Two other stimulation treatments are in the experimental phase: *vagal nerve stimulation* (VNS) and *deep brain stimulation* (DBS). These treatments tend to be available only in specialized centers. If you opt for VNS, there will be a stimulator device (about the size of a wristwatch) implanted under your skin that sends electric signals to your left vagal nerve (located in your neck). One small study (Marangell et al., 2008) found that people with rapid cycling bipolar disorder who had not responded well to other treatments showed an improvement in depressive symptoms over 1 year of VNS treatment. Like all treatments, VNS has side effects, including a decrease in your respiratory flow during sleep and a high risk of sleep apnea (an intermittent closing of the throat while sleeping). Some people report snoring, changes in their voice, coughing, and sore throat as side effects.

DBS involves the surgical implantation of a "brain pacemaker," which sends electrical impulses to various areas of the brain believed to be important in depression. One such area is the subgenual cingulate, a small area of the prefrontal cortex (Mayberg et al., 2005); another is the nucleus accumbens, which helps regulate the brain's responses to reward (Schlaepfer et al., 2008). A few small studies have found that people with treatment-resistant unipolar depression who have not responded to other treatments improve and stay well with DBS (Oldani et al., 2016). Side effects include blurred vision, soreness from the surgery, and an increased risk of hypomania or mania. The evidence to guide treatment in bipolar disorder is minimal.

In summary, ECT remains one of our best treatments for treating severe and treatment-resistant depression and should be considered if you are finding that neither antidepressants nor mood stabilizers/SGAs have worked. The other electrical stimulation treatments need more experimental evidence before they can be recommended as alternatives. Nonetheless, this field is advancing rapidly.

Light Treatment

Changes in exposure to light during the different seasons—and in different geographic locations—have long been known to affect people's mood states. You may have noticed that your moods vary considerably with the season of the year. Many people have seasonal mood disorders, which usually means they have depression in the fall or winter months and, less commonly, mania or hypomania in the spring or summer. As a result there has been quite a lot of enthusiasm for bright light treatment. It is now commonplace to find homes and office buildings that are outfitted with "mood lighting."

There are relatively few controlled trials of light therapy for bipolar disorder. One recent, small-scale randomized trial indicated that individuals with bipolar depression who were assigned to bright light therapy (7,000 lux) as well as mood stabilizers or antipsychotics had a higher rate of remission from depression over 6 weeks (68%) than patients who were assigned to a 50-lux red light (a placebo) plus medications (22%) (Sit et al., 2018). Importantly, the bright white light was administered for about 45 minutes in the middle of the day rather than in the morning.

Light treatment can interfere with your sleep if you are not protected by a mood stabilizer or SGA. Nonetheless, you should discuss this alternative with your physician if you have winter depression with excessive sleepiness, overeating, and lethargy or feel that your mood is very reactive to changes in daylight hours.

What Psychotherapy Can Do for You

"I cannot imagine leading a normal life without both taking lithium and having had the benefits of psychotherapy . . . ineffably, psychotherapy heals. It makes some sense of the confusion, reins in the terrifying thoughts and feelings, returns some control and hope and possibility of learning from it all. . . . It is where I have believed—or have learned to believe—that I might someday be able to contend with all of this. No pill can help me deal with the problem of not wanting to take pills; likewise, no amount of psychotherapy alone can prevent my manias and depressions. I need both."
—Kay Redfield Jamison, *An Unquiet Mind* (1995, pp. 88–89)

Many doctors will recommend that you combine your medical treatment with some form of psychotherapy. Ethan, a 19-year-old man who had been hospitalized during a manic episode (see details in Chapter 7), came to some important decisions about his illness and his need for medications as a result of psychotherapy. He originally refused all medications, but through the support of his therapist he eventually agreed to a trial of lithium. In turn, the combination of psychotherapy and lithium helped him recover from a relatively intractable depressive illness.

Learning to accept medication is only one reason to seek psychotherapy. Like Kay Jamison, many people with bipolar disorder say that therapy was an essential part of their recovery from mood episodes, on a par with medications. Psychotherapy can't cure you of bipolar disorder, nor is it a substitute for medications. Nonetheless, psychotherapy can help you learn to recognize the triggers for your mood swings and what to do about them. If you can afford it (or your insurance covers some part of it) and if you can find a good therapist in your community who knows about bipolar disorder, I would highly recommend that you pursue and stick with it for as long as you find it useful. In my experience, most people are satisfied with weekly hour-long visits to an individual, couple, or family therapist, or a weekly 90-minute group. More frequent sessions may be needed in the intervals following an acute illness episode.

Why Try Psychotherapy?

There are several compelling reasons to seek psychotherapy (see the box on page 155), even if you don't think you have significant personal problems. A major reason is to get some guidance in managing your disorder. You may want to dis-

---

Effective Treatment:
7 Reasons to Seek Psychotherapy for Bipolar Disorder

■ To help you make sense of environmental factors that contributed to your current or past episodes of illness

■ To identify warning signs of new episodes and develop prevention plans

■ To help you accept and adapt to a medication regimen

■ To develop strategies for coping with stress in school or the workplace

■ To deal with the social stigma of bipolar disorder

■ To deal with comorbid disorders like substance abuse, chronic anxiety, or medical illnesses

■ To address long-standing interpersonal or family problems

---

cuss the role of stressful events in eliciting your mood cycles, why you feel "set off" by certain interactions with your spouse or other family members, your difficulties accepting the illness or its social stigma, or your ambivalence about medications (see Chapter 7). You may wish to discuss the impact that your illness is having on your work life or friendships or how to talk about it with other people. These are all good reasons to seek therapy.

You may also seek therapy to address long-standing personal problems that may be unrelated to your disorder or that seem to continue whether your mood is stable or not. These issues are probably not being addressed in your medication sessions with your psychiatrist. For example, many people with bipolar disorder have had very traumatic experiences of physical or sexual abuse and regularly have flashbacks to these events (Palmier-Claus et al., 2016). Some people with bipolar disorder feel that they've never had a successful romantic relationship or job experience. Some feel chronically suicidal, even when they are not in an episode of depression. Some have experienced painful childhood losses (for example, the suicide of a parent) and need to make sense of their feelings of abandonment and rejection. Even if these psychological issues were not a primary cause of your bipolar disorder, they may become more salient to you when your mood changes. Gaining insight into the nature of these conflicts and developing skills for coping with them have the potential to make you less vulnerable to current stressors, and less susceptible to new illness episodes.

Hannah, a 27-year-old woman with bipolar II disorder, suffered from comorbid obsessive–compulsive disorder that had become severe enough that she had quit her job as a court reporter. She was bothered by intrusive thoughts that she might kill her husband, Carl, also age 27. These thoughts were especially disturbing to her because "I deeply love him . . . he's the best thing that's ever happened to me, maybe the only really good thing." When she had violent thoughts, she often cycled into depressive or suicidal states. She was consistent in taking her regimen of valproate and sertraline, but her thoughts caused her significant distress. Carl was aware of her impulses but said he wasn't worried about them. She had never acted on them, and "Besides, I'd rather she had fantasies about killing me than somebody off the street."

During a course of interpersonally oriented psychotherapy (see the next section), Hannah came to realize that she was quite angry at her husband for what she termed his "treating me like his little doll." She recounted how her various attempts at independence were met with vitriolic tirades from Carl, in which he would reassert his dominion over her. In one particularly emotional session she realized that her violent thoughts usually appeared within a few hours of having a frustrating confrontation with Carl regarding her desire to get a job or go back to school.

Later in therapy, she became more comfortable with the idea that she had legitimate reasons to be angry with Carl. She became less frightened by her violent thoughts and decided to work on being more assertive about what she wanted in her interactions with Carl. Carl finally agreed to support her in applying for a part-time job at a health club and enrolling in an evening sign language course. Her violent thoughts gradually receded.

Hannah's problems with her husband did not stem directly from her bipolar disorder, although they contributed to her mood cycling patterns. Notice that her symptom improvement stemmed from two factors: her *insight* into the reasons behind her violent thoughts and her *decision to do something differently* in her marital relationship. Most therapists nowadays believe that psychotherapy is most effective when people combine insight (a fundamental aspect of psychoanalytic therapy) with learning the needed skills for changing thinking patterns or behaviors (cognitive-behavioral therapy).

Choosing the Right Therapy

Like medications, psychotherapy comes in different sizes, shapes, and dosages. Depending on the size of your community, you may be able to locate professionals who practice individual therapy from a variety of theoretical viewpoints. Some of these may be baffling (for example, "therapeutic touch"). You may also have access to family therapy, couple therapy, or psychoeducational support groups. If you live in a rural area or a small town, you may be limited to the types of practice available in your immediate locale.

Almost all therapy goes better if you're with a therapist you respect and trust and who you feel genuinely cares about you. *But it is also important to find a thera-*

pist who understands the syndrome of bipolar disorder. Avoid being in the position of educating your therapist about your symptoms or having your behavior labeled as "acting out" or "low self-esteem" when the real issues have to do with manic or depressive symptoms. Good questions to ask your prospective therapist include whether he or she (1) works regularly with persons with bipolar disorder, (2) will integrate his or her knowledge of the disorder into the therapy, and in what ways, (3) places importance on understanding the effects of your disorder on your relationships, and the reverse, (4) will communicate regularly with the physician who is managing your medications, and (5) will focus on the present as well as the past.

For How Long?

At the first or second session, you should ask how long your therapy is likely to last, although your therapist may not be able to give you a precise answer. Following a major illness episode, it is reasonable to expect weekly or twice weekly sessions for 4–6 months, with an agreement to evaluate your progress from time to time. Avoid agreeing to open-ended, long-term contracts with no clearly articulated goals. Avoid therapy approaches in which all disorders—whether bipolar disorder, depression, anxiety problems, or substance/alcohol abuse—are ascribed to traumatic "repressed memories" (that is, memories of negative childhood experiences that are buried and presumably must be uncovered). Despite the fact that these long-term treatments have been around for some time, they are largely unproven by research, and their effectiveness in treating bipolar disorder has not been evaluated systematically. What's more, they tend to downplay or even deny the importance of the biological and genetic origins of the disorder and the need for medications. This is not to say that examining painful childhood events will not help you, but it should be done in the context of a therapy that acknowledges the likely genetic and biological bases of your disorder, helps you develop strategies for coping with it, recognizes the important role of medications, and deals with your present as well as past difficulties. You and your therapist should not forge ahead with painful "uncovering work" when you are still symptomatic and feeling fragile.

The assumptions and purposes of therapies appropriate for bipolar disorder are discussed on the following pages, as well as the research evidence for their effectiveness in stabilizing mood symptoms when combined with medications.

Individual Psychotherapy

Individual therapy is most often recommended once you have started to recover from an episode of mania or depression, so it is mostly a maintenance rather than an acute episode treatment. When you are in the process of recovering, you may still have significant mood symptoms, negative or overly pessimistic thinking, or behavior patterns that interfere with long-term stability (for example, excessive drinking); these are the "targets" of individual therapy. Consider finding a psychotherapist who can work with you in a *cognitive-behavioral therapy* (CBT) or *interpersonal therapy* (IPT) framework. These are the types of individual therapy that have research support in terms of improving the course of bipolar disorder when given alongside medications (Salcedo et al., 2016).

A therapist who specializes in CBT will encourage you to identify and evaluate patterns of negative thinking about yourself, your world, and your future. By keeping a daily thought record (see Chapter 10), you can learn to identify your assumptions about certain critical events (for example, "I lost my job because I'm just not capable of holding one"). Your CBT therapist will encourage you to recognize the impact of such assumptions on your mood states and conduct "experiments" in your day-to-day life to determine whether these assumptions are valid. As therapy proceeds, the therapist will encourage you to consider more adaptive and balanced interpretations of events and rehearse new cognitions (for example, "Maybe I lost this job because I was still recovering from my depression and couldn't function at the level I know I'm capable of"). When used to treat depression (for which CBT was developed), it usually includes a plan for structuring your day so that you get more exposure to activities you've found rewarding in the past.

People with bipolar disorder who receive CBT with medications have less severe depressive symptoms and fewer days with depression during maintenance care than those who take medications only, although not all studies find this (Goodwin et al., 2016). CBT may be especially useful if you have a comorbid anxiety disorder such as panic disorder, social phobia, or obsessive–compulsive disorder (Deckersbach et al., 2014). In numerous studies, CBT treatments such as prolonged exposure to feared stimuli, breathing retraining, relaxation, and mindfulness meditation have been shown to be effective for anxiety disorders. Chapter 10 offers a more thorough discussion of the CBT approach and a selection of cognitive restructuring exercises you can try out on your own.

IPT is geared toward helping you understand the role that your illness is playing in your close relationships or work life and in turn how your relationships and work life are affecting the stability of your moods. Interpersonal therapists encourage you to focus on a particular interpersonal problem and consider how it relates to your mood disorder. For example, some people develop manic or depressive episodes after loss or grief experiences such as the death of a parent; some after a life transition such as losing a job or a relationship breakup; and some after significant disputes with family members or partners. For others, mood states are related to habitual problems in romantic relationships, friendships, or working peaceably with others. IPT focuses on your habits in relationships and how to alter them to help stabilize your mood.

A form of IPT called *interpersonal and social rhythm therapy* (IPSRT; Frank, 2007) is more geared toward bipolar disorder and includes an additional element: monitoring your sleep–wake rhythms, patterns of daily activity, and levels of daily social stimulation. This method, called social rhythm tracking, is discussed more in Chapter 8. Working with a therapist who specializes in IPSRT may be quite helpful to you in implementing sleep–wake and other strategies for stabilizing daily and nightly routines. In one carefully designed study, IPSRT with medications was shown to delay recurrences of bipolar disorder, improve vocational functioning, and increase the stability of daily routines and sleep–wake cycles when compared to supportive therapy and medications (Frank et al., 2005).

Family and Couple Therapy

Sometimes bipolar disorder is best treated in a family or couple context. The advantage of therapy with your close relatives is that they can be educated about your disorder and taught coping skills for managing stress at the same time as you. People with bipolar disorder often have high levels of family or relationship conflict or tension during and following episodes (see Chapter 5). Family interventions can provide ways of improving your communication with your spouse, parents, or kids. Chapter 13 offers detailed instructions on how to use effective family communication strategies.

The family/couple approach that I developed with Michael Goldstein of UCLA, called *family-focused therapy* (FFT), is a psychoeducational therapy in which people with bipolar disorder and their spouses or parents are acquainted with information and illness management strategies relevant to the disorder—its symptoms, causes, prognosis, and treatment (much like the content of this book). In contrast to programs that focus exclusively on learning facts about the illness, in FFT sessions individuals with bipolar disorder and their close relatives discuss their feelings and beliefs about the illness, what coping strategies have and haven't worked, and how to adopt illness management strategies that have been effective for others. For example, you and your partner, spouse, or parent(s) can learn to collaborate in recognizing your early warning signs of recurrences and knowing who to call for help; or in modifying aspects of the environment that may be interfering with your recovery (for example, too many social demands).

Later stages of FFT focus on family or couple communication and problem-solving strategies, including how to listen, negotiate, clarify one's position and acknowledge another person's, and give an even balance of positive and negative feedback to others. Problem solving rounds out the treatment as families learn steps to identify and define problems, generate and evaluate solutions, and develop a plan for implementing one or more solutions. To learn more about this therapy, see *Bipolar Disorder: A Family-Focused Treatment Approach* (Miklowitz, 2010). Over a number of different randomized trials, we have found that adults or adolescents with bipolar disorder who get FFT with medications recover from depressive episodes faster, have less severe manic and depressive symptoms, and have fewer recurrences over 2 years than those who get medications with case management or individual psychoeducational therapy (Miklowitz & Chung, 2016).

CBT, interpersonal, and family treatments for bipolar disorder may be hard to find in your community, but look for them anyway. Several national organizations have online "therapist locator" listings. Check out the website for the Association for Behavioral and Cognitive Therapies (*www.abct.org*; go to the "Find Help" link), the Beck Institute for Cognitive Behavior Therapy (*www.beckinstitute.org*), the American Association for Marriage and Family Therapy (*www.aamft.org/Directories/ Find_a_Therapist.aspx*), or the American Psychological Association (*http://locator. apa.org*). For family-focused therapy, you can also contact the Child and Adolescent Mood Disorders program at UCLA (*www.semel.ucla.edu/cap/service/family-focused-therapy-fft*). IPT therapists are especially hard to find (for some reason, there are a lot of them in Iowa), but try searching under the International Society for Interpersonal Psychotherapy (*www.interpersonalpsychotherapy.org*) or contact the organization by email (*info@interpersonalpsychotherapy.org*).

Psychoeducational and Mutual Support Groups

"Meeting other bipolar people and hearing their stories has made me feel less isolated. It gives me hope that I can learn to control these mood swings and have a more fulfilling life."

—A 66-year-old support group participant

Many people benefit from educational support groups, either led by a trained clinician (see, for example, Bauer & McBride, 1996; Colom et al., 2009) or conducted as *mutual support* groups by persons with bipolar disorder or their caregivers. In groups, people with bipolar disorder get together and discuss feelings, attitudes, and experiences related to the disorder. When the groups are educational and skill oriented (my recommendation), you will come away with concrete strategies for doing things differently (for example, good ways to keep track of your moods or sleep–wake cycles, or who the best doctors are in your area). Several studies indicate that people with bipolar disorder who attend structured psychoeducational groups have fewer recurrences over time, are more adherent to their medications, and spend less money on their care than people who get less structured, less directive support groups (Colom et al., 2009; Salcedo et al., 2016).

Many people feel that others with bipolar disorder are the only ones who can truly understand them and give them viable solutions. People in mutual support groups talk about medications they've tried and which ones have or haven't worked; which therapies they've had; how they have dealt with problems in the work, family, or social settings; and what they do to prevent themselves from getting ill again. Of the more than 2,000 respondents to the National Depression and Manic–Depressive Association (now called the Depression and Bipolar Support Alliance) Support Group Compliance Survey (Lewis, 2000)—all of whom had been active in local support groups—95% said that their group experience helped them become more willing to take medications, communicate with their doctors, and cope with side effects. In my earliest days at UCLA, I ran a support group for people with bipolar disorder and was continually impressed with how effective the members were at helping each other.

Not everyone feels comfortable in a group setting. If you have doubts, try going for one session and see if you can relate to the other people in the group. Can you imagine feeling supported and understood by them when talking about your own problems? Do they seem to have had the kinds of life difficulties or illness management problems you've had? To see if there are groups available in your community, try calling the local mental health center in your city or town, local psychiatrists who specialize in mood disorders, or the phone numbers listed in the next paragraph.

Family Support Groups

Your spouse or parents may also want to attend a support group. They may benefit from a group in which they can confide in other relatives of persons with mood disorders. Good options for your relatives—which you may want to check out as well—include the Depression and Bipolar Support Alliance (800-826-3632; *www.dbsalliance.org*), the associated Balanced Mind Parent Network (*www.dbsalliance.org*), or the National Alliance on Mental Illness (800-950-NAMI; *www.nami.org*). Each of these organizations runs family support groups in various cities throughout the United States, Europe, and Asia. Your relatives can also join online support organizations such as the International Bipolar Foundation (*www.ibpf.org*), which has wonderful educational resources and a complete guide to finding group support in your area.

Try not to be anxious about your spouse's or other family member's desire to join such a group. You may fear that these groups will be composed of angry relatives who will badmouth you and encourage your relatives to give up and leave. In my experience, this is not the case. Rather, these groups provide useful information and support to make family members feel less isolated. Sometimes your relative may have his or her own mood problems to discuss. If you are uncomfortable, ask your relative to take you along. In most cases, these groups are open to persons with the disorder as well as their family members. And, usually, they're free.

Moving Forward

As you can see, there are numerous treatments available to people with bipolar disorder. These treatments are far from perfect, but many can effectively treat your acute symptoms and, in all likelihood, even out the course of your illness over time. Adding psychotherapy or support groups to your medication regimen helps ensure that you, the person, are treated, not just your symptoms; that you develop strategies for coping with stress; and that you feel less isolated or misunderstood.

You and your doctor may need to experiment with a number of different medication options before you find a combination that is effective and minimizes your side effects. Likewise, the first therapist you see may not be the one you end up with. This trial-and-error process will certainly be frustrating at times, but there is every reason to be hopeful that you will eventually find treatments that are optimal for you.

Committing to a long-term program of medications or therapy involves important personal decisions. You may have significant doubts about whether you should take any of these medications, even if you are suffering from debilitating mood swings that interfere with your functioning. These doubts are understandable. But when people with bipolar disorder stop taking medications, particularly if they do so abruptly and have no therapist available to help them, they often end up relapsing and worse off than they were before they stopped. To hear more about how people have resolved this dilemma, read on: Chapter 7 is devoted to the issues you will face in coming to accept a regimen of medications and their daily management.

Coming to Terms with Your Medications

> Accusing me of mania, my elder sister's voice has an odd manic quality. "Are you taking your medicine?" A low controlled mania, the kind of control in furious questions addressed to children, such as "Will you get down from there?" . . .
>
> As if by going off lithium I could erase the past, could prove it had never happened, could triumph over and contradict my diagnoses; this way I would be right and they would be wrong. It had always been the other way; they were right and I was wrong. Of course I had only to take the lithium in order to be accepted back . . . on lithium I would be "all right." . . . But I am never all right, just in remission. If I could win this gamble. . . .
>
> —KATE MILLET, *The Loony-Bin Trip* (1990, p. 32)

The nature of bipolar disorder is such that even when you feel better, you still have an underlying biological predisposition to the illness. This predisposition requires you to take medications even when you're feeling well. Often, though, when you feel better, you will be tempted to stop your medications, because you won't see the need for it. That's an understandable reaction.

Unfortunately, stopping your medications against medical advice—and sometimes even just taking inadequate dosages or missing dosages regularly—puts you at a much higher risk of having a recurrence of your disorder. In my experience, people are most likely to consider stopping their medications once they have partially recovered from a manic or depressive episode. During this recovery phase they may feel good or even hypomanic but are more in control of their moods than during the height of their illness. Taking medication feels like spoiling a good party. These reactions are especially true of younger people who have had only one or two episodes—inconsistency with medications can stem from feelings of youthful invulnerability. But I have also worked with middle-aged and older adults who acknowledge having had many, many depressive or manic episodes throughout their lives and still doubt that they need medication. Understandably, they want to know what life would be like without the pills. They may also be worried about the long-term effects of medications on their kidneys or metabolic systems.

In the last chapter, I discussed the various drug treatments available to people with bipolar disorder. In this chapter, let's consider the various reasons that people with bipolar disorder give for discontinuing their drug regimens. Many of these reasons have been offered by my own patients, including those who have been stable for quite some time but question whether their medications are really working.

I have also surveyed the research literature for the reasons people with bipolar disorder stop their medications, which are quite varied. Sometimes the issues surrounding inconsistency or *nonconcordance* are related to feelings or beliefs about the disorder, such as disagreeing with the diagnosis or missing the pleasure of the high periods. Inconsistency can also be a response to unpleasant side effects (for example, weight gain), difficulty relating to a particular physician, or dislike of having one's blood drawn. Sometimes people just forget to take their medicine. People also go off medications because of practical matters like prescriptions that lapse (and difficulties getting a new one) and the high costs of paying for medications. Not surprisingly, people with bipolar disorder stay on their medications when they perceive their physician to be empathic, collaborative, and accessible; the doctor's level of experience or list of credentials is less important in determining concordance (Sylvia et al., 2013).

In this chapter, I offer tips for making medications feel more acceptable to you (if you're having doubts) as well as ideas for discussing side effects with your physician, so that you can get the greatest possible gain (and the least possible pain) from treatment. You may recognize your own experiences in the personal stories of people struggling to accept long-term treatment with medications. I will also touch on the factors that affect people's willingness to get long-term psychotherapy, some of which overlap with medication usage and some of which do not.

What Is Medication Concordance?

Concordance with medication refers to the degree of consistency between the plans recommended by the physician and the plans carried out by the patient (Reilly-Harrington & Sachs, 2006). *Nonconcordance* means that you have not followed the physician's recommendations in taking your medications or have stopped taking them altogether, against your doctor's advice. But people can become nonconcordant in any number of ways. For example, some people take their medications correctly for several weeks and then stop all of them abruptly. Some stop only one medication in a "cocktail" of medications: they are on lithium, valproate, and quetiapine and decide to discontinue everything but the valproate (or take a higher dosage of this medication than prescribed). Other people drop their dosages or take medications intermittently (for example, take only half of their recommended olanzapine tablets, miss their evening dosages, or skip Saturday nights). For others, nonconcordance takes the form of substituting unproven remedies (for example, medicinal herbs like St. John's wort or omega-3 fatty acids) for mood stabilizers or trying to use alcohol or marijuana to control their mood states.

Why the term *concordance*? Many alternative terms have been proposed in the medical literature, the most common of which are *adherence* and *compliance*. In my experience, persons with bipolar disorder don't usually like either of those terms. *Nonadherence* feels critical and judgmental and can be associated in the mind with tape or glue (one patient asked, "What am I? A Post-it note?"). It implies that the person with the disorder is unwilling or unable to stick to an agreed-on program. Even worse is the term *noncompliance,* which implies a paternalistic stance: the patient with bipolar disorder is *not going along with* what others insist that he or she must do.

I prefer the term *concordance* because it underlines the importance of an alliance between you and your physician. Stopping medications or taking them inconsistently can often be traced to physicians, who may have failed to (1) articulate the purposes of the various medications in your regimen, (2) alert you to possible side effects or their intensity, or (3) communicate appreciation, caring, and respect for you as a person. The term *nonconcordance* suggests differences in how patients and their physicians think about treatment.

How Common Is Nonconcordance?

Estimates vary, but the consensus is that more than half of people with bipolar disorder quit taking their medications at some point in their lives (Colom, Vieta, Tacchi, Sanchez-Moreno, & Scott, 2005). A recent study found that, of 873 Swedish people with bipolar disorder treated with lithium, 54% discontinued it, usually due to adverse effects like diarrhea or tremor (Öhlund et al., 2018). You are more likely to be nonconcordant with medications if you are male, younger rather than older, had an early age of illness onset (teen or preteen years), have rapid cycling of episodes, have been hospitalized recently, are prone to alcohol or substance abuse disorders or comorbid anxiety disorders, or lack a supportive family structure, a spouse, or friends to rely on (Colom et al., 2000; Perlis et al., 2010).

People with bipolar disorder are not the only ones who have trouble accepting a long-term regimen of medication. Those with diabetes, heart disease, hypertension, glaucoma, cancer, osteoporosis, sleep apnea, epilepsy, migraine headaches, or any other chronic medical condition that requires ongoing pharmacotherapy are up against the same challenges you are. People are equally inconsistent in taking antibiotics and birth control pills! You're not alone in this type of struggle.

What Are the Consequences of Nonconcordance?

People with bipolar disorder are often told to take medications without being given compelling reasons for doing so or a full understanding of what might happen if they don't. *The main reason that stopping your medications is inadvisable is that it is associated with a high risk of recurrence.* Not taking medications as prescribed is the greatest single factor contributing to when and how often people with bipolar disorder have recurrences. Nonconcordance also greatly increases the risk of suicide. As Jamison (1995) explains: "That I owed my life to pills was not, however, obvious to me for a long time; my lack of judgment about the necessity to take lithium proved to be an exceedingly costly one" (p. 89).

When medications are discontinued by the person very abruptly (which is usually the case), the chances of relapsing—or of committing suicide—are higher than when mood stabilizers or antidepressants are discontinued slowly (Suppes, Dennehy, & Gibbons, 2000; Baldessarini, Tondo, Ghiani, & Lepri, 2010). If you are on lithium and suddenly stop taking it, and then start up again, it will take a while before you reach a stable blood level and have its full protection against recurrences. If you take medicines inconsistently, you can also end up with inadequate blood levels that lead to the same negative results.

Many people want to go on "drug holidays," thinking that if they get worse, they can always go back on the drug and return to normal—just like that. This is like when people are told to take an antibiotic daily for 10 days to treat a sinus infection. They may feel better after 5 days and just stop taking the antibiotic. But that leaves you in a state where you no longer have active symptoms, but the underlying episode of infection is still going on. During this state, you are at high risk of having a relapse of symptoms.

Because the consequences of discontinuing mood-stabilizing medications are not always immediate (that is, you can temporarily feel better after stopping your medications), you may feel that you are in the clear and can go on living your life without them. Unfortunately, your good feelings can be due to the hypomania that often develops shortly after mood stabilizers are stopped. This hypomania is often the first stage in the evolution of a more serious manic episode. If you go off a drug such as lithium and then have a relapse of your illness, there is a very real possibility that you won't respond as well when you resume taking it. In fact, starting and stopping medications can lead to a pattern of continuous cycling in which illness episodes beget other illness episodes, and the periods of feeling well between periods of illness get shorter and shorter (the "kindling effect"; Post, 2007). On the positive side, getting medical treatment early in the course of your disorder (that is, when you are first diagnosed) and staying with it can prevent these patterns of continuous mood cycling.

Why Do People Stop Taking Their Medications— and Why Should You Resist Doing So?

Ethan, a 19-year-old college student, had his first manic episode while at university. He became belligerent, inappropriately sexual, giddy, and grandiose, claiming that his artwork and writing were soon to make him millions. His thoughts raced and he became hyperverbal. He was given lithium and an antipsychotic medication while an inpatient at the university's hospital. He showed a partial response but was still hypomanic when he returned to his parents' house after dropping out of school. He abruptly stopped his medications without telling his parents. He sank into a deep depression, marked by insomnia, lethargy, slowed thinking, suicidality, and thoughts such as "I suck . . . I don't deserve to live . . . I've done nothing for anyone in this universe." He eventually agreed to see a therapist, rather than a psychiatrist, under the proviso that "whoever he is needs to know that I'm philosophically and spiritually opposed to medications of any sort."

Ethan did not rule out the possibility that he had bipolar disorder. He made it clear, however, that he wanted to address his individual struggles with identity, sexuality, moral values, and family relationships, rather than having his therapist treat him as a "manic–depressive case." The therapist spent a number of sessions developing an alliance with Ethan and helping him understand the onset of the depression from two standpoints: its psychosocial triggers (events in college, such as rejection by a girlfriend) and its biological and genetic bases, including a history of suicide and bipolar disorder in his maternal grandfather. The therapist did not challenge the idea that Ethan's depression was "existential and spiritual" but gradually introduced the notion that it might have a chemical basis as well. After six individual sessions, his father and stepmother were brought in for conjoint sessions where Ethan explained his position and treatment options were discussed. Over the next 2 months, Ethan's mood improved somewhat, but he remained moderately depressed and complained of insomnia.

After he and Ethan had developed a solid alliance, the therapist reintroduced the idea of trying lithium. Ethan agreed to try it again for 3 months. The therapist referred Ethan to a psychiatrist, who took time to develop a rapport with him and listen to his story. The psychiatrist recommended he begin with a dose of 1,200 mg. Ethan responded quickly: his depression lifted, his suicidal thoughts disappeared, and his sleep improved.

After 6 months of twice-weekly individual plus family therapy, and regular maintenance lithium treatment, he decided to return to college. Despite initially planning to discontinue lithium "as soon as I'm on my own," he remained on it once back in college, where his treatment was managed by a doctor at the student health service. Contact with the therapist several years later revealed that his mood disorder was stable, he remained in school, and he was still taking lithium.

Accepting a regimen of pharmacotherapy to treat bipolar disorder is a very important personal decision. Naturally you will have questions. If you have just been diagnosed with bipolar disorder or are at an early point in its course, questions about the long-term implications of taking medicines may be particularly salient for you, as they were for Ethan. But you may have strong feelings about medications even if you have been taking mood stabilizers for a long time. In this section, I discuss some of the reasons people stop taking their medications and some counterarguments to consider if you find yourself agreeing with these reasons.

"I Miss My High Periods"

"Does a fish know when it's wet? Hypomania felt good to me. I felt like I was finally getting there in my life. It didn't feel at all like there was anything wrong to me; it felt great, and I'd been feeling bad for so long. So I went off my medication, and then I started getting higher and higher. People told me to go back on, but it felt patronizing. I resented their lack of recognition that I was accomplishing things. I told them, 'You don't understand, you've got me in a box, you're sticking me in one of your categories.' But then I cycled into a depression and got suicidal. I went back to my doc and—wouldn't you know it?—back on lithium."

—A 38-year-old man with bipolar I disorder,
reviewing his most recent mood cycle

The hypomanic or manic periods of bipolar disorder, especially if they are accompanied by euphoria and grandiosity, can feel quite good. When in this state you feel productive, driven, on top of things, cheerful, and invulnerable. Who wouldn't enjoy this state, and why spoil it with pills?

One of my clients compared mania to being in love. When you fall in love, you feel giddy, happy, and driven, and you sleep less; you feel more confident, attractive, and sexual; you want to talk to more people and do more things. My client said, "If you were in love, and someone came along with a tablet that would cure you of the feeling, where would you tell that person to go?"

Not everyone experiences mania as a happy state. It can also be a wired, pressured, irritable state. But even when people experience mania negatively, they resent the idea that their moods are under the control of a substance. As I've said in earlier chapters, no one likes the feeling of being under the control of another person or thing, and in my experience people with bipolar disorder are particularly sensitive to this issue. They often have a love–hate relationship with their moods: they hate the fact that their moods fluctuate so wildly and particularly resent the lows, but mood variations are also central to who they are and how they experience life.

There is no mincing words about it: mood stabilizers do take away the high periods. When people take lithium or any of the other mood stabilizers or SGAs, their moods become more stable. Some people complain that they become *too* stable. Stability puts you in the driver's seat and gives you actual control over your fate rather than the illusion of control that mania gives you. *But stability also means giving up the intensity of the roller-coaster ride that bipolar disorder provides.* In other words, taking medicines can mean increased stability at the cost of the exciting, positive features of the disorder.

Nonetheless, the excitement and drama of the high periods often bring debilitating depressions in their wake. The 38-year-old man just quoted experienced an almost immediate crash after his mania crested. This is also true if you have the bipolar II form of the disorder: even if your hypomania is not particularly destructive in itself, preventing hypomanic episodes can help prevent the severe depressions that often follow (see Chapter 9).

"I Feel Fine Now, So Why Do I Need Medicine?"

Many people with bipolar disorder realize that they need medications when they're cycling into an episode, but don't see the need for "prophylaxis"—the use of medications when they're healthy to *prevent* future episodes. When their manic or depressive episode has resolved, they wonder, "Why should I keep taking medications and dealing with these side effects?" Some people think of mood stabilizers in the same way they might think of painkillers: you take them only when you're hurting, and you stop taking them once the pain disappears. It's the same logic people (like me) use when they're on diets. Once they have met their initial goal of losing, say, 15 pounds, they see no reason to continue dieting, even though continuing to diet is the key to weight maintenance.

This confusion is understandable, but remember one of the key points in Chapters 5 and 6: people with bipolar disorder have underlying biological predispositions that require them to take mood stabilizers on an ongoing basis for prevention purposes. There is no guarantee that you'll be free of episodes even if you do take mood stabilizers or antipsychotics, but the chances that you'll remain well over long periods and have less severe episodes are greatly improved.

"Medications Take Away My Creativity"

One of the most fascinating aspects of bipolar disorder is its association with artistic creativity. Many famous artists, writers, poets, and musicians probably had bipolar disorder or a variant of it. Examples include Sylvia Plath, Anne Sexton, Robert Lowell, Ernest Hemingway, Delmore Schwartz, Vincent van Gogh, and Ludwig van Beethoven. Kay Jamison (1993) has written extensively about this issue in her book *Touched with Fire: Manic–Depressive Illness and the Artistic Temperament.* I can also recommend a recent review of creativity studies in bipolar disorder by Sheri Johnson and her colleagues (Johnson et al., 2012).

The link with creativity can put the person with bipolar disorder in a bind. What if you pride yourself on your writing, artistic talent, or musical ability and fear that taking medicines will destroy your creative output? If having mood swings can improve the quality of your art by investing it with emotion and passion, why take them away? Does mood-stabilizing medication actually interfere with creativity? Not many research studies have been done, and most are case studies that have examined a select group of artistic people to observe what effect lithium had on their work. None of these studies on creativity involve people on anticonvulsants or antipsychotics, so we don't know if those medications are better or worse.

Do people with bipolar disorder become more creative when they stop their medications? The literature does not provide a clear answer to this question either, at least where lithium is concerned. Kocsis and associates (1993) tested 46 people with bipolar disorder who were on long-term lithium treatment. They found that patients' scores on memory, associative productivity, and motor speed (finger tapping) improved once they went off lithium. The people who improved the most on these measures were those who had the highest levels of lithium in their bloodstream before going off the drug, suggesting that higher dosages may lead to more interference with mental functioning.

What do these findings mean for people who have artistic talent? First, lithium can have effects on your cognitive or motor performance, but it isn't at all certain that it interferes with your creativity. In fact, the opposite may be true. Among eminent writers, the bipolar II form of the disorder (depression with hypomania) is more common than full bipolar I disorder (Carreno & Goodnick, 1998). In another study, people with bipolar II were more likely to draw or play musical instruments and to have greater focus and clarity during their highs than people with bipolar I disorder (McCraw, Parker, Fletcher, & Friend, 2013). In other words, milder manic or hypomanic states (for example, positive emotions combined with high energy but little impairment) may be more clearly linked to creativity than full manic states (Johnson et al., 2012).

> **Effective treatment:** Most professionals believe that people with bipolar disorder do better in their art, music, or writing when they're in remission from their disorder, or perhaps slightly hypomanic, but not fully manic or depressed.

If you have bipolar I disorder, reducing severe manic symptoms with medications may actually *enhance* your creativity (Andreasen, 2008). In this sense, medication may even be helpful to your work if it successfully controls your more severe manic swings. But if you are convinced that lithium or your other medications are affecting your creativity or focus, talk to your doctor about reducing the dosage before you decide to go off it. Perhaps he or she will think it's safe for you to experiment with a lower dosage, especially if you have been stable for a while. Your doctor may also recommend you try a different mood stabilizer.

"Medications Give Me Unacceptable Side Effects"

As discussed in Chapter 6, all of the major mood stabilizers, antipsychotics, and antidepressants have side effects, which can range from the mild (for example, thirst on lithium) to the severe (toxic reactions, kidney clearance problems, rapid cycling, agranulocytosis). In many cases, medication side effects are transient and will disappear or at least become milder after you've been on the medication for a while. Other side effects are not so easy to ignore and can be ongoing.

Many people go off their medicines because they find the side effects too unpleasant and disruptive. This is also true when people are prescribed medications for traditional medical conditions. Blood pressure medications, for example, can make people fatigued. Allergy medications can make people feel sleepy or "dried up." Even natural or herbal substances have side effects. For example, St. John's wort, once touted as an alternative antidepressant, can give you stomachaches, make you sun sensitive, and, if not taken alongside a mood stabilizer, cause switches into mania (Dalwood, Dhillon, Tibrewal, Gupta, & Bastiampillai, 2015).

Taking a medication is a cost–benefit decision. There are clearly benefits to mood stabilizers and SGAs. But they also have costs, including side effects and actual financial outlays (see the cost–benefit exercise on pages 179–181). Most people with bipolar disorder, if able to weigh the costs and benefits objectively, come down on the side of continuing to take their medications, especially if they've been through some painful mood disorder episodes. But that doesn't mean you should have to live with terrible side effects or loss of your creative abilities as a trade-off for health and mood stability.

"How Should I Work with My Doctor Regarding Side Effects?"

Optimally, managing your side effects is a collaborative process between you and your physician in which you discuss each medication's effectiveness and adverse effects. To enhance this process, keep a record of which side effects you experience each day and tell your physician about them. The form on page 172 will help you organize your thoughts on this. Copy the completed record, take it to your next medication visit, and go over it with your doctor. (The blank form is also available to download and print; see the information at the end of the Contents.)

Many side effects can be managed with a simple dosage adjustment (for example, dropping the number of lithium tablets so that you feel less sluggish mentally) or by taking your pills at different times. For example, if you take lithium in one dose rather than several, you may have less need to urinate frequently. If you take the extended-release form of valproate (Depakote ER), you may have less gastrointestinal distress. Other side effects can be controlled with adjunctive medications. For example, hand tremors or migraine headaches can be helped by adding a beta-blocker, propranolol (Inderal), to your medication regimen. The hair thin-

Keeping Track of Your Side Effects

Day of week	Medications taken	Dosage	Side effects experienced*
Monday	_____	_____	_____
	_____	_____	_____
	_____	_____	_____
Tuesday	_____	_____	_____
	_____	_____	_____
	_____	_____	_____
Wednesday	_____	_____	_____
	_____	_____	_____
	_____	_____	_____
Thursday	_____	_____	_____
	_____	_____	_____
	_____	_____	_____
Friday	_____	_____	_____
	_____	_____	_____
	_____	_____	_____
Saturday	_____	_____	_____
	_____	_____	_____
	_____	_____	_____
Sunday	_____	_____	_____
	_____	_____	_____
	_____	_____	_____
Example: Monday	Lithium	1,200 mg/day	Thirst, shaking hands
	Lamictal	300 mg/day	Nausea, dry mouth
	Seroquel	400 mg/day	Overeating, sedation

Weight at beginning of week _____   End of week _____

*Side effect examples: dry mouth, urinating frequently, rash, acne, stomachaches, insomnia, headaches, fatigue, hair loss, problems with concentration, hand tremor, hunger/weight gain. If you're not sure which medication causes which side effect, simply list each side effect you experience and put a question mark (?) next to each one.

PERSONALIZED CARE TIP:
Reporting side effects

Side effects represent a problem for which there are solutions other than simply stopping your medicines. Informing your doctor at each visit of your side effects will help the doctor evaluate with you the alternatives to your current treatment plan. If you have unusual side effects that aren't in the list of expected effects associated with each medication, report them anyway.

You may feel angry at your doctor because he or she should have alerted you to the side effects you'd be experiencing. Your anger is understandable, but keep in mind that the physician may not have been able to predict your individual profile of adverse effects. Discuss your feelings with your doctor; he or she needs to know how important these issues are to you.

---

ning associated with valproate can sometimes be managed with zinc or selenium supplements. Avoid trying to adjust your medications on your own, which can lead to a worsening of mood symptoms.

You and your doctor may also decide to switch to another medication entirely. For example, if you have problems with memory or motivation on lithium, you may want to switch to valproate, which is less likely to produce these side effects (Malhi et al., 2009). If you have problems with weight gain on valproate, then lamotrigine, carbamazepine, or one of the more weight-neutral SGAs (ziprasidone, aripiprazole) may be better alternatives for you.

"Taking Medications Is a Sign of Personal Weakness, Sickness, and Lack of Control"

"For me, it's all about control. I have always had trouble with authority, and medication feels like just one more authority figure. Someone comes along and says, 'Here, just take this salt and you'll feel better and be like the rest of us.' I think it's garbage, and it makes me feel like the person doesn't know me very well. I can handle things by myself just fine, thank you."

—A 19-year-old man shortly after his hospitalization for mania

Many people feel that taking medicines is a sign of personal weakness. It feels like admitting that you're sick, defective, or mentally ill. Certainly, taking medications daily can remind you of your troubles and make you resent the illness even more than you do already. But many people take this perspective further and claim that they can get along without medications just by exerting self-control. If you are in a hypomanic phase, you're particularly likely to feel this way. Unfortunately, bipolar disorder cannot be controlled by sheer willpower. Neither can other biologically based illnesses.

There are many ways to think about control. In some people's minds, control is about not needing help from anyone or anything. For others, control means availing yourself of opportunities to further your life goals. It is true that taking a medicine now means giving up a certain amount of control in the short run. But taking care of yourself in this way can also give you more control in the long run. Maintaining mood stability translates into a greater likelihood of staying out of the hospital, not having to schedule so many doctor visits, saving money on additional treatments, being able to plan ahead for things you want to do, enjoying better family and romantic relationships, and leading a more productive work life. *In other words, taking medications can give you the kind of control you crave, rather than eliminating it. Not taking medications, in contrast, can mean giving up control if it leads to becoming ill again.*

Later chapters discuss self-management strategies such as sleep–wake monitoring, mood charting, cognitive restructuring, and coping with family stress. Implementing these behavioral strategies can contribute to feeling in greater control of your fate. But these strategies will work much better if you are simultaneously being protected by medications.

"Taking Psych Medications Stigmatizes Me"

Bipolar disorder carries much of the unfair societal stigma (social rejection or shame) that all forms of mental illness carry, and taking medication can feel like a proxy for this stigma. You may worry about what employers, friends, and romantic partners will think if they know you're on mood stabilizers or antipsychotics.

This is not an easy issue, and it is a very real concern for many people. There may be jobs you can't take because of being on medication (for example, a job that requires fine motor control over your hands). Employers' reactions upon learning of an employee's psychiatric disorder have been known to range from complete sympathy to finding ways to fire the person (although such discrimination is illegal, as discussed in Chapter 13). But the situation is improving. My impression, especially over the last 30 years, has been that our society is becoming more and more understanding of the biological bases of psychiatric disorders and the need for psychiatric medications. More and more writers, movie celebrities, and public figures are admitting to being treated for bipolar disorder. Few people would reflexively dump a potential romantic partner or employee simply because that person admits to taking mood stabilizers or antidepressants.

Of course, you are not obliged to tell your employer or other significant people in your life about your mood disorder or its treatments. You may also want to be selective in what you tell them. As I discuss in Chapter 13, there are constructive ways to educate others about your need for medications and support or understanding so that the stigma is minimized.

"The Medications Don't Work"

Some people with bipolar disorder complain that their medications are just not effective. They wonder why they should take medications when they don't feel their symptoms are being controlled but they still have to deal with side effects.

The reality is that your bipolar disorder is only partially controllable by medicines (see Chapter 6). But almost everyone with the disorder does better on mood medications than off them. You will continue to experience mood fluctuations on mood stabilizers, but if you examine the course of your illness carefully, you'll probably find that there has been some improvement. Keeping a mood chart (Chapter 8) will help you determine how your medicines are affecting your sleep and moods in a relatively objective way.

A question to ask yourself is "Is my medication truly ineffective, or does it just not work as well as I would like it to?" Depending on your answer, you may want to discuss the matter with your doctor. It is possible—especially if you are trying mood stabilizers for the first time—that you are not improving as much as you could. You should not hesitate to tell your doctor if that is what you believe. The doctor may agree with you and suggest a different mood stabilizer or SGA or various adjunctive medications to enhance your current regimen (Chapter 6).

"My Problems Are Psychological, Not Biological"

If you feel that your mood problems have only a psychological origin (for example, related to childhood trauma or disturbed family relationships or the absence of

---

PERSONALIZED CARE TIP:

Determining whether you're benefiting from medications

If you have been taking mood stabilizers or SGAs for at least 3 weeks, try to be objective about whether there has been any improvement. In addition to keeping a mood chart (Chapter 8), ask relatives for their opinions about the impact of your medications on your functioning. They may have seen effects that you aren't aware of (for example, being less easily provoked to anger, smiling more often, being less irritated by changes in your environment, seeming like your old self). Sometimes the benefits aren't as straightforward as mood stability. For example, Neil, age 18, did not think that his quetiapine had any effect on his moods. He did believe, however, that he was getting along better with his parents and friends since starting it.

a romantic relationship), then it may not be obvious to you what role medication has in your treatment. You may feel that your underlying vulnerabilities have more to do with a negative view of yourself than with biological or genetic factors.

Take another look at Chapter 5, in which I talk about the vulnerability–stress model. Psychological stress, such as interpersonal or family conflicts or loss experiences, can interact with your biological and psychological vulnerabilities (for example, low self-esteem or self-defeating beliefs, such as "I'll never accomplish what I set out to do"). This is one of the reasons we recommend medications and psychotherapy *in combination,* rather than as substitutes for each other. Remember, your problems needn't be biological *or* psychological. They can be both.

Medications may actually make your psychotherapy more successful. Most psychotherapists say that they can't accomplish much when a person with bipolar disorder is in a severely depressed, manic, or mixed state. If medicines make your mood stable, or at least stable enough for you to make it to regular therapy appointments and carry through on homework assignments, you'll benefit a great deal more from psychotherapy. You'll be able to deal more productively with the underlying issues that may be contributing to your unhappiness or distress.

"Taking Medications Means I'm Giving in to My Parents (or My Spouse)"

"I'm a product of what I learned from my parents, but I've also learned things from other people in college, after college, in various work situations, in relationships, and from the hard knocks of life. If I go on lithium, it can't be their decision. Whether I go back on it, when I go back, how much I go back on it, and who will be my doctor are all things I've got to decide by myself. If they make the decision for me, even if I agree with it, I won't be able to follow through."

—A 23-year-old woman with bipolar I disorder

As this woman says, and as Kate Millet says in the quote at the beginning of this chapter, taking medications can mean feeling like you're giving in to your family's demands. If you are a young adult and live with your parents, you can quickly get tired of hearing them nag you to take your pills, interpret your emotional responses to everyday things as signs that you need more medicine, or remind you that you're the sick one in the family. You may believe that others in the family also have the disorder and that they should be the ones taking medicines, not you.

Most young adults want independence from their parents, and having a psychiatric disorder can make it seem like the clock has been set back by a few years. Likewise, swallowing pills, seeing doctors, and getting your blood levels tested may feel like you are under your parents' thumb. The reality is that taking medications, while perhaps initially reflecting your acquiescence to your parents' plans, greatly increases your chances of independence from them later. If your mood is stable, there is a much greater chance that you'll be able to function away from home. But it's hard to take this long-term view when taking pills makes you feel like you're a child again.

If you're married or partnered, you may have the same feelings about your spouse. Your spouse may be taking a hard line with you; some of my clients' spouses have even threatened to leave if their partner didn't remain consistent in taking medications. Your spouse's insistence that you take your pills can make the option feel all the more unappealing to you.

How do people resolve this dilemma? Many of my patients eventually come around to recognizing the role of mood stabilizers in maintaining their own health and their relationships with their family members. But it is important that you feel the decision to take medicines is largely your own. Chapter 13 gives you some tips on how to communicate with family members on illness-related problems, including how to negotiate the sometimes volatile issue of taking medications.

Many of my patients have reported feeling better about taking medicines once they began to view drug treatment as important for furthering their personal goals. Some have made the transition from engaging in power struggles with their parents or spouse to taking more responsibility for managing their own drug treatment (for example, keeping to the regular dosing schedule so that reminders from others become unnecessary, monitoring their side effects, remembering to fill prescriptions, arranging their own doctor visits). This transition helped them feel that medications were less of a threat to their autonomy and identity.

"I Can't Remember to Take My Medications"

This is a very real problem and one that physicians often underestimate. Sometimes people forget whether they have taken a morning or an afternoon dosage and then end up taking an extra dose in the evening, which can increase their chances of experiencing severe side effects. Others mistakenly remember taking a tablet they haven't actually taken.

If you are using alcohol or street drugs regularly, including marijuana, you're going to have particular problems remembering to take your pills as prescribed. This is probably one of the reasons that substance abuse is so highly correlated with medication nonconcordance. If you are able to get your substance use under control (see Chapter 8), you'll have a much easier time remembering to take your mood stabilizers, and they will almost certainly be more effective.

If you are having trouble remembering to take your tablets, ask your physician whether you can be given your medications in their least complex dosing pattern. Some medications, including lithium, can be taken all in one dosage. Sometimes the regimen can be simplified to morning and evening dosages only. Don't be ashamed of forgetting—it's a more common problem than you think.

Some people try to time their dosages around events that will cue them, like meals or their morning or bedtime routines. Others keep spare pills in their desk drawers at work in case they forget to bring them. Still others acquaint their spouse with the medication routines and ask for reminders. If you are comfortable with your spouse taking this role, it may help you stay on schedule.

Effective solution: If you have trouble remembering to take your medications, try one of these devices:

- Pill boxes that divide up the day's doses
- Key chains with an attached container that holds one day's pills
- Alarms on cell phones or watches
- Online calendar reminders
- Reminders next to your toothbrush or breakfast cereal

In Chapter 8, on maintaining wellness, you'll be introduced to the daily mood chart. On the chart you'll see places to record the amount of each medication you've taken. Keeping a daily mood chart will not only remind you but may help you see the relation between your medication habits and the stability of your mood states. One of my clients related the following: "Breakfast and medications were always connected for me. But then when I got my new job, I forgot to eat breakfast and also missed my morning medication dose—I took it to work with me and would completely forget about it. When my mood started dropping and I started keeping a mood chart, I discovered I wasn't taking my morning dose as frequently as I thought I was. Keeping track made me more conscious of remembering my morning dose and also helped me make breakfast more of a priority."

Summarizing the Pros and Cons of Medications

After you've thought through some of the issues just discussed, it may be useful to summarize the costs and benefits of medications in your own terms. The forms on pages 179–181 will help you organize your thinking about pros and cons and things you can do to make medications feel more acceptable. You may want to copy these forms and take them with you to your doctor's office—they can provide a format for discussing issues of concern to you. It may also be helpful to review the information on these forms if you have the impulse to discontinue your medications, to be reminded of your reasons for taking them in the first place and the other alternatives available to you. (The blank form is also available to download and print; see the information at the end of the Contents.)

Try to individualize this exercise as much as possible: you may know of advantages and disadvantages of the medications that I have not listed here. Your family members may be able to help you identify the costs and benefits of different drugs in your regimen.

The Pros and Cons of Taking Medications

<u>REASONS TO TAKE MOOD MEDICATIONS</u>

(*Examples:* they help control my manic symptoms, help with my depressed mood, improve my sleep, make me better able to focus, decrease my anxiety, improve the way I relate to other people, decrease my conflict with family members, improve my energy level, make me feel more confident, help me concentrate better at work, keep me from spending too much money, help me avoid traffic tickets)

1.

2.

3.

4.

5.

(continued)

DISADVANTAGES OF MOOD MEDICATIONS

(*Examples:* side effects [give specifics], miss my high periods, cost of medications and psychiatry visits, dislike having my moods controlled, dislike my doctor, dislike making medical appointments, feel less sexual or less creative, medications carry a stigma, medications aren't that effective)

1.

2.

3.

4.

5.

(continued)

THINGS I CAN DO TO IMPROVE THE SITUATION

(*Examples:* discuss side effects with physician, consider other medications or dosing strategies, take more responsibility for renewing my prescriptions, change my doctor, change my insurance plan, educate others about my disorder, create reminders to take my tablets, cut down my use of alcohol or drugs)

1.

2.

3.

4.

5.

Future Directions

The decision to commit to a regimen of medications—especially over the long term—is a very difficult one. As you can see from this chapter, people with bipolar disorder struggle with many practical and emotional issues when coming to terms with their medications. You are certainly not alone in your struggles to accept the disorder and its required treatments.

New drugs for bipolar disorder are being developed and tested all the time. In all likelihood, some will prove successful and others will come into vogue for a while and then disappear. But there is good reason to believe that you will find a medication regimen that works and that won't require you to tolerate debilitating side effects.

Above all, remember the meaning of the term *concordance*: a collaborative process between you and your physician. It is very important to communicate your concerns to your physician and see if anything can be done to adjust your regimen so that it is maximally effective as well as tolerable. Most physicians are open to this kind of communication and even welcome it, particularly if you talk to them before you stop on your own or make decisions about changing your dosages. The exercises in this chapter can help you organize information about your drug treatment so that you can work with your physician more efficiently within the limited blocks of time that managed care allows.

Fortunately, managing bipolar disorder is not just about taking medications. There are self-management strategies you can use during periods of wellness (Chapter 8), when experiencing the beginning signs of mania (Chapter 9), and when depressed or suicidal (Chapters 10 and 11). Try to think of medication as one element in a collection of strategies for managing your disorder.

PART III

Practical Strategies for Staying Well

Tips to Help You Manage Moods

Amy, age 33, had a 6-year history of bipolar disorder. Three years after being diagnosed, she began a period of rapid cycling that seemed to be provoked, in part, by an on-again, off-again relationship with her boyfriend. When she abruptly relocated out of state due to his business, her rapid cycling intensified. She obtained part-time work in her new city and sought psychiatric treatment. Her psychiatrist gave her a combination of lithium and valproate, which helped even out her cycles, but she still experienced unpleasant ups and downs. Her sleep was quite variable from night to night.

Her psychiatrist suggested that she supplement her medication treatment with therapy from a psychologist with whom he worked. The psychologist encouraged Amy to start a mood chart, in which she kept track of her moods on a daily basis, the number of hours of sleep she had each night, her medication consistency, and any events that she found stressful, whether positive or negative. At first she found this assignment boring and a hassle. She complained to her therapist that she didn't like being reminded of her illness so frequently. Her therapist acknowledged the discomfort of the assignment but reminded her that tracking her moods was a first step toward gaining more control over them. After some discussion she agreed to continue with the chart but decided not to track events until she was sure the rest of the chart would be useful. She made no commitment to keep it on a regular basis.

Amy and her therapist began examining her charts during their weekly meetings. Over a period of several months, they began to identify certain behavioral patterns associated with Amy's mood swings. For example, her therapist pointed out that Amy's mixed mood states often began with a rejection by her boyfriend (such as being ignored or slighted by him in the company of others). Rather than directly confronting him about these experiences, she would usually go out drinking with her female friends that night or the next.

Her sleep then became more disturbed, and her mood took on an irritable, anxious quality. Her mood usually stabilized once she reestablished a regular bedtime and wake time.

She asked her friends whether they would feel any differently about her if she went out with them but didn't drink. None seemed particularly bothered by this, although one expressed surprise. Amy did not stop drinking entirely, but she did find that limiting her alcohol intake helped her sleep better, which in turn made her feel less irritable, anxious, and depressed the next day. She made clear to her therapist that she had no intention of giving up her "outrageous side." But with time, she became more consistent with these lifestyle changes, pleasantly surprised by their beneficial effects on her mood.

What can you do to maximize your intervals of wellness and minimize the time you spend ill? Many people go for long periods of time without having significant symptoms, but virtually everyone with the disorder has recurrences of the illness at some point. Research studies are telling us that the people who do the best over time are those who take medications regularly, have a good and consistent relationship with their doctor(s), and successfully implement self-management strategies.

What does it mean to manage bipolar disorder successfully? In Chapter 5 we talked about risk factors in bipolar disorder (things that make your illness worse). There are also protective factors: things that keep you well when you are vulnerable to mood swings. You are already familiar with some of these protective factors from earlier chapters—for example, consistency with your medications, keeping regular routines, and having social supports.

In essence, maintaining wellness means minimizing your risk factors and maximizing your protective factors to the extent possible (see the table on page 187). Sometimes risk and protective factors are simply opposite sides of the same coin. For example, sleep deprivation is a risk factor, whereas maintaining a regular sleep–wake rhythm is a protective factor. In other cases, protection involves introducing a new element into your daily life, such as keeping a mood chart.

Minimizing risk and maximizing protection will almost certainly improve the course of your illness and your quality of life. But doing so can be difficult. It can require giving up things that you have come to depend on (for example, drinking alcohol to relax, eating certain foods, or staying up late at night). It will be next to impossible for you to avoid every risk factor and take full advantage of every protective factor in the table. For example, some people can scrupulously maintain their medication regimen and get enough exer-

> **Effective prevention:** *Know yourself.* If you know your strengths and limitations well, you may be able to decide which risk factors you can and cannot realistically avoid and which self-management strategies are possible to implement within your current lifestyle.

cise but are unable to give up alcohol or smoking. Others can keep relatively consistent daily and nightly routines but find it difficult to regulate their exposure to family stress or interpersonal conflicts.

This chapter will acquaint you with practical "Maintaining Wellness" strategies that roughly fall into four broad categories:

- Tracking your mood with a daily chart
- Maintaining regular routines and sleep–wake cycles
- Avoiding alcohol and other mood-altering substances
- Developing and maintaining family and external social supports

Risk and Protective Factors in Bipolar Disorder

Risk factors that increase your chances of becoming ill	
Risk factors	Examples
Life changes (positive or negative) that cause stress	Loss of a job, starting or ending a relationship, birth of a child
Alcohol and drug abuse	Drinking binges; experimenting with cocaine, LSD, or Ecstasy; excessive marijuana or opiate use
Sleep deprivation	Changing time zones, cramming for exams, sudden changes in sleep–wake habits
Family distress or other interpersonal conflicts	High levels of criticism from a parent, spouse, or partner; provocative or hostile interchanges with family members or coworkers
Inconsistency with medications	Suddenly stopping your mood stabilizers; regularly missing dosages

Protective factors that help keep you from becoming ill	
Protective factors	Examples
Observing and monitoring your moods and fluctuation triggers	Keeping a daily mood or social rhythm chart
Exercise	Jogging, yoga, long walks, gym workouts, hiking, biking
Maintaining regular daily and nightly routines	Going to bed and waking up at regular hours; having a predictable exercise and social schedule
Relying on social and family supports	Clear communication with relatives; asking your significant others for help in emergencies
Engaging in regular medical and psychosocial treatment	Staying on a consistent medication regimen, obtaining weekly psychotherapy, attending support groups

None of these will seem surprising to you given what you already know about maintaining your health. You probably also know how hard it is to implement these strategies. Of course, they'll be easiest to implement when you are feeling well or experiencing only mild mood swings, but implementing them may help protect you from more severe mood episodes. Throughout the chapter, I'll show you how other people with bipolar disorder have used these strategies in their daily lives and how they have avoided some of the pitfalls associated with sticking with them. Chapters 9, 10, and 11 give you tools to use to stop a developing manic, depressive, or suicidal episode from spiraling beyond your control.

Maintaining Wellness Strategy No. 1: Keeping a Mood Chart

If you've been seeing a psychiatrist for a long time, you're probably familiar with some form of mood chart. If this is your first episode, your psychiatrist or therapist may not have suggested this assignment yet. A mood chart is simply a daily diary of your mood states, with dates indicating when these moods start and stop. The chart can also incorporate information about your sleep, medications, and life stressors. Most of these mood charts are available online.

Why should you keep a mood chart? First, becoming aware of even subtle changes in your mood and activity levels will help you recognize if you are having a mood disorder relapse and determine whether you should contact your doctor to see if a change in medications would be helpful. Many people have been able to catch their episodes early by observing the minor fluctuations recorded on their mood charts, which often herald the onset of a major manic, mixed, or depressive episode. A picture is worth a thousand words!

Second, your doctor will find the chart useful, in that he or she will be able to see how well your medications are working or, alternatively, know when they are making you feel worse (such as when antidepressants bring about an increase in anxiety or agitation). He or she may also want you to monitor symptoms other than elevated or depressed mood, such as pessimistic thoughts, sleep disturbance, or irritability.

Third, you can use your mood chart information to identify environmental triggers of your mood cycling, which may suggest stress management strategies to lessen the impact of these triggers. With time and practice, many of my patients have become effective at identifying triggers, such as the onset of their menstrual cycle, arguments with particular family members, or work stress. Amy, for example, came to recognize through mood charting that conflicts with her boyfriend were a trigger for her down moods. She also found that her usual strategy for coping with distress—going out drinking—was contributing to her irritable mood states for several days after. This realization did not stop her from drinking altogether, but it did make her weigh the pros and cons of excessive alcohol use as a means of "self-medicating."

The chart that Amy filled out (see page 190) was used in the National Institute of Mental Health's Systematic Treatment Enhancement Program for Bipolar Disorder (STEP-BD; Sachs et al., 2003). There is a blank version of this chart on page 191 (also available to download and print—see the information at the end of the Contents or go to *https://reports.ccihub.com/public/downloads/daily_mood_chart. pdf*). Each chart allows you to track your moods every day for up to 1 month. So, if you have started the chart in the middle of the month, continue to use the same sheet until the middle of next month and then begin a new sheet. In other words, "day 1" need not be the first of the month. It could be the 10th, and day 10 could be the 20th.

People with bipolar disorder find this to be a user-friendly chart for recording the cycling of their moods over time, even though it looks annoying at first. Once you get used to it, you can usually fill it out in a few minutes each day. I usually suggest that people keep the chart on an indefinite basis, but if this seems daunting, try it for a month or two to see if it proves useful. After that, you may decide to chart your moods in a different way, or your doctor may suggest a different kind of chart.

For now, let's consider Amy's mood chart, which she completed during a month in which she experienced significant mood fluctuations. Her "X" marks indicate her mood states on any given day, rated on a –3 (lowest, most depressed mood) to +3 (highest, most elevated mood) scale. Notice that on some days she entered two ratings, one for mania and one for depression (her mixed mood states).

Amy identified some of the life events that contributed to her mood swings, starting with her dog's illness. Her mood had been relatively stable (note the absence of peaks between the argument with her dad and the rejecting event with her boyfriend), but then she stayed out late at a concert and experienced a few days of hypomania. By day 16 of the month, she'd had 7 consecutive nights of poor sleep and began to experience mixed mood symptoms. Her medication was not changed during this interval, but she was inconsistent with her regimen during days 10 and 11. So, she identified four things that may have correlated with her mood shifts during this particular month: events involving her pet, problems with her boyfriend, sleep deprivation, and medication inconsistencies.

We don't know for sure whether these variables would have affected Amy's moods during a different month. This is one of the reasons it is important to keep the chart on an ongoing basis—to determine whether you have a predictable set of *mood triggers* (for example, arguments with family members, final exams, changing time zones, a specific pattern of sleep deprivation). Identifying mood triggers is an important step in gaining control over your moods, which you'll learn more about in this and subsequent chapters.

Mood Chart

Name Amy

TREATMENTS
(Enter number of tablets taken each day)

Month/Year August 2010

MOOD
Rate with 2 marks each day to indicate best and worst (if applicable)

0 = none
1 = mild
2 = moderate
3 = severe

___ mg	Antipsychotic ___ mg	___ mg	Antidepressant ___ mg	Anticonvulsant Depakote 1000mg	Benzodiazepine ___ mg	Lithium 1200mg	Verbal Therapy	Daily Notes	Irritability	Anxiety	Hours Slept Last Night	Depressed: Severe — Significant Impairment NOT ABLE TO WORK	Depressed: Mod. — Significant Impairment ABLE TO WORK	Depressed: Mild — Without significant impairment	WNL — MOOD NOT DEFINITELY ELEVATED OR DEPRESSED; NO SYMPTOMS; Circle date to indicate menses	Elevated: Mild — Without significant impairment	Elevated: Mod. — Significant Impairment ABLE TO WORK	Elevated: Severe — Significant Impairment NOT ABLE TO WORK	Psychotic Symptoms Strange Ideas, Hallucinations
				4		4		argument with Dad	1	1	7			X	1				
				4		4			1	1	6			X	2				
				4		4	√		0	0	8				X 3				
				4		4			0	0	6				X 4				
				4		4			0	0	6				X 5				
				4		4			0	0	6				X 6				
				4		4			0	0	6				X 7				
				4		4			0	0	6				X 8				
				4		4		boyfriend was rejecting	2	1	10			X	9				
				2		2		concert, stayed out until 3am	0	1	5				10		X		
				2		2			0	0	3				11		X		
				4		4			1	0	6				12	X			
				4		4			0	0	5				13	X			
				4		4	√		0	0	6				14	X			
				4		4			0	0	6				15	X			
				4		4		dog got sick, went to hospital	2	2	4			X	16	X			
				4		4			1	2	6			X	17	X			
				4		4			1	2	6			X	18	X			
				4		4			1	2	6			X	19	X			
				4		4			1	2	6			X	20 (circled)	X			
				4		4	√	dog out of hospital	1	0	7			X	21 (circled)				
				4		4			1	0	7			X	22 (circled)				
				4		4			1	0	7			X	23 (circled)				
				4		4			1	0	7			X	24 (circled)				
				4		4			1	0	6			X	25				
				4		4			1	0	6			X	26				
				4		4			1	0	6			X	27				
				4		4	√		0	0	6				28				
				4		4			0	0	6				29				
				4		4		friend's wedding	1	0	5			X	30	X			
				4		4		cooking most of the day	1	0	5			X		X			
								Weight: 127											

Note. WNL = Within normal limits. Adapted by permission of Gary Sachs, MD (Copyright 1993).

Amy's Self-Rated Mood Chart.

Mood Chart

MOOD

Rate with 2 marks each day to indicate best and worst (if applicable)

Psychotic Symptoms Strange Ideas, Hallucinations		
Elevated	Severe	Significant Impairment NOT ABLE TO WORK
	Mod.	Significant Impairment ABLE TO WORK
	Mild	Without significant impairment
WNL	MOOD NOT DEFINITELY ELEVATED OR DEPRESSED	NO SYMPTOMS / Circle date to indicate menses
Depressed	Mild	Without significant impairment
	Mod.	Significant Impairment ABLE TO WORK
	Severe	Significant Impairment NOT ABLE TO WORK
		Hours Slept Last Night

0 = none
1 = mild
2 = moderate
3 = severe

Anxiety

Irritability

Month/Year

Daily Notes

Weight:

TREATMENTS
(Enter number of tablets taken each day)

Verbal Therapy

Lithium _____ mg

Benzodiazepine _____ mg

Anticonvulsant
Depakote _____ mg

Antidepressant _____ mg

_____ mg

Antipsychotic _____ mg

_____ mg

Name

Note. WNL = Within normal limits. Adapted by permission of Gary Sachs, MD (Copyright 1993).

From *The Bipolar Disorder Survival Guide: What You and Your Family Need to Know, Third Edition*, by David J. Miklowitz. Copyright © 2019 The Guilford Press. Purchasers of this book can photocopy and/or download enlarged versions of this material (see the box at the end of the Contents).

Step 1: Rating Your Mood Each Day

The first step in mood charting is to become familiar with a numerical scale that corresponds to various levels of mood disturbance. The box that follows gives you guidelines for making judgments about your daily mood, using a scale from –3 (severe depression) to +3 (severe mania). It gives examples of how people with bipolar disorder feel and think (and what they say) when they're in these various states. Not every example or descriptive label in the box need apply for you to be able to use the corresponding scale number. Rather, try to figure out which category of depression or elevation best describes how you feel on a given day.

Mood Descriptors

(0) *"WNL" (within normal limits).* This is your baseline: Your mood is not elevated or depressed, your energy level is normal for you, you are not irritable, sleep is normal, and you're able to carry out your daily work and other tasks with little or no difficulty. You have no other obvious symptoms of your mood disorder.

Elevated Mood

(+1) *Mildly elevated.* You are feeling giddy, cheerful, or energized, or somewhat more irritable or anxious or nervous than usual, but you are not really impaired; you have more energy and more ideas, and you feel more self-confident but have been able to work effectively and relate normally to others. People in this category may say any or all of the following: "I'm more restless/animated/talkative today than usual," "I'm making more phone calls," "I'm getting by with a little less sleep" (for example, 1 or 2 hours less than usual), "I'm more easily distracted today," "I'm snapping at people more," "I'm more frustrated by little things," "I'm somewhat revved up or wired," "My mind is clicking along a little faster," "I'm feeling sexier," "I'm more optimistic," "I'm hypomanic."

(+2) *Moderately elevated.* "High" or moderately manic; your mood is elevated, giddy, euphoric, or very irritable and anxious, and people have told you it seems inappropriate. You feel like breaking things, you feel heavily goal-driven and hypersexual, and your thoughts are going very fast; you have significant difficulty focusing on your work; you are having run-ins with people (they seem to be moving and talking too slowly); people are complaining that you seem angry or grouchy, that you seem silly, are laughing too loudly or too much, or are moving way too fast. You have yelled at others inappropriately. You are sleeping as little as 4 hours per night and not feeling tired. Common statements may include "I'm feeling very impatient today," "I think I can get by with a lot less sleep,"

(continued)

Mood Descriptors *(continued)*

"I'm very preoccupied with sex," "My mind is working faster than ever," "I have so much to say and I hate being interrupted," "I'm feeling irritated, angry at everything."

(+3) *Severely elevated/manic.* In this category are uncontrolled euphoria or aggressiveness; you are laughing constantly or your irritability is out of control; you have had loud verbal or physical fights with people; you feel like you are exceptionally talented or have special powers (for example, the ability to read people's minds, to change the weather); you are constantly moving about and cannot sit still; you cannot work or get along with others; you have gotten in trouble in public, have been stopped by the police, or have been taken to the hospital; you are sleeping little or not at all.

Depressed Mood

(−1) *Mildly depressed.* You are feeling somewhat slowed down or sad; you have trouble keeping certain pessimistic thoughts out of your head; you feel more self-critical; you want to sleep more or are having trouble falling or staying asleep, and you feel somewhat more fatigued; things don't seem as interesting as they usually do. However, you can still work effectively and are relating normally to others, even though you may feel less effective; your depression is not obvious to others.

(−2) *Moderately depressed.* You are feeling very sad, down in the dumps, hopeless, moderately slowed down, or uninterested in things for most of the day; you are sleeping more or having a lot of trouble falling asleep or staying asleep (for example, waking up regularly in the middle of the night and not being able to fall back to sleep); fewer and fewer things are of interest to you; you are ruminating a lot about current or past failings; you are feeling grouchy, easily annoyed, or irritable; you have significant difficulty getting your work done (missing days at work or school or being less productive); your concentration is impaired; others comment that you seem morose or slowed down or that you're speaking slowly. You have considered suicide and may have even thought of various methods.

(−3) *Severely depressed.* You feel deeply sad or numb; things look drab, and you have lost interest in almost everything; you are experiencing severe suicidal feelings; you wish to die or have made an attempt on your life; you feel extremely hopeless; you believe you have sinned terribly and should be punished; you can't work, concentrate, interact with others, or complete self-care tasks (for example, bathing, washing clothes); you stay in bed most of the day but cannot sleep, and have severe problems with lack of energy.

Sources: Williams (1988); Young, Biggs, Ziegler, & Meyer (1978).

Mood charting requires a bit of practice. You may be a person who is naturally able to judge whether you are feeling manic or depressed, and you may be easily able to describe the experience to others. Alternatively, the descriptive labels *manic* or *depressed* may not capture the way you feel. If this is the case, take time to learn the mood chart and numerical scales and try to see if you can equate the terms used in the chart with your particular way of describing moods. For example, *depressed* can mean the same thing as "crashed"; *elevated* can mean the same thing as "wired," "amped," or "buzzing."

Practice by seeing if you can apply a mood descriptor to your mood today and yesterday, using the scale of –3 to +3. If you feel that your mood varies considerably during the day, make a "best" and a "worst" rating (for example, you may be at a –2 in the morning and a –1 or 0 by evening). If your mood has been mixed—both elevated and depressed on the same day—make two ratings, indicating the highest and lowest points.

> **Effective solution:** If you are not sure if your mood chart rating is reasonable, ask someone who knows you well (perhaps a family member or your partner) if he or she would agree with your rating on any given day.

In choosing your level, try to think about the least and most depressed or manic you've ever been in your life and determine where these states fit on the scale. For some people, the worst period ever might have been a –1; for others it might have been a –3. If your mood has never gone above or below a 2, use these as benchmarks for judging your mood today and throughout the week.

Compare your depression level today against that of a typical day (your baseline, or how you feel most of the time, which would rate WNL). Then compare your mood to other days when you felt blue or out of sorts but not impaired (–1), days when you have felt impaired but could still function with significant difficulty (–2), and, if applicable, days when you felt so down that you could not work at all or interact with others (–3). These comparisons should help you determine today's rating. Likewise, try to think of the most manic or hypomanic you've ever felt. If you were ever severely manic and in the hospital, your rating at that time would have been a +3. If you have ever been elevated and/or irritable to the extent that you were having trouble functioning at work, your rating would be a +2. If you have been wired and "upbeat," but this state did not cause run-ins with others or make it difficult to sleep, a +1 (hypomanic) probably applies. In other words, think in terms of your own personal benchmarks.

Step 2: Recording Your Anxiety and Irritability

You'll notice that the mood chart also asks you to rate your anxiety and irritability levels on a 0–3 scale. There are two reasons to do this. First, anxiety and irritability can be the first signs of a new manic, mixed, or depressive episode. Second, some medications may produce these symptoms as side effects (for example, SSRIs). So, it's a good idea to track these symptoms, even if you're not sure how they are related to the cycling of your bipolar disorder.

Examples of "1" levels of irritability include feeling somewhat snappish or grumpy, but not to the extent that you can't relate to other people. A "2" would mean moderate irritability that causes problems for you at work or at home. A "3" would mean that you were so severely irritable and angry that you were having real trouble functioning. People at a "3" are having intensive verbal or even physical altercations with others, are destroying property, or have been threatened with arrest. Likewise, a "1" anxiety rating would mean you feel mildly jittery, apprehensive, and perhaps scared but able to get along without extra effort. A "2" would mean moderate anxiety that makes it difficult to work, read, socialize, or perform daily chores; however, you can still function with extra effort. A "3" would mean you have overt panic and severe, incapacitating anxiety.

Step 3: Recording Your Hours of Sleep

Along with your mood rating, make a daily rating of how many hours of sleep you had the previous night. If you're rating your mood for, say, Thursday, record the hours you slept from Wednesday night to Thursday morning. If your sleep is intermittent, try to estimate the actual number of hours you were asleep, not the number of which you were in bed. Your recall of your prior night's sleep may be most accurate when you first wake up in the morning.

If you take naps regularly, separately recording nighttime and daytime sleep will allow you to investigate whether napping in the afternoon makes it harder to sleep that night or makes your mood worse or better by the end of the day.

After a week or more of charting, you may begin to see how your sleep and mood are related. Many people are surprised at the result. Amy, for example, had always assumed that lack of sleep caused her to get more depressed, yet she found from her mood charting that sleep loss was more consistently associated with her hypomanic periods (note the shift on day 10 of her chart).

Step 4: Taking Daily Notes on Life Events and Social Stressors

If you feel that your mood has been influenced by one or more events or interactions with people, record these on your chart under "Daily Notes." Some of these may be significant (for example, breaking up with your partner, quitting your job), and others may seem minor (having a change in work hours; racing to the airport to catch a plane; getting stuck in a traffic jam). Record all events that you feel may be important, even if they seem as if they would be inconsequential for many people. For example, Amy found that even relatively routine quarrels with her father were associated with a mild drop in her mood (to a –1). The purpose here is to observe the connection between specific events and specific mood changes. When reviewing the day and filling out your chart, consider questions such as the following:

- ■ "What happened right before I began feeling irritable or hypomanic?"
- ■ "What happened right after my irritable mood set in?"
- ■ "What happened right before my mood spiraled downward?"

When you're recording stressors, recall one issue raised in Chapter 5: it can be difficult to tell whether stress was the cause or the effect of your mood. Over time, mood charting may help you determine the timing of events in relation to changes in your mood. For example, did you race to the airport and then feel a surge in your energy level and mood, or were you feeling speedy before you raced to the airport? Did you get into an argument with your father and then feel down about yourself, or were you feeling down on yourself and irritable before you got into the argument? Don't worry for now if you're not sure which caused which. Instead, just try to identify the factors that coincide: stressful events, mood states, and sleep patterns.

The "Daily Notes" section is also a good place to record your alcohol or drug use. If you drank or smoked marijuana on a specific day, record that information as an event even if your intake seemed trivial (for example, "drank a beer" or "smoked half a joint"). Then you can observe for yourself whether, and to what degree, alcohol or marijuana affects your mood the next day. You may also learn whether you are using substances, in part, to alleviate a negative mood state from the previous days or week.

Step 5: Recording Your Treatments

Record all of the medications and dosages you are supposed to take at the top of the left columns of the chart, including medications that are not specifically for your bipolar disorder (for example, blood pressure pills). In the boxes corresponding to the day of the month you're rating, record the number of pills of each medication that you actually took. This will help you, your physician, and other members of your treatment team know if medication inconsistencies are affecting your day-to-day mood. Amy missed her evening dosages on the night she went to the concert and the next evening as well, which probably contributed to her mood instability. As discussed in Chapter 7, most people miss a medication dosage once in a while, but it's important to keep track of these seemingly minor inconsistencies. Likewise, place a check mark next to any days when you attended a psychotherapy session. As with medication, some people are quite regular and others are quite irregular in their therapy attendance.

You may be taking some of your medications "as needed." For example, some people take a medication like clonazepam (Klonopin) only when they can't get to sleep or they feel unusually anxious. Indicate "as needed" on the top left column of your mood chart next to medications that fit this description. Some people find that their mood is lower on the day after they have taken an as-needed medication. Others find that certain as-needed medications (for example, the allergy medication pseudoephedrine) make them feel temporarily energized, wired, or hypomanic and interfere with their sleep.

Your physician will be able to use your medication records in a number of ways. Let's imagine that he or she has prescribed valproate and an SSRI antidepressant. Let's also imagine that your chart indicates improvements in your mood a week or two after you started the SSRI, but then you began to report "roller-coastering" or rapid cycling of your emotions and energy levels. If all of these changes are documented on your chart, your physician may suggest discontinuing the antidepressant or adjusting your dosage as a way to stabilize your mood.

Step 6: Recording Your Weight and Menstrual Cycle

Two other pieces of information will help round out your mood chart. First, record your weight at least once during the month. It's best to weigh yourself on the same day each week so that you can see whether your medications, stress, or mood cycling are connected with short-term changes in your weight. If you are gaining weight on an SGA (for example, quetiapine [Seroquel]), your physician may choose to switch you to a different medication within the same class (for example, risperidone [Risperdal]) or adjust your dosage. If you are a woman, circle the days on which you had your period. You and your doctor may wish to examine whether your mood cycles begin before, during, or after the onset of your menses (also see Chapter 12).

Evaluating Your Mood Chart

Share your completed mood chart with your therapist and physician during each visit. Together, you can evaluate the influence of certain stressors on your mood, the influence of sleep disturbances, the effects of various medications, and your consistency with them. Even if you're not meeting regularly with your doctor or therapist, make a point of examining the chart at the end of each week to see if any patterns jump out at you. Keeping the chart over a year or more will enable you to develop longer-range hypotheses about which biological or social factors are provoking shifts in your mood (for example, periods of greater alcohol or marijuana use, the onset of winter or spring, the Christmas holidays, periods of increased work, beginning of the school year).

Problems with Mood Charting

Mood charting can feel reductionistic: it does not do justice to the many varied experiences you probably have on a daily basis. It is also very present-focused. Some people feel that their mood shifts are related to factors that can't be recorded easily on the chart (for example, traumatic events in the recent past or in childhood). Even with these limitations, however, mood charting is a very efficient way of summarizing a great deal of information succinctly for yourself and your doctor. If you are using mood charting as a supplement to your personal psychotherapy, think of it as a point of departure for exploring larger issues that affect your mood. For example, events such as minor disagreements with a partner can have profound effects on your mood if they trigger fears of separation or loss.

Mood charting can also be difficult to remember to do every day. Try to pick one time each day to complete your chart and stick to this time on a day-to-day basis. Some people fill it out right before getting ready for bed; others tie mood charting to a specific daily activity (for example: after finishing dinner, after walking the dog, before watching the evening news). Avoid choosing the worst moment of the day to fill out the chart if that moment does not represent how you've felt for the whole day. So if you usually feel quite unhappy when you first wake up but feel better within an hour or so, pick another, more representative time of day than the beginning of the morning.

Avoid trying to fill out a month's worth of mood charts just before your doctor appointments, as people sometimes do. The more accurate the information you convey to your doctor, the more informative the chart will be for guiding treatment decisions.

PERSONALIZED CARE TIP:
Getting the most out of mood charting

- Fill out the chart at the same time every day to make it a habit.
- Don't pick the worst moment of your day.
- Don't try to fill out days' worth of charts right before your doctor appointments.
- Evaluate whether your depressed feelings are chronic and stable (as many people report) or whether they vary over a single week or month.
- Look for linkages between the daily stressors that affect your mood (for example, being provoked to anger by someone's seemingly judgmental stance) and the longer-term issues you are discussing with your therapist (for example, why you sometimes overreact to critical comments made by your parents).

Maintaining Wellness Strategy No. 2: Maintaining Regular Daily and Nightly Routines

"I really feel that I benefited from psychoanalysis. I was in it four times a week. But I don't think it had anything to do with talking about my childhood. There was something very therapeutic about getting on the subway and having a place to go to in the morning, seeing the same therapist every day, seeing the same attendant in the parking lot, getting back in my car at the same time . . . I found all of that structure very comforting."

—A 40-year-old woman with bipolar II disorder

In Chapter 5, I discussed the beneficial effects on your mood of external "time keepers" and the potentially negative effects of events or social demands that disrupt your daily routines and sleep–wake cycles. *Actively maintaining daily and nightly routines is one of the most important behavioral changes you can undertake—aside from regularly taking your medications—to help keep you in the driver's seat in managing your disorder.* In this section, I discuss the *social rhythm stability* approach to maintaining wellness.

Keeping a Social Rhythm Chart

The Social Rhythm Metric (SRM; Monk, Kupfer, Frank, & Ritenour, 1991; page 200) is a more time-consuming device than the mood chart, but it is also potentially more informative. In this chart, you keep track of when you eat, sleep, exercise, and socialize and make ratings of your daily mood. With time, you can work on stabilizing your daily routines as a means of stabilizing your mood. This involves planning your regular activities for predictable times of the day or night.

The SRM was developed as a central component of Ellen Frank and David Kupfer's work on interpersonal and social rhythm therapy (IPSRT). As discussed in Chapter 6, Frank and her colleagues have shown that the combination of IPSRT and pharmacotherapy is effective in improving the course of bipolar disorder when compared to supportive psychotherapy and pharmacotherapy (Frank et al., 2005). I was trained in Frank's IPSRT approach some years ago and have become convinced of the value of daily rhythm tracking and stabilization for persons with bipolar disorder.

The purpose of social rhythm tracking is to allow you to discover the relationship between changes in your daily routines, levels of interpersonal stimulation, sleep–wake cycles, and mood. Over several weeks or months, you will begin to see certain patterns emerge (as Amy did). For example, you may find that changes in your activity levels or sleep patterns presage the development of new episodes. In the beginning phases of mania you may observe a gradual decrease in the time

Please fill this out at the end of the day.

Day of Week: **Date:**

MOOD RATING (Choose one): _____

Scale

−5 −4 −3 −2 −1 0 1 2 3 4 5
Very Depressed   Normal   Very Elated

Describe your mood today:

PEOPLE
1 = Just Present
2 = Actively Involved
3 = Others Very Stimulating

ACTIVITY	Check If DID NOT DO	CLOCK TIME	A.M.	P.M.	Check If ALONE	Spouse/ Partner	Children	Other Family Members	Other Person(s)
SAMPLE ACTIVITY (for reference only)		6:20	√			2			1
Out of bed									
First contact (in person or by phone) with another person									
Have morning beverage									
Have breakfast									
Go outside for the first time									
Start work, school, housework, volunteer activities, child or family care									
Have lunch									
Take an afternoon nap									
Have dinner									
Physical exercise									
Have an evening snack/drink									
Watch an evening tv news program									
Watch another tv program									
Activity A									
Activity B									
Return home (last time)									
Go to bed									

(TIME spans the CLOCK TIME, A.M., P.M. columns; Check spans A.M. and P.M.)

Reprinted by permission from Monk et al. (1991). Copyright © 1991 Elsevier Science. Reprinted by permission in *The Bipolar Disorder Survival Guide: What You and Your Family Need to Know,* Third Edition, by David J. Miklowitz (2019, The Guilford Press). Purchasers of this book can photocopy and/or download enlarged versions of this material (see the box at the end of the Contents).

you spend sleeping and an increase in the time you spend exercising. Likewise, you may find that as you recover from a manic or depressive episode, your activity and sleep patterns naturally go back to the way they were before you became ill. In other words, your sleep and activity patterns can be a sign of whether your mood problems are getting better or worse.

As with the mood chart, it's best to fill out the SRM every day and review it each week by yourself and with your therapist or psychiatrist. Keeping the social rhythm chart on a regular, ongoing basis will enable you to spot shifts in your daily routines and sleep–wake cycles that may be of subtle importance in determining your mood. (The chart is available to download and print; see the information at the end of the Contents.)

The chart on page 202 was completed by Leslie, a 40-year-old woman with bipolar II disorder. First notice the upper left-hand corner, where she has chosen a daily mood rating of –2 on a scale that ranges from –5 to +5. In this respect it is like the mood chart. But notice that there are 17 activities listed on the left side; most people will do some portion of these every day. Indicate in the boxes what time you did the following activities: woke up, had your first cup of coffee, went to work, went to school or did some other daily activity, ate lunch, exercised, came home, ate dinner, and went to bed. These daily routines, in part, drive your sleep–wake habits. For example, if you have a shifting work schedule that demands that you work from 8 A.M. to 4 P.M. one day and then 4 P.M. to 12 A.M. the next, your bedtime and wake time will be correspondingly altered from day to day, and your mood may change (up or down) in the days that follow. In contrast, if you eat, exercise, work, and interact with others at fairly regular times of the day or evening, you will come to expect sleep at a certain time (Frank, 2007).

The SRM also asks you to record *who did each of these activities with you and how stimulating the person or persons were.* The degree to which your interchanges with others are provocative, conflict ridden, or otherwise stimulating, versus low key or laid back, can be important determining factors in the degree of stability you experience in your emotional states and possibly even your sleep. Say you ate dinner with your spouse or partner but had an argument, and then the two of you went to opposite ends of the house (rated a "3" on stimulation); you would probably have more trouble falling asleep that night. Compare that night to another night when you and your spouse had a relaxing dinner together (which might be rated a "1"—"others just present").

High levels of stimulation from other people can feel quite positive but still affect your mood or sleep–wake cycle. Deborah, age 26, found that her evening waitressing job, which she enjoyed a great deal, contained highly stimulating bursts of activity (usually 3-hour blocks in which she was in great demand by the patrons). She consistently had more trouble falling asleep after getting home than she did on nights when she wasn't working. She had an easier time when she was assigned the early evening shift.

THE SOCIAL RHYTHM METRIC (SRM)
MacArthur Foundation Mental Health Research Network I

Please fill this out at the end of the day.

Day of Week: Sun   Date: 5-28

MOOD RATING (Choose one): _-2_

Scale

–5 –4 –3 –2 –1 0 1 2 3 4 5
Very Depressed   Normal   Very Elated

Describe your mood today:
agitated, nervous, irritable

PEOPLE
1 = Just Present
2 = Actively Involved
3 = Others Very Stimulating

ACTIVITY	Check If DID NOT DO	CLOCK TIME	A.M.	P.M.	Check If ALONE	Spouse/ Partner	Children	Other Family Members	Other Person(s)
SAMPLE ACTIVITY (for reference only)		6:20	√			2			1
Out of bed		9:30	√		√				
First contact (in person or by phone) with another person		10:00	√						2
Have morning beverage		9:30	√						1
Have breakfast		10:00	√						2
Go outside for the first time		10:45	√						3
Start work, school, housework, volunteer activities, child or family care	√								
Have lunch		12:00							3
Take an afternoon nap	√								
Have dinner		7:30		√	√				
Physical exercise		5:30		√	√				
Have an evening snack/drink		9:00		√	√				
Watch an evening tv news program		10:00		√	√				
Watch another tv program	√								
Activity A Phone conversation		9:30		√					3
Activity B									
Return home (last time)		7:00		√					2
Go to bed		10:00			√				

Leslie's social rhythm chart.

Reprinted by permission from Monk et al. (1991). Copyright © 1991 by Elsevier Science.

Katherine, age 42, enjoyed the intensive contact with people she had through her job in the clothing section of a department store. However, the social stimulation rose to almost intolerable levels during the weekends prior to the Christmas holidays, and she found herself becoming increasingly irritable. She learned not to schedule any social activities on the weekend evenings following these workdays as a way of modulating her exposure to stress and stimulation.

Leslie's Example: Evaluating a Social Rhythm Chart

Although only 1 day is shown in Leslie's example on page 202, we can develop some hypotheses about factors that affected her mood states. For her, a mixed mood state is a day of depression, along with agitation, nervousness, and irritability. Note that even though the sample day occurred during the spring, when daylight hours were longer, she had a relatively short day (woke up at 9:30 A.M. and went to bed at 10 P.M.). She was sleeping too much. She also had several high-stimulation interactions during the day (including an argument over the telephone with her ex-husband about their child and a confrontation with a roommate whom she felt was being inconsiderate). She had at least one alcoholic drink when alone. In addition to her biological predispositions, these factors may have partially determined her agitated, depressed mood.

It is possible that these events and activities resulted from her mood state (for example, she might have been anxious and irritable and therefore more prone to confrontations). To help determine which caused which, Leslie collected social rhythm and mood information on herself over a period of several months. She began to see how provocative interactions with certain people, sleep patterns, and alcohol combined to change her mood, as well as how her mood states affected the timing and frequency of these events and habits. She became increasingly certain that alcohol before bedtime and sleeping more than 9 hours combined to make her nervous and irritable and more prone to run-ins with people.

"How Can I Regulate My Daily Routines?"

The next step is to devise strategies that help you regulate your daily routines. Keeping regular routines sounds straightforward, but if you've ever tried to do it, you know that significant challenges are likely to arise. You can do this alone, but you might also want to ask people who know you well (partner, spouse, close friends) what they think gets in your way of regulating your routines (examples: TV programs come on that you hadn't meant to watch but find yourself drawn in by; you put off exercise until everything else is done). Then you can develop target times for various activities (for example, sleep and exercise) with awareness of some of these challenges.

The first, most important ingredient is to go to bed around the same time every night and wake up around the same time every morning. Try to maintain this pattern on weekends, even when you'd rather sleep late—keep within 30 minutes to 1 hour of your regulated weekday times. Of course, there will be times when getting to bed at your target hour or waking up at a specific time is impossible, such as when you travel, have social plans on a weekend, have a sick child, or need to get up extra early to pick up someone at the airport. Some of these events will be controllable by you (for example, whether to go to the early or late showing of a certain movie) and some will not (for example, a change in shifts at work; the timing of an airline flight). If your schedule is shifted by an hour or two on a given night, try to reinstate your original sleep–wake target times as soon as possible.

Try to maintain your sleep patterns even if events conspire to make you change them. For example, if you have lost your job, try to get up at the same time you would have gotten up when you were going in to work. If your new job requires different hours (say, getting to work by 8 A.M. instead of 9 A.M.), adjust your bedtime to an hour earlier. It's best to ease into your new schedule gradually rather than suddenly.

You can also work with your therapist to *anticipate events that will change your daily routines* and plan ways to regulate yourself once these events occur. For example, if you know that you may be changing jobs soon or traveling in the near future, you can anticipate that your sleep will be disrupted. Make plans in advance to go to bed and wake up at consistent times even after these disruptive events have occurred.

Second, if you have been having trouble sleeping (see the section on sleep starting on page 206), try to avoid *sleep bingeing,* in which you catch up from all the lost sleep during the week by sleeping more on weekends. You'll probably find that sleep bingeing makes your depression and anxiety worse. It also makes it harder to sleep the next night.

Third, try to see if you can maintain the same hours each day at work or school. For example, try to take classes during the same interval each day (for example, Tuesday and Thursday mornings, without mixing in evening classes). Try to avoid having all of your classes on one or two days and none on the other three. To parallel your regular job hours, try to exercise at the same time (just after work or school is often a good time) rather than late in the evening on one night and then early in the morning the next day. Try to have a regular period to unwind before going to bed. Avoid having your most stimulating interactions with partners, friends, or coworkers right before you go to sleep.

Practical Challenges to Maintaining Regular Routines

There are practical problems to be solved, of course. The courses you want to take may be offered at all different times of the day or night. You may have a job that requires a lot of travel, necessitates long shifts on weekends, requires work at home in the evening on some nights but not others, or involves changing shifts. An example is a contract nursing job, in which people are often called for a full 8-hour shift only an hour before the shift is to start. Restaurant jobs often have shifting schedules as well. In Chapter 13, you'll find some suggestions for negotiating work hours with your employer in light of the limitations your disorder can impose.

Here are examples of how some of my patients have kept regular social rhythms even when facing the demands of school or job. Walter had an open discussion with his employer about his mood disorder. His employer agreed to keep him on the 8–5 daily shift at his computer programming job, rather than the constantly variable shifts that were typical. Juanita, who traveled frequently, always tried to get the same number of hours of sleep each night, even when she was in a new time zone. Maintaining her sleep habits required a degree of assertiveness, given that she was often encouraged by her traveling coworkers to stay out late.

Candace (see also Maintaining Wellness Strategy No. 4, on page 215) found that her weekends involved long intervals with little contact with others, and her depressions usually became worse then. Scheduling low-key activities with friends or acquaintances during weekend days gave her a greater feeling of consistency in routines from the week to the weekend and helped improve her mood. Likewise, Wesley, who became depressed after breaking up with his girlfriend, found that scheduling activities with other people each morning or, at a minimum, taking trips to a coffee shop to eat breakfast helped get him out of bed by a certain time.

The SRM can help you design a daily schedule of sleeping, eating, exercising, and socializing that is comfortable and feasible, given the demands of your current social, family, and work life. Try to set goals for when you plan to go to bed and when you want to wake up and try not to deviate from these plans by more than 30 minutes to an hour, even when there are rewarding activities (for example, parties, late-night movies) that you feel would improve your mood. A partner/spouse or roommate you live with may be able to help you stick to the program.

Resistance to Social Rhythm Tracking and Regulating Routines

Some people complain that social rhythm tracking is tedious and reminds them of doing homework assignments for school. Like most treatment and self-management techniques, the SRM is not without its costs in terms of time and effort. But as you get used to it, you will find that you can do it at the end of the day in about 5 minutes. With time, you may find that certain items on the chart are more important to record than others. For example, your bedtime, wake time, job hours, and exercise times may be critical in determining your mood stability, but your mealtimes or TV habits may be less important.

In my experience and that of other clinicians, the bigger issue that people with bipolar disorder face is the trade-off involved in regulating their routines: it means giving up a degree of spontaneity. People sometimes wonder, "Why can't I have the same kind of 'devil-may-care' attitude that others have? If everyone else is staying up until 2 A.M. to party, why can't I?"

These reactions are understandable. For Amy, keeping a regulated routine made her feel that she was different from everyone else. On the other hand, she came to realize that the unpredictability and social stimulation she craved was like a drug. She usually had a "mood hangover" the next day.

There is comfort in knowing that you are doing something proactive to manage your disorder. You will almost certainly see benefits in terms of your mood stability and productivity when you structure your days and nights. With time, a regulated routine will give you a sense of security and control over your fate.

Even apart from the issue of mood stabilization, some of my clients find that social rhythm tracking helps them manage their disorder and lifestyle in ways they hadn't expected. For example, Carmen, age 29, found that SRM tracking helped her become more consistent in her medication-taking habits, which until that point had been haphazard and unpredictable. After filling out his chart for several weeks, Mandeep, 35, observed that "I have a habit of jamming in too many things to avoid depression, but then I get like a car that's run out of gas. I want contact with people, but I can get to the point where I'm doing too much. I need some more consistency, and I need not to be constantly overstimulated and running away from myself."

It is not only people with mood disorders who have to stay on regular, regimented schedules. Parents usually need to follow very predictable routines to manage the daily activities of their children. Athletes need to stick to well-regulated training schedules. People who become expert performers, such as accomplished professional musicians, have often developed highly regimented routines to help them accomplish their craft.

Nonetheless, if you're finding a regimented routine too stifling, discuss this with your therapist or physician. There may be compromises that can be made. Perhaps you can identify the point at which fluctuating routines negatively affect your mood. For example, a 30-minute departure from your bedtime may make no difference, but 90 minutes might make a big difference. Try to see if you can identify the range of fluctuation in routines within which you can function and still feel stable.

"OK, Now That I'm Going to Bed on Time, How Do I Fall Asleep?"

"I toss and turn, look at the clock, sneer and snort through my nose, walk around the house . . . do my yoga, do my meditation, turn on Poker After Dark . . . but I still can't sleep. It irks me to no end that my wife can just lie down and she's out. I almost want to wake her up to make her suffer like I am, but I don't . . . It goes like this every night, and then, of course, I'm a wreck at work the next day."

—A 51-year-old man with rapid cycling bipolar II disorder

For some people with bipolar disorder, getting to bed at the right time isn't the main problem. The problem is falling asleep and staying asleep. There is nothing more frustrating than lying awake and trying to fall asleep. Sleep disturbance is a key symptom of bipolar disorder and sometimes can be a side effect of antidepressant or psychostimulant medications. It can also be due to substances like caffeine, excessive sugar, tobacco, or alcohol, especially if these are ingested close to your bedtime.

You and your physician may decide that a sleeping medication is the best alternative to keep sleep disturbance from contributing to your worsening mood state. Examples of sleep medications include clonazepam (Klonopin) and zolpidem (Ambien). Although these medications often work well, not everyone likes to take them (and doctors are sometimes unwilling to prescribe them) because you can become tolerant (that is, you may need a bigger dosage over time to fall asleep), or you may become unable to sleep without them. Many physicians are instead prescribing a low dose of quetiapine (Seroquel) for sleep. It is nonaddictive but, like the other SGAs, can be associated with weight gain (see Chapter 6).

Fortunately, there is a literature on behavioral interventions for sleep problems. Michael Otto and his colleagues at Harvard Medical School and Massachusetts General Hospital (Otto et al., 1999) have developed recommendations for ways to improve sleep if you're suffering from bipolar disorder (see the box on this page). Some of these sleep techniques would be applicable to people without bipolar disorder as well.

Examples of "stress in the bedroom" include having arguments with your spouse, preparing work assignments for the next day while in bed, examining your next day's work schedule, checking the stock market pages, checking your email or text messages or Facebook page one last time, eating a large meal, and making last-minute phone calls. These activities should be avoided right before bedtime. More generally, try to keep the last hour just before sleep free of stressful or stimulating activities so that you can unwind and relax.

If possible, try to arrange your bedroom so that noise is blocked out (for example, the smartphone is off, no TVs or radios are playing) or wear earplugs. Paradoxically, activities that

> **Effective solution:** Coping with sleep disturbance
>
> - Avoid doing stressful work or having stressful conversations in your bedroom before sleep.
> - Make sure your room is dark and facilitates falling asleep.
> - Use earplugs or white noise machines as needed.
> - Give yourself time to unwind before sleep.
> - Never "compete" with others to get to sleep.
> - Use muscle relaxation techniques or breathing meditations (for example, counting your breaths).
> - Adjust your sleep cycle before traveling.

people often take for granted as necessary for falling asleep may actually contribute to sleep disturbance. For example, many people watch the evening news in bed before turning out the lights, but the news overstimulates them and cranks them up. Likewise, many people feel they can't fall asleep without reading a book, yet sometimes reading, even if it's only a novel, can get the brain running in all sorts of different directions. If you've been reading a good murder mystery, it may be hard to put down and stop thinking about! Likewise, most people believe that regular exercise contributes to good sleep because it tires you out and relaxes your muscles. But it can also keep you awake if you exercise right before bedtime—try to give yourself as much as 3 hours between finishing your exercises and going to bed.

If you want to investigate which activities are contributing to your sleep problems, try nights with and without these activities and record the changes on your mood chart or SRM (for example, write "no TV" on Thursday night and "yes TV" on Friday night and record your sleep for each). Try to see if you can detect whether doing or not doing certain activities affects your sleep and mood.

Some people feel that falling asleep is like an athletic competition, like running a race in a certain time. Being unable to sleep makes them feel inadequate or incompetent, and performance anxiety begins to accompany their attempts to sleep. Try not to think of your sleep problems as something you're doing to yourself, but rather as a biological sign of your disorder. Rather than wrestling with yourself about being unable to sleep, experience the physical sensations of being in bed, including how your body feels, how you experience the covers over you, or how the pillow feels against your head. You can often get into a meditative state by observing your breathing: count your breath intakes (without trying to speed them up or slow them down) or watch the upward and downward movement of your stomach. If you have access to a relaxation tape or meditation exercises, use these to help you experience the physical sensations that lead to sleep (Ehrnstrom & Brosse, 2016).

Many people have trouble sleeping when they travel. If you fly from the West Coast of the United States to the East Coast, you may arrive when everyone else is going to sleep, but for you it is 3 hours earlier. Transatlantic travel (for example, flying from Chicago to Paris) is particularly difficult for people with bipolar disorder because there is such a dramatic shift in circadian rhythms. But travel is often unavoidable.

One way to combat travel disruption is to gradually adjust your internal time clock to the new place you're going before you actually leave. So, over the course of the week before you travel to a later time zone, go to bed an hour earlier than usual, then an hour and a half, and then 2 hours earlier, and so forth. By the time you arrive, it may be easier to adjust to the hours of the new time zone. This procedure usually works best if you'll be in the new time zone for more than a few days.

There are other strategies you can use to improve your sleep, some of which go beyond the scope of this book. If you've been having difficulties, consider reading self-help books specifically oriented toward sleep issues, such as Paul Glovinsky and Art Spielman's (2006) *The Insomnia Answer: A Personalized Program for Identifying and Overcoming the Three Types of Insomnia,* Gregg Jacobs's (2009) *Say Goodnight to Insomnia,* or Colleen Ehrnstrom and Alisha Brosse's (2016) *End the Insomnia Struggle.*

Maintaining Wellness Strategy No. 3: Avoiding Alcohol and Recreational Drugs

Ruth, a 32-year-old woman who had just been diagnosed with bipolar I disorder, had a severe problem with drinking that usually began when she was relatively free of bipolar symptoms. Typically, romantic relationships with men or conflict-ridden business entanglements were the background of these episodes. Her drinking binges were so severe that she often had to be hospitalized and detoxified. She eventually was court-ordered to undergo an Antabuse program, in which she was required to come in twice a week to take a medication that made her vomit if she drank.

Her own view was that her bipolar disorder was making her drink. Many observers, including her doctors and family members, felt that it was the other way around: that her drinking came first and led to her mood cycling. She constantly complained of the pain of the mood swings and their associated anxiety, but her symptoms co-occurred so consistently with drinking that it was difficult to tell which were due to the mood disorder and which to the alcohol. In fact, her family wasn't even convinced that she had bipolar disorder and thought it was one of many excuses for drinking she had given over the years.

During one interval about 3 years earlier, Ruth became convinced that she should give up alcohol and stayed abstinent for almost 6 months. Her mood swings were much improved during this interval: she still had a mild depression but no mania or mixed symptoms. She was able to obtain a regular waitressing job and was functioning better than she had in a long time. During this period of recovery, however, Ruth came to the conclusion that she had no real problem with drinking. She began to reinterpret her past almost exclusively in terms of her bipolar diagnosis, denying any causal influence of alcohol. For example, she labeled her past alcohol binges as "rapid cycling" and "self-medicating." She reasoned that she wouldn't again lose control of her drinking since her mood disorder had become stable with valproate and citalopram (Celexa, an antidepressant).

About 5 months into her period of abstinence, she traveled to Palm Springs for a weekend with her new boyfriend. Quite deliberately, she discontinued her Antabuse 5 days before the trip. Within 1 week she was back in the hospital and needed detoxification. Her depression was much more severe upon her hospital discharge, and she was court-ordered, once again, into the Antabuse program.

You have probably heard long, somewhat preachy diatribes from mental health professionals, teachers, or your parents about how you shouldn't smoke marijuana, drink, or use drugs (other than psychiatric medications, that is). Their position can seem overly simplistic and noncognizant of the emotional pain you are in on a daily basis. Using substances when you have bipolar disorder is certainly understandable, especially if you don't think your prescription medications have been working properly.

I have no moral qualms about people drinking alcohol or using marijuana; my concerns stem entirely from watching too many people with bipolar disorder destroy themselves with substances. People with bipolar disorder are more strongly affected—in terms of their mood stability and behavior—by small amounts of alcohol or substances than their age-mates. This is especially the case if they indulge in alcohol or drugs when their mood states are already unstable and starting to fluctuate. My main piece of advice is to go into it with your eyes open, being aware of the risks you face.

Alcohol and Drugs: What Are the Risks?

Most psychiatrists and psychologists agree that if you have bipolar disorder, you should avoid alcohol and recreational drugs altogether. As discussed in Chapter 5, if you drink regularly or use drugs, your medications will be less effective and you are likely to be inconsistent about taking them and will have a more difficult course of illness as a result. Worst of all, alcohol and drug use puts you at a much greater risk for committing suicide (Carrà, Bartoli, Crocamo, Brady, & Clerici, 2014; Schaffer, Sinyor, Reis, Goldstein, & Levitt, 2014; see also Chapter 11).

Some doctors will tell you that you can drink alcohol in very small quantities (for example, a single glass of wine with dinner). There do seem to be people with bipolar disorder who can do this and stay stable, but in my experience it's the minority. The risks posed by alcohol or drugs are at a maximal point during the phases leading up to and including the acute manic or depressive episode and during the recovery interval following it. It's best to avoid alcohol and drugs (including marijuana) entirely during these buildup and recovery periods.

Many people with bipolar disorder, like Ruth, have a codiagnosis of alcohol or drug abuse or dependence (the *dual diagnosis* situation). People with dual diagnoses must learn to become abstinent, because the two disorders can worsen each other, much as they did for Ruth. If you have previously had problems with alcohol or drugs, consider joining a 12-step program such as Alcoholics Anonymous (as Ruth eventually did) or Narcotics Anonymous. These groups can serve as powerful resources in helping people maintain abstinence. If you don't like AA groups, individual 12-step or cognitive-behavioral programs for addictive behavior (for example, motivational enhancement therapy; Miller & Rollnick, 2012) are often available.

> Spencer, age 45, struggled with his desire to drink for many years. Through couple therapy sessions about his disorder and mood charting, he learned to recognize his prodromal signs of mood episodes: subtle increases in irritability and anger, lethargy, and insomnia. During these cycling intervals, he learned to drink nonalcoholic beer when he was with his wife and friends who were drinking. He eventually gave up drinking. He summarized his experience this way:

> > "I used to be a two-drink-a-night person, every night, for many years. I finally came to the conclusion that I just couldn't do it. It wasn't some moral thing; it was actually just a simple decision that drinking created a state in me that was miserable. For 2 days after drinking even just small amounts I would feel irritated with everybody, emotionally exhausted, and want to sleep all day. The price I was paying was too high. But before I could quit, I had to have hard evidence that alcohol was worsening my life, that it was something I didn't need to do to myself. I finally saw alcohol as a big contributor to my anger and my problems with people. Without alcohol, I can decide if I want to work on my anger; it's within my power to do so. With alcohol, the anger just takes me over."

Beliefs about Drinking, Drug Abuse, and Bipolar Disorder

People often have mistaken beliefs about alcohol, drug substances, and bipolar disorder. Some of these are listed in the box at the bottom of this page.

I've heard people with bipolar disorder claim that marijuana or cocaine is just as effective as a mood stabilizer such as lithium or valproate in controlling their mood states. They argue that alcohol calms them down, reduces their anxiety, or improves their depression; they argue that marijuana boosts their mood when they

---

Mistaken Beliefs about Bipolar Disorder and Alcohol or Drug Abuse

- Alcohol or marijuana can be used as mood stabilizers.
- Harder drugs like methamphetamine, LSD, or cocaine can be used as antidepressants.
- Alcohol or substances cannot worsen your disorder if your mood has been stable.

are depressed. One patient said, "For me, alcohol is like the ropes that keep the hot air balloon from going up . . . and on the other side is like a disguise covering over the depression."

Some people do drink or use drugs to make themselves feel better, but whether these substances are really doing the trick—as opposed to making their moods worse—is another question. We know that alcohol worsens depression (as in the examples given on pages 209 and 211). People who have both bipolar disorder and alcohol problems also have more rapid cycling, mixed symptoms, and anxiety or panic than those who do not drink (B. I. Goldstein et al., 2014). Alcohol can also interfere with sleep, which can worsen mania.

People often assume, as Ruth did, that their depression always comes first and that they use alcohol or marijuana or cocaine for the purpose of self-medicating this depression. For many people with bipolar disorder, however, the alcohol abuse precedes the depression rather than the reverse (Strakowski, DelBello, Fleck, & Arndt, 2000). For some, a vicious cycle takes over: They drink heavily and get depressed and anxious, then stop drinking and experience a recurrence of depression or panic symptoms that is attributable to the alcohol withdrawal. Then they try to self-medicate these mood symptoms with more alcohol. This pattern makes the course of both disorders much worse.

There is currently no evidence that the medical uses of marijuana extend to bipolar disorder. Although marijuana is not as toxic as alcohol for persons with bipolar disorder, it can still be detrimental to your mood stability. In Strakowski and colleagues' study (2000), marijuana use was most closely associated with manic symptoms, whereas alcohol use was more closely associated with depressive symptoms. One patient put it this way: "Weed makes me think and think and think, and then it keeps me from sleeping. It's like a catalyst for something in me." Marijuana can also interfere with your attention and concentration (as well as your ability to remember to take your medications). Some people find it makes them lethargic and unmotivated. Others feel paranoid and anxious and physiologically overaroused.

Rationalizing their heavy drug use, some people claim that LSD (acid), amphetamine (speed), methamphetamine (meth), cocaine (crack), and Ecstasy are really antidepressants. They argue that these drugs can help their depression more than a standard antidepressant such as Prozac. Some even know about studies showing that LSD stimulates the action of certain serotonin receptors or that amphetamine prolongs dopamine activity, as some antidepressants do. But they are misinterpreting the clinical implications of these studies. Even though many street drugs do affect the same neurotransmitter systems as antidepressants, street drugs do not produce true mood stability. Instead, they produce short-term bursts of neuronal activity accompanied by elation or irritability (much like mania or hypomania), rather than truly alleviating depression. When the drug wears off, you will feel the same or, in some cases, worse.

Some people with bipolar disorder use substances to intensify the elated and grandiose aspects of their hypomanic or manic states. They feel driven toward further stimulation and novelty. Cocaine, marijuana, and amphetamine are especially likely to be used in this way. The result is often a severe increase in manic symptoms or the initiation of rapid cycling states, sometimes leading to hospitalization.

You may believe that taking alcohol or drugs is fine as long as you have been feeling well for a period of time. This was Ruth's logic, and she tested it frequently by going "off the wagon" whenever she had a couple of weeks of mood stability. For her, ordinary life seemed very drab. The up-and-down periods that alcohol brought were preferable to feeling that life had become ordinary and boring. Many people whose mood is stable report that alcohol and drugs provide a temporary respite from feelings of emptiness. It is true that substances often activate the reward circuitry of the brain. But the relief is temporary at best, and the same substances can trigger negative mood states that are far more unpleasant than boredom.

The Maintaining Wellness Exercise (page 214) may help you identify what makes you want to drink or use drugs (McCrady, 2007). Try to identify:

- Triggers for use (for example, being with people whom you want to impress)
- The feelings you want to alleviate (for example, depression or anxiety)
- Your expectations of what will happen (for example, you will feel less socially inhibited)
- The actual and immediate consequences of using the drug/alcohol (for example, feeling relaxed or more confident, or feeling anxious, paranoid, or disoriented)
- The extended or delayed consequences of use (for example, sleep disturbance, being late to work the next day, feeling irritable, drowsy, or anxious for several days afterward)

Amy learned to avoid certain situations and people who, she believed, made her drink more. Earl, who smoked marijuana heavily, learned to plan distracting activities for those times of the day when he was most likely to get high (typically late afternoons after he finished his classes). Bethany learned to challenge her belief that alcohol alleviated her depressions. When she systematically evaluated the results of her drinking, she concluded that she felt better at first but more irritable and depressed later. She began to think of alcohol as a cause rather than an effect of her depression.

> **Effective solution:** Think of drinking or drug use as one event in a sequence of events rather than as a singular, isolated act. Then you'll be in a position to think about changing this sequence.

A Maintaining Wellness Exercise
Identifying Triggers for Alcohol and Drug Abuse,
Your Responses to Those Triggers, and the Consequences

List the type of alcohol or the drug you use most frequently (*examples:* beer, wine, marijuana/cannabis, Vicodin, cocaine).

_____

_____

_____

List the *situations* in which you are most likely to get drunk or high (*examples:* being alone; being out with friends; parties; Friday afternoon after work; being with specific people).

_____

_____

_____

List the *feelings* you ordinarily have right before you drink/get high (*examples:* depressed, anxious, irritable, excited).

_____

_____

_____

Describe your *expectations* about what this drink/drug will do for you (*examples:* it will make me relax and ease up with people; help me deal with difficult situations; decrease my depression; help me sleep; make me think more clearly).

_____

_____

_____

Describe the *actual consequences* of your drinking/drug use the last few times. Try to distinguish (1) what actually happened immediately after you drank or got high (*examples:* relaxed me, got me into an argument, alleviated my depression, made me feel more social) versus (2) the delayed effects (I felt more depressed the next day, had a hangover, got to work late).

Immediate effects:

_____

_____

Delayed effects:

_____

_____

Maintaining Wellness Strategy No. 4:
Relying on Social Supports

Candace, a 49-year-old woman with bipolar II disorder, suffered from an ongoing depression that was not alleviated by antidepressants or mood stabilizers. After becoming frustrated with the myriad medications she had tried, she consulted a psychotherapist, who observed that she was quite socially isolated: she had broken up with her boyfriend 2 months earlier, she had few new friends or even acquaintances, and she had become disconnected from her parents and her two sisters. She corresponded with a few people online but hadn't met most of them. Her therapist encouraged her to try some new activities that might help her build a friendship circle, which she strongly resisted doing. Her weekends were largely spent alone in her apartment, where "my thoughts eat me alive."

Candace had few hobbies in her current life but had played soccer in college. With some reluctance, she joined a group that played soccer on weekends. She felt awkward at first. "They're not my kind of people," she observed. At the beginning she had to force herself to go. Little by little, however, she found that her weekends became more structured because of the soccer practices. Although she never admitted to enjoying the company of members of the team, she did notice that her mood brightened when she participated in an activity with them. At first she thought this was due to physical exercise, but she found that her mood also brightened when she went to potluck dinners or movies at the team members' houses.

She eventually disclosed her illness to a few of her teammates, who "weren't fazed like I thought they'd be." One of them even described her own periods of depression and what antidepressants she had taken. With time, the group became like a second family to her, and she began dating one of the men. After playing with the team for 6 months, she acknowledged in one of her therapy sessions that her chronic depression, while still present, was not as bad as it had been before she had made these connections.

Social support—feeling emotional connections with people with whom one regularly interacts—is an important protective factor against depression. Having a group of people you know well, whom you trust with knowing about your bipolar disorder, and whom you see with some regularity, will help you do better in terms of the cycling of your disorder.

You may be a person who seeks out others naturally, or you may prefer spending time by yourself. Either way, when you're depressed, it is hard to interact with anybody. Unless you have a social support system in place when you're well, you may find it hard to reach out for the very help you need when depression strikes. Likewise, maintaining regular contact with your social support group when you're well will do much to prevent future depression. When you encounter the inevitable conflicts that come up with family members or coworkers, your friends and supportive relatives can be like a landing pad of comfort and steadiness. They provide a counterpart to, and minimize the impact of, other stressful conflicts. Sheri Johnson and colleagues (Johnson, Winett, Meyer, Greenhouse, & Miller, 1999) found that after an episode of depression, people with bipolar disorder who had good social support systems recovered more quickly and had less severe depression symptoms over 6 months than those with small or nonexistent support systems.

I don't want to oversimplify things by implying that having people around you is all that counts. As I discussed in Chapter 5, high levels of conflict with certain members of your core circle, particularly family members or partners but also with close friends, can be associated with a more difficult course of your illness. It is empathic, give-and-take relationships with members of your core circle, and just plain low-key social or family time, that will best protect you from depression. Needless to say, that won't always be possible. Chapter 13, on family and work relationships, will acquaint you with skills to help you maximize the positive influences of your social support system.

Your Core Circle

As you'll see in the next chapters, your social supports can be crucial in keeping your illness from cycling out of control. But first, let's identify who these people are.

Fill out the form on page 217, Identifying Your Core Circle. You may be surprised at your list! For some people, the core circle consists of members of a church or temple, a group devoted to a particular pursuit (as was the case for Candace), or people at school. It is not uncommon to socialize with just a few friends or family members. It isn't simply the number of people in your life that protects you from a drop in your mood but the quality of these relationships, the degree to which you feel good about yourself when with them, and the regularity of the contact.

Maintaining Friendships While Avoiding Alcohol or Drugs

What if your social circle is one that relies heavily on alcohol or drugs? Dispensing with alcohol, marijuana, or hard drug use can indeed have negative social consequences. For example, some people find it hard to go out with their friends without drinking. Some say that their friends devalue their efforts to stay sober. If these problems apply to you, consider discussing your dilemma with one or more trusted friends. Do they understand about your disorder and the likely impact of alcohol or drug use?

If you're not comfortable disclosing the disorder to any of your friends, consider giving other justifications for why you don't want to drink. Many people today respect measures taken to improve one's physical and mental health and fitness, so saying you're trying to lose weight, or that drinking at night discourages

Identifying Your Core Circle

List all the people you consider *friends*—those you feel you can confide in (talk to, get emotional support from) and whom you see or have phone contact with at least once a week. List their phone numbers or email addresses in the second column.

_____   _____

_____   _____

_____   _____

_____   _____

_____   _____

List which *family members* you see regularly and feel comfortable confiding in. List their phone numbers or email addresses in the second column.

_____   _____

_____   _____

_____   _____

_____   _____

_____   _____

If you were ever in trouble (for example, had a medical emergency) and needed somebody to help you, whom would you be most likely to contact and in what order (list them in order of preference, from first to fourth)? List their phone numbers or emails in the second column (if these are not already listed above).

_____   _____

_____   _____

_____   _____

_____   _____

Are there any *groups* of people who could help you feel less lonely or assist you if you were having mood problems (*examples:* church or synagogue groups, support groups like Alcoholics Anonymous, groups dedicated to certain activities—art, cooking, foreign languages, meditation, or sports)?

_____   _____

_____   _____

_____   _____

_____   _____

you from getting up and working out when you want to, or that when you drink you don't have the mental sharpness you need at work the next day might keep them from pushing you further.

Many of my clients report that giving up alcohol or drugs does make socializing with certain people more awkward. Very few, however, experience outright rejection if their friends understand their motivations: They are abstaining out of a desire to take care of their health—rather than to judge or place themselves above others.

• • • • • • • • • • • • •

Think about managing your disorder in stages. Some techniques are best applied when you're well (this chapter) and others during various phases of illness (Chapters 9–11). In previous chapters I emphasized the importance of maintaining consistency with your medications and your psychotherapy and physician appointments. The strategies covered in this chapter for maintaining wellness—mood charting, keeping regular sleep–wake routines, avoiding or minimizing use of alcohol and drugs, and relying on social supports—can enhance the effects of your psychiatric treatments in keeping your mood stable. In the next three chapters you'll see how the lifestyle management techniques discussed here can be adjusted when you feel your moods start to spiral upward or downward.

CHAPTER 9

Heading Off
the Escalation of Mania

Robert, 45, managed a successful landscape architecture firm. He'd had three manic episodes in the 4 years since he had been dating his current girlfriend, Jessie, with whom he was now living. Two of his episodes involved hospitalizations. He maintained close contact with his two kids, 18-year-old Angie and 22-year-old Brian. Jessie had no children.

His most recent manic episode, which had led to a hospitalization, involved an identifiable set of warning signs. According to his report, his first sign was becoming disinterested in his job and irritable with coworkers, about whom he had become mistrustful. This was a difficult time to become disinterested; his business was flourishing due to a new housing development project he had been involved in planning. During the earliest stages of his manic episode, he described being aware that something was wrong: his thoughts began to race and he was full of great plans and innovations. He had still been able to sleep for at least 4–5 hours per night, however, and saw no need to call his psychiatrist.

According to Jessie, Robert became "overly expressive" and "took on this physical dominance stance" during the 1-week interval prior to his hospitalization. He attended one of Angie's basketball games and "was the loudest one in the bleachers. At some point the coach asked him to leave." On another evening Jessie and Robert had gone to a fast-food restaurant in which he had "barked" his order at the waitress. He later apologized. Jessie and Robert discussed his escalating behavior and Robert admitted that he was being "hyper" but also felt good: "I'm seeing things more clearly than ever before."

They finally agreed to call his doctor, whom he hadn't seen face-to-face in almost a year. Robert's doctor talked with him by phone but didn't really ask questions about his mood state, focusing instead on his feelings about his work situation. She concluded that "you need some rest. You sound exhausted." No changes were recommended in his medication regimen, which consisted of relatively low dosages of valproate (Depakote) and verapamil (Isoptin, a calcium channel blocker).

Things took a turn for the worse when Robert, irritated that his son, Brian, had not returned his calls, went down to the record store where Brian worked. He and Brian had a verbal showdown next to the cash register, involving much profanity. Brian's boss angrily told Robert and Brian to "take it somewhere else." Brian was quite upset and told Robert never to come see him at work again.

In the next few days, Robert's behavior escalated dramatically. His movements became rapid and frenetic. He became angry, paranoid, and fixated on grandiose notions about a music career, even though he had been playing his guitar only occasionally, as a hobby. He bought an expensive Fender Stratocaster but then impulsively traded it for an instrument worth much less money. He and Jessie began to have bitter arguments in which, according to Robert, "she took on this angry, resentful, and removed tone but also got controlling and know-it-all." He impulsively moved out of their apartment and went to live at his office. One night, he called her in tears to say he had begun to panic because he thought he was dying or that he might kill himself. To Jessie, he sounded drunk but also highly reactive to anything she said. Jessie called the police, who found him in his office staring fixedly at the ceiling. They escorted him to the emergency room of a local hospital. He was treated on an inpatient basis for 2 weeks before being discharged on a new regimen of valproate (at a higher dosage) and the antipsychotic risperidone (Risperdal).

A manic episode can wreak havoc with a person's life. It can drain finances, ruin marriages and long-term relationships, destroy a person's physical health, produce legal problems, and lead to loss of employment. It can even lead to loss of life. The fallout can be long-lasting. In a now-classic study, William Coryell and his colleagues at the University of Iowa Medical Center (1993) found that the social and job-related effects of a manic episode are observable for up to 5 years after the episode has resolved.

If you think back to your last manic (or hypomanic) episode, you will probably recall that it was quite exhilarating at the time. Part of you may want to re-create the manic phases for the euphoric, energized, confident feelings that often accompany them (see also Chapter 7). When your mood is escalating, your thought processes may seem very directed, creative, and brilliant to you, even if others find them bizarre. Perhaps you even knew you were getting manic but didn't want to shut off the intoxicating feelings. Perhaps you enjoyed the feeling of being highly energized and goal driven and coming up with ideas others had trouble comprehending. This is true for many of the people with bipolar disorder with whom I've worked.

In retrospect, you probably feel that, if it had been possible to prevent or at least minimize the damage associated with your manic episodes, you would have done so. After his hospitalization, Robert expressed a great deal of remorse at the toll his manic episodes were taking: Jessie was threatening to leave him, and his son Brian was not talking to him. His relationships with his employees had been damaged as well.

If you have not had full manic or mixed episodes, but only hypomanic ones (that is, you have bipolar II or unspecified bipolar disorder), little damage may have been done during your activated states. Nonetheless, you may have found that hypomanic episodes—much like their more severe counterparts—bring on major depressions in their aftermath. The adage that "what goes up must come down" applies only too well to bipolar disorder.

Because of their biological bases, you can't prevent manic or hypomanic episodes from occurring altogether. *But you may be able to control how severe they get and limit the damage they cause. You can learn to "head them off at the pass" by recognizing when they are starting to occur and then putting into motion plans for preventing yourself from spiraling upward even further.* In Robert's case, there was a brief window of opportunity in which his early warning signs were apparent and more could be done to prevent his escalation into a full-blown episode. You'll learn more about how Robert and Jessie learned to anticipate and derail his worst manic symptoms later in this chapter.

If you can successfully implement a plan to prevent or decrease the severity of your manic episodes, then your family, job, and social functioning will almost certainly improve. Some aspects of this plan will involve things you do on your own, and other aspects will involve the actions of your family members or significant other. Still other aspects will involve your doctor and therapist (if you have one). *When mania is escalating, you will need the help of others because it will be hard to rein yourself in.* It's best to make relapse prevention plans when you're well, because when you are becoming high, you will have a difficult time recognizing the potential dangers associated with your behavior and what to do to curtail the upward cycle.

I think of a developing manic episode as a train leaving a station. When the train is starting to move and someone wants to get off, the conductor still has time to stop the train before it reaches full speed. But if he waits too long, the train will be on its own trajectory and passengers will be stuck on the train until it stops or crashes on its own. Manic episodes can feel like this train. The key is to be able to tell when the train has started to move and to try to get off it before it's barreling down the tracks.

The Relapse Prevention Drill

How important is it to know when you are getting manic? One study indicated that there were two predictors of rehospitalization in bipolar disorder: not taking medications and failing to recognize the early signs of relapse (Joyce, 1985). On a more hopeful note, people with bipolar disorder who receive educational interventions with their relatives, such as learning to identify early warning signs of mania and then seeking mental health services, are less likely to have full recurrences of mania over 2 years or more than those who do not receive this kind of education (Miklowitz & Chung, 2016; see the box on this page). As Robert said, once he and Jessie had begun to implement a successful relapse prevention plan, "I used to think I was in the driver's seat when I was manic, but that was just the illness talking. Now I think I'm in the driver's seat when I can stop myself from getting higher."

In this chapter, you'll learn a three-step strategy for getting off the train before mania runs its full course. The method, called a relapse prevention drill, was used successfully in our studies of family-focused treatment for people with bipolar disorder (see Chapter 6). A relapse drill is like the fire drills you took part in back in school. Like fire drills, relapse drills are formulated when everything is safe and going well so that you know exactly what to do should an emergency occur. The relapse drill involves a series of steps you take to try to prevent the damage that could be done by full recurrence of mania:

- Identify your prodromal symptoms.
- List preventive measures.
- Create a written plan or contract detailing the prevention procedures.

New research: A study of community mental health teams in the United Kingdom indicated that care-coordinating clinicians can easily learn strategies to help patients identify and intervene with early warning signs of depressive or manic recurrences (Lobban et al., 2010). A total of 23 teams of clinicians treated 96 patients with either routine care or enhanced relapse prevention treatment—which focused on identification of triggers (proximal causes), early warning signs of new episodes, and action plans (coping strategies for managing mood states). On average, patients who got the relapse prevention treatment stayed free of new episodes 8½ weeks longer than patients who received routine care. Social and occupational functioning scores were also significantly better in the enhanced relapse prevention group.

As we have observed in our research (Rea et al., 2003; Miklowitz, George, Richards, Simoneau, & Suddath, 2003), Lobban and colleagues found that involving family members and friends can do much to derail new episodes because they are often the first to recognize when you are becoming ill. It is much harder to do that on your own.

In the first step, *identifying your prodromal symptoms,* you make a list (usually with the help of a family member or friend) of early warning signs that signal the beginning of a manic or hypomanic period. Identifying warning signs may also involve identifying the circumstances that elicit these symptoms (for example, drinking heavily or using drugs, missing medication dosages, encountering stressful work or family situations).

In the second step, *listing preventive measures,* you brainstorm about what actions to take if one or more prodromal signs appear (for example, go in for an emergency psychiatry appointment, arrange for others to take care of your children). These actions involve you, your doctor, and members of your core circle (see also the examples in the sections that follow).

In the third phase you, your significant others, and your doctors put the first and second steps together and *develop a written plan, which is a kind of contract, for what to do when you feel a manic, mixed, or hypomanic episode coming on.* It's important that all key players have ready access to the contract so that they can help you put it into action when you are beginning to escalate, since that is when you're least likely to seek help.

This chapter focuses only on the prevention of manic or mixed episodes. This material is also relevant to preventing hypomanic episodes, which, while doing less damage, often have a similar set of warning signs and can be arrested with some of the same preventive strategies. The two chapters that follow this one discuss ways to prevent or minimize the downward spiral of depression. But before I get into the actual mechanics of developing a contract, let me say something about a sensitive issue that may have already occurred to you: *the discomfort of relying on others when you are becoming ill.*

A Little Help from Your Friends

"I start yelling, and then I'm suddenly happy again, my sleep goes all haywire, my thoughts go so fast I can't grasp them. I get high-spirited and strong-willed. But the weirdest thing to me is that I don't even know I'm ill, and why would I take my medications if I'm not ill? My husband always knows first, my sister next, and then my best friends. I'm always the last one to know when I'm getting manic."
—A 33-year-old woman with bipolar I disorder

The loss of insight into yourself is a neurological sign of mania—people don't see anything abnormal about their behavior when at the height of an episode, and sometimes even when they're cycling upward or coming out of an episode (de Assis da Silva et al., 2017; Ghaemi, Sachs, & Goodwin, 2000). It's much like when someone has a stroke but is unaware of the memory deficits that follow, or when someone is hypnotized or in a dream state and doesn't realize he or she is acting differently. Because of this lack of insight, close relatives (your parents or siblings), a spouse or romantic partner, or your friends may be the first to recognize your mania, seeing things in your behavior that you cannot (see the quotations from relatives on pages 226–227). For that reason, it's essential to involve them in the three steps of the relapse prevention process. Refer back to the exercise in Chapter 8 in which you were asked to list those family members and friends whom you feel you could trust in an emergency (that is, your core circle).

Close relatives should be involved in the care of any person with a chronic illness, whether it is a psychiatric disorder or a traditional medical disorder like heart disease or diabetes. We know from research in health psychology that people who have the most successful long-term health care practices have learned to involve their family members from the start. For example, their family members encourage them to eat healthy foods, stop smoking or getting into situations where smoking feels inevitable, or get exercise. However, involving others is a double-edged sword: accepting the help or oversight of another person will probably cause you a certain amount of psychological distress (Lewis & Rook, 1999).

What is this distress about? Most people resent the idea of having others— particularly their parents—in a position of authority when they start to become ill. In the extreme, it can feel like agreeing to have someone else take away your independence. These are understandable reactions shared by people with many other medical illnesses. For example, people with insulin-dependent diabetes dislike the idea that someone else might have to inject them if they go into shock. People with high blood pressure or cardiovascular diseases dislike the idea that a spouse might control their food or salt intake.

Keeping in mind the issues listed in the personalized care tip on page 225, consider various ways to make the involvement of others feel more acceptable. *First, remember that you're asking them to step in when you get sick, not when you are healthy and competently running your day-to-day life.* You may fear that if you let others control one difficult interval in your life, giving up control in other areas will soon follow. You may fear that your wife, husband, or partner will always be hovering over you and making sure you eat, sleep, work, and socialize according to his or her rules. But the truth is that you are giving up control over only a fragment of your life, and for only the brief period during which you are escalating into mania. In fact, you may want to make this point clear to them: that you are asking for help *only* when you become ill, not when you're well.

Second, try to involve people with whom you do not have a long history of control battles. If you have a history of severe conflicts with your mother or father over independence, involve your siblings or close friends instead. There may be members of your core circle whom you see frequently who would know if something was going wrong and whom you would trust with a degree of decision-making capacity during a time of crisis.

A practical problem that can come up when relying on social supports is that no one in your core circle may see you often enough to know, within a brief time,

> ## PERSONALIZED CARE TIP:
> # Involving your family members in prevention plans
>
> People with bipolar disorder are especially prone to anger and resentment when control is being taken away from them. I have heard the statement "I hate the idea of giving up control to anyone" from many clients, whether the control is being given up to a lover, a spouse, a doctor, or (especially) a parent. Why is this issue so salient to people in the manic phases of bipolar disorder? First, when you experience the internal feelings of chaos that mood fluctuations cause, it can become especially important to feel like you're at least in control of your outside world. Second, the feelings of confidence and power associated with the early and later stages of mania make you especially prone to rejecting the advice, opinions, or direct help of others. Third, many people with bipolar disorder have had bad experiences in the past when others—however well intentioned—tried to exert control over them during emergencies.
>
> If your reaction to involving others is negative, think about why you feel this way. What bothers you most about leaning on others? Is the issue really about control or personal autonomy? Is it about competition? Do you fear that there will be "strings attached" to the help? Alternatively, do you feel that you already ask too much of that person? In addressing the issue of whom to choose to help in emergencies, my clients have said: "The only person who would probably do this for me is exactly the person I don't want to have any more control over my life—my mother"; "My relationship with my wife is such that there's always a price to pay. If I lean on her, she'll slam me in some other way"; and "My brother and I have always been competitive. If he were to step in when I got manic, it would be kind of like saying, 'You won.'" It's important to try to understand what issues are at stake for you when you seek help from family members.

whether you are showing the early warning signs of mania. If your relatives live far away or speak to you only by phone, they may not observe the subtle changes that constitute your manic escalation, or they may not have the practical resources (for example, access to your physician) to be able to help. Clients have handled this by relying more heavily on local friends or roommates to perform the same functions or by giving long-distance relatives the phone numbers of their therapist or physician, with instructions to call if the relative has concerns.

If you do not have local connections with significant others, then it becomes all the more important to observe your own mood and behavior and seek help from your doctor when you need it. Some people use the fluctuations on their mood charts (Chapter 8) to determine when to increase contact with their thera-

New research: My colleagues at Oxford University (Amy Bilderbeck, Guy Goodwin, John Geddes, and others) and I conducted a randomized trial comparing two forms of psychosocial treatment for people with bipolar disorder. All participants completed a weekly online mood-tracking diary called "True Colours," responding to text messages sent by our research team requesting that they complete depression and mania rating scales (via smartphone or email) (Bilderbeck et al., 2016). In the first psychosocial treatment condition, participants also received an informational workbook with exercises for them to do concerning the management of bipolar disorder. In the second treatment condition, participants responded to True Colours weekly mood-monitoring queries but also had five sessions of individual therapy with a lay counselor, focusing on learning about the illness and developing a relapse prevention plan. For example, participants would observe changes in their moods or sleep–wake patterns and develop plans for what to do should prodromal symptoms of mania occur, such as attempting to regulate their sleep–wake patterns, avoiding drugs and alcohol, or discussing medication changes with their doctor.

The two treatments were associated with similarly severe depression scores and comparable hospital readmission rates over the 12 months of the study. However, the combination of psychoeducational therapy and mood tracking had one special advantage: participants who received this treatment had acquired greater knowledge about their illness after 3 months compared to mood tracking with the self-care workbook. Moreover, greater illness knowledge at 3 months was related to being well (without significant mania or depression symptoms) for a higher proportion of weeks over the next 9 months. In other words, people in the combination treatment learned more about their disorder and how to manage it, leading to greater stability over time. This study underlines the importance of mood tracking and relapse prevention planning in a therapy or counseling context as key components in the management of bipolar disorder (Bilderbeck et al., 2016).

pist or physician. You may observe very minor increases in your mood as the episode is building, even over intervals as short as a few days. Although subjective, these observations can still inform your treatments and are far preferable to ignoring your illness and letting it take its own course.

Step 1: Identifying the Early Warning Signs of Mania

"He gets disconnected and into himself, kind of overwhelming, irritable . . . in your face, loud, insensitive. He almost sounds like someone else in his body. But at this point I know what it looks like."

—The wife of a 50-year-old man with bipolar I disorder

"I start thinking that I made mistakes at my job [as a refrigerator repairman] . . . I start wondering if I wired things incorrectly and then thinking that the refrigerator in some-one's house will blow up and burn them . . . I start wondering whether I've just thought things or said them out loud. It makes me pull away from everybody. I get tight-lipped."
—A 60-year-old man with bipolar I disorder describing
his manic phases with psychotic features

"She's shy about 95% of the time, but when she's getting high she gets in people's faces, like telling her whole life story to a bank teller; she gets imposing, overly emotional and effusive, kind of sappy or even starts crying . . . I can see other people backing off and sort of looking at me, like, 'Why don't you do something?' She doesn't know that's how she's coming across."
—The husband of a 37-year-old woman with bipolar I disorder

Defining the Prodromal Phase of Mania

Recall that in Chapter 2, I described the manic syndrome as involving changes in mood, energy or activity levels, thinking and perception, sleep, and impulse control. Think about the beginning phases of a new episode of mania (whether it's your first or your 50th) as involving any or all of these (we will discuss the beginning phases of depressive episodes in the next chapter). The *prodromal phase,* usually defined as the period from the first onset of symptoms to the point at which symptoms reach the height of their severity, can last a day or two to several months (the study by Correll et al., 2014, discussed on the next page found an average of 10.3 months for this interval). During this prodromal phase, your symptoms will probably be mild and not necessarily troublesome—and therefore difficult to detect. They are usually muted versions of the symptoms of a full manic episode. Nevertheless, I encourage my patients to err on the side of caution: the appearance of even one or two mild prodromal symptoms is a signal to seek help.

In a study of the prodromal phases of manic episodes, Emily Altman and our group at UCLA (1992) observed people with bipolar disorder over a 9-month period following a hospitalization and rated their symptoms every month. Some had manic episodes during the observation period. The patients who developed mania showed very mild increases in *unusual thought content* in the month before their full episodes. These unusual thoughts were reflected in statements the patients made during clinical interviews regarding their beliefs in the influences of spirits, psychic powers, or the occult; their overly optimistic schemes for making money quickly; their feeling that others were staring or laughing at them; or the belief that their mind was sharper than everyone else's (in other words, grandiose symptoms). These changes in thinking were mild, and in some cases even the person expressing them admitted the ideas sounded odd or unrealistic. *So, observable changes in the content of your thinking and speech may be a clue that you are beginning to escalate.*

A review of 28 studies of the bipolar prodrome (Malhi, Bargh, Coulston, Das, & Berk, 2014) indicated some broad consistencies as to the symptoms people experience before their *first* manic episode. The most frequent signals included *mood lability* (frequent and unpredictable changes between depressed, irritable, anxious, and elevated mood), nonmood symptoms (for example, inattention), and either subthreshold mania or cyclothymic temperament (short hypomanic episodes alternating with short, subthreshold depressive episodes). None of these precursors is surprising, as they reflect key attributes of the illness in less extreme form.

A detailed study of 52 teens (mean age 16) and young adults with bipolar I disorder clarified the parameters of the manic prodromal period (Correll et al., 2014). First, most had a long and "slow burn" buildup to mania characterized by subthreshold high and low symptoms rather than a rapid deterioration in mood or behavior. Second, irritability, racing thoughts, increased activity/energy, and depressive mood were reported by at least 50% of the participants; 65.4% reported decreased school or work functioning and 57.7% reported frequent mood swings. You can use these findings to help define the feelings, thoughts, or behaviors that constitute your own prodromal period.

> **Effective prevention:** It is during the prodromal phase that you have the most control over your fate. That's why it's important to prepare yourself to recognize even the mildest symptoms of mania. Be especially attuned to when your mood is swinging a lot, your energy level increases, or you find that people are reacting to your irritability or crankiness.

List Your Prodromal Symptoms

It appears that many people with bipolar disorder can describe how they behave when they're getting manic, at least when they're asked after the fact. The harder question is, how do you know ahead of time what symptoms you should be looking for? *One way to increase the probability that you or others will recognize a developing episode is to make a list, when you're well, of early warning signs recalled from your last few episodes.* In other words, take advantage of the greater insight you have into your illness when you are well. This kind of objectivity will be harder to summon when you are heading into an episode, but having the list available may help you view your escalating mood, thoughts, and behaviors in a different light. Soon I'll talk about what you can actually do when these prodromal signs appear.

The form on page 229 will help get you started recording your prodromal symptoms. Your early warning signs, of course, may be different from the ones listed in the form. Nancy experienced the onset of her hypomanic episodes as an increase in anxiety and worry. Pete reported that, despite feeling speedy and internally stimulated, he withdrew more when he was escalating because he knew that he would alienate other people once he became fully manic. Heather became obsessed with a certain movie star and began "seeing things out of the corner of my eye."

Listing Your Prodromal Signs of Mania or Hypomania

With the help of your close friends or relatives, list a couple of adjectives describing what your *mood* is like when your manic or hypomanic episodes first begin (*examples:* up, happy, more aware, willful, more reactive, cranky, irritable, euphoric, anxious, wired, cheery, like a yo-yo, pumped up).

_____

_____

Describe changes in your *activity* and *energy* levels as your manic episode is developing. Include changes in how you relate to others (*examples:* call lots of people, make lots of new friends, take on more projects or start multitasking, talk more and faster, get in people's faces, tell people off, feel "horny" or very sexually driven).

_____

_____

_____

Describe changes in your *thinking* and *perception* (*examples:* thoughts race or at least go faster, sounds get louder, colors get brighter, I think I can do anything, I think others are looking at me or laughing at me, I get more interested in religion or the occult, I feel really smart and confident, I start thinking about many new ideas involving money, other people seem boring and closed-minded, I get extrasensory perception, I have psychic abilities, I think about hurting or killing myself, I ruminate about things, I get easily distracted).

_____

_____

_____

Describe changes in your *sleep* patterns (*examples:* sleeping 2 hours less than usual but not feeling tired the next day, waking up a lot during the night, staying up late and relying on catnaps during the day, not needing sleep).

_____

_____

Describe anything you've done in the last week that you wouldn't ordinarily do (*examples:* spent a lot of money or invested money on impulse, got one or more speeding tickets or drove recklessly, had more sexual encounters with partner or other partners, gambled money).

_____

_____

Describe the *context* (any changes, events, or circumstances) associated with these symptoms (*examples:* an increase in your work stress, stopping or becoming inconsistent with your medications, missing your doctor's appointments, starting to drink or use drugs, starting a new project, changes in your work hours, travel across time zones, more family or relationship conflicts, starting a new relationship or ending another one, changes in your financial circumstances).

_____

_____

_____

It is important to distinguish the early warning signs of mania from those of depression, which usually involve feeling slowed down, fatigued, self-critical, hopeless, or uninterested in things (see the next chapter). Holly reported periods of increased irritability and anxiety prior to manic episodes but misidentified these as signs of depression. Prior to learning more about her disorder, she used to self-medicate her irritability with over-the-counter remedies such as fish oil or SAM-e. During one period of escalation she even convinced an internist to prescribe an antidepressant, which made her manic symptoms much worse. With time, she observed that irritability and anxiety usually portended mania rather than depression, and she learned to rely on more traditional prevention methods, such as increasing the dosage of her mood stabilizer.

If you've had only one or two episodes, you may have difficulty listing your prodromal symptoms. Your family or friends may be able to help you here, as may your doctor. Chapter 2 describes how different mania can look to people who have the disorder than it looks to their family members or doctors. You may not agree with your relatives that a certain behavior (for example, aggressiveness) or thinking pattern (for example, inattentiveness or distractibility) characterizes you when you're getting manic, but it's better to list these behaviors or thinking patterns if they might in some way help your relatives recognize your episodes early. Like-

---

PERSONALIZED CARE TIP:
Recognizing the prodrome of a hypomanic episode

If you have bipolar II disorder, you may wonder whether your hypomanias really have a definable beginning and end. Hypomanic episodes can be very subtle, and, because they do not significantly interfere with your day-to-day functioning, they can be hard to distinguish from your usual state. However, even hypomania involves observable physical, cognitive, and emotional changes relative to your ordinary state. In developing your relapse prevention plan, give early warning signs of hypomania the same importance as warning signs for manic or mixed phases.

Typical prodromal symptoms of hypomania are sleep loss (sometimes a change of only an hour or two), increases in energy levels, feeling more goal-directed, increases in the speed of your thoughts or speech, a feeling of creativity or being able to "think outside the box," and irritability or impatience. Perhaps you can recall when these changes last occurred and you knew something was different. Remember that a prodrome needs to be a change from your usual self: if you are usually highly energetic, can get along with 6 hours of sleep, and habitually talk fast, you may just have a "high voltage" or "hyperthymic" temperament. For some people, increases in anxiety are a key sign of hypomania, usually combined with racing thoughts, irritability, and increased activity.

wise, record your views of your early warning signs or eliciting circumstances even if these views don't coincide with what your relatives think.

Robert, the man discussed at the beginning of the chapter, reported feeling very sexual and having racing thoughts before he had changes in his mood. His girlfriend, Jessie, saw it differently: she thought he became irritable first, then loud and physically intrusive. Another person with bipolar disorder, Tom, said that his manias almost always involved religious preoccupations and paranoia. His parents described him as "getting a certain look in his eyes" and "muttering stuff underneath his breath." The physician who treated Alan, the 60-year-old refrigerator repairman who believed that others could hear what he was thinking, felt that Alan's "bouncy, upbeat quality" was his first prodromal sign. Characterizations like these are helpful in rounding out what your prodromal phases look like from your own vantage point and the vantage point of others.

Identifying the Context in Which Your Early Warning Signs Occur

You may have an easier time describing your prodromal symptoms if you also record information about the context in which they occur. For example, Robert felt that his irritability during his last manic episode was closely tied to increases in his work demands and annoyances expressed by coworkers, who had begun pressuring him about the company's financial outlook. For Ruth (see Chapter 8), manic cycles were nearly always precipitated by alcohol usage, sometimes even in small quantities. In the form for listing prodromal symptoms (on page 229), there is a space to record any eliciting circumstances (usual or unusual) that you or any of your relatives think may be associated with your early warning signs.

Identifying circumstances associated with your prior manic episodes can help you minimize the impact of the next one. If you know that a particular circumstance (for example, an increased workload due to the Christmas holidays) was associated with your last episode (even if you don't think it caused your illness), you may want to become more vigilant about your feeling states or behavior during the next interval in which your work demands increase. This kind of vigilance can help you determine when you should ask for medical or other kinds of help, time off, or other accommodations (also see Chapter 13).

Teresa worked as an accountant. She came to realize that tax season, with its much longer work hours, was a trigger for her manic episodes. Prior to tax season, she obtained a prescription from her doctor for a tranquilizing medication (in her case, quetiapine [Seroquel]) to be started if she was unable to sleep, experienced racing thoughts, or felt overly goal driven. She was also able to arrange a few days off in the middle of tax season when she felt herself becoming exhausted from lack of sleep. As a result, she got through tax season without a full episode, although she remained aware of an underlying energized state that was only partially masked by the medication.

Step 2, Part A: Preventive Steps You Can Take Yourself or with Others' Help

What should you and your significant others do when you have one or more early warning signs? I've separated this section from the next (Part B), which concerns negotiating help from your doctor and the mental health system. Later, we'll put Steps 1 and 2 together into a written contract (Step 3).

Not all of the following preventive steps will apply to you. For example, you may be a person who has trouble with money but not with sexual indiscretions. You may have a history of making impulsive life decisions but have never driven recklessly. Your individual pattern of prodromal symptoms may dictate which of the following preventive measures are most urgent and which can wait. So, for example, if you have prodromal symptoms like irritability and a decreased need for sleep, you may want to see your physician, but asking someone else to hold on to your credit cards may not be as essential (unless irritability and sleep disturbances have, in the past, heralded a drive toward haphazard investments).

Managing Money

"One time I took a cab way downtown, tipped the driver 50%, and then bought two very expensive dresses at a department store that I thought was having a big sale. It turned out they weren't. I bought the dresses anyway, without knowing anything about the materials I was buying or whether the prices were good, without taking anyone with me, which I would have done normally. I spent over a thousand dollars, which we didn't have. I eventually took one of them back, but [when I was manic] I destroyed the other one by leaving an iron on top of it."

—A 55-year-old woman with bipolar I disorder describing her last manic episode

Bipolar disorder makes managing money much harder than it would ordinarily be. When people are becoming manic, and especially when they reach the full height of their mania, they often go on spending sprees and invest wildly. In *An Unquiet Mind*, Jamison (1995) offers good examples of the thinking behind spending sprees. But as she recounts, spending sprees and foolish business investments can damage your life and contribute to your feelings of hopelessness after the manic episode has cleared.

Mania tends to generate "hyperpositive thinking," in which you overestimate your abilities to achieve (for example, make a lot of money) and underestimate the risks (for example, going into debt) of your behavior (Mansell & Pedley, 2008). When you have hyperpositive thoughts (for example, "I can't possibly lose"), it can be hard to step back and evaluate them objectively. In fact, some people equate *imagining* being able to do something with actually being able to do it. If you can imagine making a lot of money very quickly, how much harder could it be to actually do it?

You and your significant others can become attuned to when you are overly optimistic or hyperpositive. Do you suddenly believe you have found quick answers to financial problems that have been plaguing you for years? Are you becoming more and more enthralled with "get rich quick" or "pyramid" schemes? Do you find yourself unusually preoccupied with money or merchandise, and driven to purchase expensive things (see the example of Robert and his electric guitars at the beginning of this chapter)? Do you think that you must have those things, sooner rather than later, or else you will be "ripped off"? Have you come to believe that your finances are virtually unlimited? Do you feel impatient or frustrated with your spouse when he or she tells you that you can't afford something?

You may not be able to prevent these thoughts from occurring, but here are some concrete steps you can take when they first appear:

- Have someone else hold on to your credit cards.
- Avoid trips to the bank unless you are going to take a trusted person with you.
- Stay away from your favorite stores.
- Avoid watching television stations whose primary purpose is to sell you goods.
- Don't give your credit card numbers or bank account information to telemarketers or investment counselors who call you with their special deals (an advisable practice even when you're feeling well, of course!).
- Avoid investing in the stock market altogether or making sudden changes in, or withdrawals from, your retirement accounts.
- Stay away from online stock trading.

In other words, decreasing your access to the *means* of implementing your plans makes it less likely you will actually carry them out.

Another practical maneuver is to arrange, when you're well, to make it logistically difficult for you to get ahold of large sums of money in a short time. There are several ways to do this, including keeping your money in small amounts spread across several accounts in different financial institutions or keeping the majority of your money in a joint account that requires a cosigner for a withdrawal. Karla, a 35-year-old woman with bipolar I disorder, made the following agreement with her boyfriend, Taki: Karla obtained three bank debit cards from their three shared accounts. Each of her cards was labeled with an expense category (for example, "clothing") and had a posted spending limit. The two agreed to determine, on a weekly basis, which purchases she had already made and how close she was to the spending limit in each category.

If you work closely with an investment counselor, it may be possible to entrust this adviser with information about your illness so that he or she can stop you from investing too wildly or irrationally. Consider asking your counselor to set an upper limit on how much money you can exchange within a single transaction.

Of course, maintaining these kinds of controls over your finances implies that your thinking is still fairly rational and that you can make good decisions. Rational thought is often possible during the earliest phases of mania (another reason to catch your episodes at the beginning). But as you may know, once your symptoms have accelerated, it becomes difficult to make logical decisions of any type and you may become highly resentful of anyone else's intervention. If you get your significant others involved *early* in the escalation process, and trust them enough to take your credit cards, provide final signatures on investments, or offer input into your spending decisions, you may be able to avoid a major financial collapse. Remember that most major financial decisions require a second opinion even in the best of circumstances. Finally, keep in mind that it may feel more acceptable to you to have certain people in your core circle involved in your finances and not others. If you aren't comfortable with a parent taking on this role, consider asking a close friend or an uncle, aunt, or cousin.

Effective prevention: If you think you are in the prodromal phases of mania or hypomania, consider the 48-hour rule: Wait 48 hours and get at least two full nights of sleep before making a purchase that exceeds a certain limit (Newman, Leahy, Beck, Reilly-Harrington, & Gyulai, 2001). During these 48 hours, discuss the intended purchase with as many as three trusted people (a family member, a friend, and a doctor or therapist). During the waiting period, ask yourself:

- If someone else wanted to do what I am intending to do, what advice would I give that person?
- What is the worst thing that could happen if I'm not able to follow through with my plans?
- What is the worst thing that could happen if I did carry them out?

The passage of time, your own critique of the situation, and the input of others may help you evaluate the likely success of your financial decisions.

Giving Up the Car Keys

Are your manic episodes usually characterized by reckless driving? This is the case for some people and not for others. One of my male clients put it succinctly: "My highs almost always go along with some problem involving my car." If you do have a poor driving record, your early warning signs may signal the need to stop driving for now. Mania—much like drinking alcohol—makes your driving unsafe for you and others. You are at especially high risk for an auto accident if you are in a manic state and are also drinking and driving, as some people do. This is yet another arena in which it helps to have others' input.

Your significant others can collaborate in helping you make good judgments about whether you can drive safely. While you will resent that your spouse or siblings have access to the car and you don't, remember that it is only for the limited time until your manic or hypomanic symptoms have cleared. Your doctor's input will also be valuable if he or she knows your driving history.

Avoiding Major Life Decisions

When you have one or more early warning signs, avoid making decisions that could affect your or others' futures, particularly if these decisions involve meetings with people who have a degree of "fate control." Now is not the time to ask your boss for a raise or a change in job duties—you are likely to come across as demanding and entitled (see also Chapter 13 on strategies for coping in the work setting). If you are an employer, delay your decision to assemble your employees to inform them of major structural changes in the company. Likewise, avoid making decisions about your family life that could lead to long-term consequences, such as getting married, separated, or divorced; deciding to have children; buying a new house or moving to another city; changing careers; or deciding to home-school your kids.

It's hard to make these agreements with yourself, and even harder to implement them when you feel so good, so optimistic, and so elated. The decisions you feel pressed to make may seem like great ideas at the time, even though to others—or even to yourself when you're well—they seem unrealistic and extremely risky. You may believe that you're thinking "outside the box" and that doing so can only lead to beneficial outcomes. Try to think of the pressure to make these decisions, along with your feeling of greater mental clarity, as a part of your illness (especially if you also notice other symptoms, such as distractibility, racing thoughts, or an increase in your sex drive). People with bipolar disorder almost invariably make their best life decisions when they're in the remitted, euthymic state, and they usually end up regretting those decisions they made while manic or hypomanic.

Avoiding Risky Sexual Situations

"I was getting real manic and got tired of being around Carol and the kids, so I went out to a bar. I ran into this old girlfriend and got drunk with her. We wound up in bed that night. I can't believe I did that—I'm not that kind of person! It seemed like such a great thing at the time. Of course, I felt terrible about it later, and it really hurt my relation-

ship with Carol. Even though she knows about mania and its biology and all that, she blames me for getting myself in that situation in the first place. She thought it was what I really wanted to do, and the mania just gave me the excuse to do it."
—A 46-year-old man with bipolar I disorder, recently separated from his wife

Like many rewarding endeavors, sex has a particular pull when you're getting manic. This can be true even if you're a person who is sexually conservative in your stable times. People get themselves into risky sexual situations when they are escalating, and sometimes the emotional results—which can include feelings of shame, humiliation, and anger—worsen their cycling mood state. As you know, impulsive encounters carry a high risk of contracting sexually transmitted diseases.

As discussed in Chapter 2, mania is more a goal-driven state than a happy one. When you feel strongly pulled toward rewards, it's hard to step back and ask whether you're making healthy decisions for yourself. Some people benefit from knowing that they're prone to sexual "acting out" when they're in the prodromal or active phases of mania or hypomania. Knowing this about yourself is the first step toward controlling it.

People with bipolar disorder, especially women, are more likely to have been sexually abused as youngsters than their healthy age-mates (Palmier-Claus et al., 2016). Experiences of abuse, whether from a parent, a family friend, or a stranger, can all contribute to your difficulties in regulating mood states—or setting limits with others—as an adult. Having a sexual abuse history makes some people code potentially adverse sexual encounters as expectable or even welcome. If you find that memories of abusive sexual encounters start to crop up when your mood is escalating, list these memories as an early warning sign of mania.

Of course, none of this means that you have to avoid sexual encounters altogether. Some people report that their primary romantic relationships improve when they get manic or hypomanic because they become more sexually engaged with their partners. Others feel that the increase in their sexual encounters with their partner contributes to an upward escalation of their mood states. In either case, being manic doesn't mean having to avoid sex with your regular partner.

The best way to avoid dangerous sexual situations is to spend as much time as possible with people you know and trust, who can talk you out of impulsive sexual encounters. That is, when you go out at night, go with a friend who knows about your illness

> **Effective solution:** The fact that becoming manic can increase your sex drive doesn't mean you have to avoid sexual activity. In fact, sex can be a good outlet for your energy if it is with the right person at the right time. The key is not to allow your mania to drive you toward irresponsible or risky sex with people you don't know or don't trust.

and who can "run interference" when you start to show poor judgment. Make special efforts to stay away from alcohol and street drugs: there is nothing worse than "self-medicating" an escalating mood with cocaine, marijuana, or alcohol, which will almost certainly contribute to your mood escalation and lower your threshold for acting on a sexual impulse. Encourage your friends to take you home if they think you're making foolish decisions. Ultimately the decision to have or not have sex with someone is yours alone, but limit setting from others (even if quite irritating to you at the time) can help keep you from getting into encounters that you'll regret later.

A Reminder to Use Your "Maintaining Wellness" Strategies

When you are in the early stages of mania, it is essential to implement the strategies for maintaining wellness outlined in Chapter 8. I won't reiterate them all here; suffice it to say that now is an especially important time to maintain regular daily and nightly routines. Try as hard as you can to get a full night's sleep (your doctor may be able to recommend sleeping medications) and to keep your hours consistent from the week to the weekend. Avoid stressful interactions with other people, particularly family members, to the extent possible. Stick closely to your medication regimen. Continue to chart your mood on a daily basis to identify changes in your mood status as early as possible.

Step 2, Part B: Preventive Maneuvers Involving Your Doctor

Collaborating with your psychiatrist to prevent or diminish the impact of your manic episodes is more complicated than it sounds. Most psychiatrists will tell you that you should call them for an emergency medical appointment when you think your illness is getting worse. This sounds like a "no-brainer." But the reality is that you may not believe you are really ill or that your illness is bad enough to warrant a phone call. Alternatively, you may not feel comfortable calling your doctor, especially if the doctor is new to you or if you have had bad experiences with calling him or her in the past. Some psychiatrists are nearly impossible to reach, a feature you may want to consider when choosing a doctor for medication management.

Even if you see the need for emergency care, you may have doubts about how much your doctor will really help you. You may fear that the doctor will recommend medication changes that have worse side effects than the ones you already experience. You may fear being hospitalized immediately, which would cause you social embarrassment at work or at home. Of course, you are more likely to avoid hospitalization if you call your physician early than if you wait until the point of no return. But calling during an emergency requires a certain amount of trust that the physician will approach you compassionately and take steps that will alleviate, not worsen, your symptoms. This section deals with strategies for collaborating with your physician during emergencies.

"When Should I Call, and What Should I Say?"

A good rule of thumb is to call as soon as you feel like your mood or energy level has changed upward or downward or when you believe (or if a significant other believes) that you've developed one or two prodromal symptoms. *In other words, err on the side of getting help when you or others think you might need it, rather than assuming you don't and being wrong.*

Make sure your doctor's phone numbers (or the numbers of the clinic where the doctor works) are easily accessible, including emergency contact information. There are places on your mania prevention contract (on pages 246–247) to record this information. Most physicians have a "backup" doctor available for emergencies during weekends or vacations. Usually the phone numbers of this backup physician are included in the message on your doctor's or the clinic's emergency phone line. When you do reach your physician or backup, be ready to recount any prodromal symptoms you think you have developed. Before starting, make sure you are talking to an MD, a PhD, a social worker, or a psychiatric nurse. I have known patients who went to some lengths to explain their manic symptoms, only to be told they had reached the answering service.

Following is a telephone interchange between a person with bipolar I disorder, Chad, and his psychiatrist, Dr. Eastwood.

Chad: Yeah, I think I'm going off again.

Dr. Eastwood: What's going on?

Chad: I'm taking my medication, but I'm having all sorts of thoughts and stuff.

Dr. Eastwood: Thoughts about what?

Chad: Like about the past. About my dad and his death and stuff.

Dr. Eastwood: How's your mood, Chad? Any changes?

Chad: Yeah, just more pissed off, getting grouchy, yelling at the kids. I just don't know if I wanna do the whole family thing anymore.

Dr. Eastwood: How's your sleep been the last few nights?

Chad: OK, but not great; can't stay asleep very long. I've been pacing at night and stuff. Thoughts going a mile a minute. Bed's not comfortable.

Dr. Eastwood: Sounds like a lot's going on right now. Anything else I need to know? Are you thinking about hurting yourself? Do you feel like you need to be in the hospital?

Chad: No, not there yet. Just upset and stuff. I feel mad, and I can't sleep.

Dr. Eastwood: How have things gone with your medications?

Chad: I missed my lithium this morning, took it this evening.

In this interchange, Dr. Eastwood has done a quick assessment and concluded that Chad may be in the prodromal phase of a manic or a mixed episode. At this stage, Chad's escalation can be treated on an outpatient basis, which Dr. Eastwood did by setting up an emergency medical appointment, increasing the dosage of Chad's lithium, and adding a small dose of an antipsychotic medication. A blood test revealed that Chad's lithium level was low, even though Chad said he had been taking the medication relatively regularly. These changes to his medication regimen did the trick without a host of new side effects. Within a week, Chad's mania had stopped escalating and his depression subsided, and he began to return to his baseline state.

Chad did a good job of describing his prodromal symptoms. Dr. Eastwood guided him toward describing these symptoms and his medication usage. She was fairly task oriented and kept Chad from getting off track. Notice that Dr. Eastwood did not pursue any psychotherapeutic issues over the phone, such as Chad's feelings about his father or his current family. Expect that when you call under emergency circumstances, in most cases your physician will not conduct a psychotherapy session with you. This may be frustrating because you may feel that certain personal issues are important in explaining your symptoms. Many people believe, as Chad did, that their manic symptoms are triggered by feelings of loss. But the emergency phone call to your physician is mainly for the purpose of evaluating whether a change in medication is necessary or, in more extreme circumstances, whether you need to be hospitalized. Once your symptoms have settled down, the physician (or your outpatient therapist) may be able to help you make sense of how current or past stressors or losses are contributing to your escalating mood.

"What If I'm Uncomfortable with My Physician?"

Robert, described at the beginning of this chapter, did not particularly like his physician and saw her infrequently. Perhaps as a result, this doctor was not as helpful as she could have been in preventing his manic episode. Had he been in contact with a doctor with whom he had a good relationship, a face-to-face session might have been arranged quickly, with more positive results.

Not everyone feels comfortable calling his or her doctor during an emergency, and during a manic escalation your discomfort may be exaggerated (most emotions become more dramatic during mania). One of my clients, Holly, had long-standing frustrations with her doctor. She called Dr. Nelson on a number of occasions when she felt she was cycling rapidly. Typically, Dr. Nelson did not call her back. She considered switching physicians but wasn't convinced she had given Dr. Nelson a fair try.

I encouraged Holly to talk over this dilemma with Dr. Nelson, a man whom I had experienced as very approachable. But Holly felt uncomfortable broaching the topic, fearing that he was going to "fire me as a patient." I finally interceded and called Dr. Nelson when Holly developed mixed affective symptoms and suicidal thoughts. Dr. Nelson told me that he had tried to talk to Holly on a number of occasions but that *she* hadn't returned *his* calls. He also found that when he gave Holly advice on how to control her symptoms, she would become angry and uncooperative. So there were frustrations on both sides.

Eventually, we scheduled a meeting involving Holly, Dr. Nelson, and me. We hammered out a series of agreements regarding what steps would be taken if she developed mixed or manic symptoms in the future. Dr. Nelson gave an additional phone number to Holly and reiterated his emergency and backup/vacation policies. Ultimately, Holly's treatment was made more successful by this direct contact with her psychiatrist (see also Chapter 6).

Your best option is to talk over your concerns with your physician until you feel reasonably comfortable about contacting the doctor in an emergency. Explain your fears about new medications, side effects, or the need for hospitalization (discussed more on page 243). If your bottom line is that you would never call this person when you're feeling bad, find another physician.

"Should Somebody Else Call for Me?"

When you feel exhilarated, excited, and goal driven, you may see no reason to destroy this state by taking what the physician has to offer—which is usually more medication. For this reason, it may make sense for someone close to you to make the call to your psychiatrist or primary-care physician. Give members of your core circle some leeway in deciding when to make this call, recognizing that you may not agree that your physician's help is needed. It is my strong impression—both in my clinical practice and in our research studies—that people who have allowed members of their core circle to call their doctors in emergencies have had better outcomes. For example, Paul, the husband of Lorraine, a 64-year-old woman with bipolar I disorder, routinely called his wife's doctor whenever she became giddy, delusional, or agitated. Lorraine's doctor was usually able to deal with the escalation over the phone by making adjustments to her existing doses instead of hospitalizing her.

> **Effective prevention:** Consult your physician as to whether a friend or close relative can accompany you to your medical visits. If you have become confused or distractible, your significant other or friend may be better able to recall the physician's recommendations when you need to implement them later.

Contact between your relatives and your doctor may require mutual understanding about treatment policies. Your doctor should make clear to you and your relatives the circumstances under which they should call (for example, when you are clearly escalating or are depressed; when you are refusing all your treatments). Your relatives may have a set of unrealistic expectations, such as the following: your doctor will call them as soon as you've missed an appointment or as soon as you've reported *any* symptoms; your doctor will discuss any planned medication adjustments with them before making them; they can call whenever there has been a family argument or whenever they want to know something about bipolar disorder. These are assumptions your physician will not usually share. Remember to sign a HIPAA (Health Insurance Portability and Accountability Act) release-of-information form in your doctor's office, allowing your chosen relative to exchange information with your doctor.

"What Will My Doctor Do?"

During an emergency session, your physician will probably take the steps outlined in the box on this page. He or she will start by assessing your symptoms and reevaluating your medication regimen. Your doctor may decide to make changes to your regimen over the phone if an appointment can't be arranged. A major intent of catching and treating your symptoms early is to help you avoid hospitalization, but if this is not possible, your doctor can help you arrange one.

Your doctor will usually begin by asking you the kinds of questions Dr. Eastwood asked Chad. Physicians vary on which symptoms they emphasize (some focus on mood and others on activity levels or sleep), but generally, the more you can speak to your doctor in the language of prodromal symptoms (for example, racing thoughts, goal-driven behavior, decreased need for sleep), the more your physician will know what to recommend. Your doctor will probably want to know if you have missed any dosages of your medication, and you should be as honest as possible about this. It's not at all uncommon for people to miss dosages (especially if they are expected to take a lot of pills) when they are becoming manic or hypomanic, and it should not be a source of shame.

If you are on lithium or valproate, your doctor may ask you to get your

---

Effective prevention: Steps your physician will take to arrest the escalation of mania:

- Assess the severity of your symptoms.
- Evaluate blood levels of certain of your medications (lithium, valproate).
- Make changes to your regimen, including adding or subtracting certain medications or increasing the dosage of current agents.
- Initiate more frequent contact with you and your family members.
- Arrange a hospitalization if necessary.

blood level tested. He or she will most likely be interested in your "trough" level, which is usually collected 10–14 hours after your last dose (people who get their blood level checked just a few hours after taking their last dose may appear to be getting enough medication when, in fact, they are not). For example, if you have been taking lithium and your trough level is 0.6 mg/ml or less (see Chapter 6), the doctor may conclude that you've missed dosages or that your dosage is too low to be therapeutic. Then he or she may recommend that you increase your lithium dosage as a way of preventing further escalation. Because it may take a few days before your blood level is processed, your doctor may decide not to wait for that information before changing your dosage, especially if he or she has been collecting blood level information from you all along. If possible, your doctor may increase the frequency of your treatment sessions during the interval in which your symptoms are worsening.

If your physician increases the dosage of your primary mood stabilizer, you and your significant others will want to become familiar with the signs of neuro-toxicity (see also Chapter 6), which are the medical complications associated with getting too much of a medication. For lithium, these symptoms include drowsi-ness, severe nausea, abdominal discomfort, severe diarrhea, blurry vision, slurred speech, muscle twitching, or being confused as to where or who you are. For val-proate, they include severe dizziness, drowsiness, irregular breathing, and severe trembling. If you show any of these symptoms, your doctor should be notified immediately—by you or a member of your core circle—so that he or she can adjust or even take you off these medications.

Your doctor may add some of the medications discussed in Chapter 6, includ-ing second-generation antipsychotics with mood-stabilizing properties such as quetiapine or risperidone, or benzodiazepines such as clonazepam (Klonopin) or lorazepam (Ativan). These medications may help bring you down from an acti-vated, agitated state, improve your sleep, and treat delusional thinking (for exam-ple, paranoia). If you are on only one mood stabilizer, your doctor may add a second one (for example, adding valproate to lithium). These decisions are often based on physician choice rather than research data. For example, we do not know whether simply increasing the dosage of lithium or valproate is more or less effective in pre-venting relapses of mania than adding one of these mood stabilizers to the other.

Don't be surprised if your physician believes that the best treatment for your escalating mania is to stop taking one of your current medications rather than to start on a new one. If you are getting manic and have rapid cycling (four or more episodes in the prior year), the most effective intervention may be to discontinue your antidepressant (if you are on one). Your physician is unlikely to start you on an antidepressant when you are escalating into mania or hypomania (see Chapter 6). Your physician may also recommend that you discontinue your periodic use of caffeine or bronchodilators such as Proventil.

"When Is Hospitalization Required?"

Many people with bipolar disorder never need to be hospitalized. In addition, alternatives to inpatient hospitalization—such as partial hospital, day hospital, or intensive outpatient programs—have emerged in recent years as short-term strategies for emergencies. These programs provide close monitoring of your symptoms and treatment response without the need to enter an inpatient facility. But if your manic symptoms escalate to a certain point of disruptiveness, or if you are actively suicidal or dangerous to others, there is a good chance that your doctor will recommend that you be hospitalized for a period of time. You are more likely to be hospitalized if you are manic (or mixed) than if you are hypomanic or depressed.

It is very common for people in manic episodes to believe that they don't need to be hospitalized. Often they insist on leaving very soon after they are admitted, thinking they are closer to recovery than their doctors or others think. Perhaps you have had some of these experiences. But if your doctor believes that you are at imminent risk of hurting yourself or someone else, or are otherwise unable to take care of yourself, it is his or her professional, ethical, and legal responsibility to seek permission from a judge to continue inpatient treatment, under a court order if necessary. You won't feel good about this course of action, but it may be necessary to preserve safety for yourself and others.

If your doctor does recommend hospitalization, it is usually easiest if he or she calls the hospital to arrange for an inpatient bed. In some cases, you or your family members may have to make the arrangements (for example, if your doctor hasn't seen you in some time or doesn't have hospital admitting privileges). As a relapse prevention measure, keep the phone number of the recommended hospital's emergency room and your insurance cards in easily accessible places (see the Contract for Preventing Mania exercise on pages 246–247).

Nowadays, many people have managed care health insurance plans that stipulate which hospitals can or cannot admit them and for how long. Before signing up for a new insurance policy, it is important to find out if the psychiatrist whom you see is "in network" and if the hospitals at which he or she has admission privileges are providers within the plan. Otherwise, your health insurance policy could require you to be admitted to a different hospital from the one your doctor might recommend.

"What Will Happen to Me in the Hospital?"

If you do have an inpatient hospitalization, you will probably meet on a daily basis with an inpatient psychiatrist (who is probably not your regular doctor). You should expect some individual or group counseling sessions concerning life issues, relapse prevention, and posthospital adjustment. In the best-case scenario, family or spousal visits are encouraged and become an integral part of the treatment plan.

Hospitalization can be a scary proposition. Many people fear that psychiatric hospitals are like snake pits—a place where things are dirty, people are violent, the nurses are cruel and malevolent, shock treatment is used as a punishment, and little help is delivered. Although this is largely a distortion based on the past, hospitals do vary considerably in quality, just as do the doctors and nurses who work within them. Many hospitals are excellent and provide state-of-the-art mental health care. Others are underfunded, employ out-of-date models of intervention, and are not oriented toward treatment as much as the protection of others. If you have been in a hospital more than once, you probably have had diverse experiences, depending on which hospital you went to and the condition in which you were admitted.

Consider the following if you need to be hospitalized. First, many people confuse being hospitalized with being institutionalized. The latter usually means that people are kept in a hospital for months or years at a time, under court order, because they are a danger to themselves or others. In contrast, psychiatric hospitalizations are usually short, averaging about a week long in the United States.

Second, the treatment you receive in the hospital is usually geared toward controlling your acute symptoms (including suicidal thoughts or intentions) to reduce the immediate risk to you and those around you. Hospitalization also allows you to "dry out" if you have been drinking or using drugs during your manic escalation. Your inpatient stay will enable you to start a new regimen of medications or newly adjusted dosages, "wash out" your existing medications, or try other treatments (for example, electroconvulsive therapy or, in some hospitals, ketamine if you are acutely depressed and not responding to mood stabilizers, antipsychotics, or antidepressants). However, your stay will probably not be long enough for you to know if your new regimen is effective in the long term.

Third, hospitalization is not a personal failure. You have a biological vulnerability to manic or depressive episodes that is not fully under your control, and it is not your fault if you

---

Effective treatment: If your doctor, therapist, and family members believe hospitalization will help you, you may find it less frightening and more acceptable if you remember the following:

- Being hospitalized is not the same as being institutionalized; it lasts a very short time.
- Hospitalization can be the best way to get acute symptoms under control.
- Hospitalization is an opportunity to have your medications reevaluated and, if necessary, washed out.
- Agreeing to be hospitalized does not signal the end of your control over your disorder or your own life.
- Hospitalization can provide a needed break from daily stresses and family conflicts and give you a chance to gain a new perspective.

need hospitalization. Being hospitalized does not mean that others have to run your life from now on. Instead, it signifies the temporary giving up of control for a short period of time. You will have your life back soon enough, especially if you are able to collaborate with your doctor and the inpatient team to develop an effective posthospital plan.

Finally, hospitalization can provide you with a much-needed rest or break from the stressors of your day-to-day life. Although you'd no doubt rather spend a week in the Bahamas, a short or even a longer hospital stay can give you time to think through what is and isn't working about your treatment plan, your current relationships, or your career. It can also give you distance from your relatives, which you (and they) may need from time to time. Robert's hospitalization helped him rethink his feelings about Jessie and his children, and upon being discharged, he felt more resolved to make things work. It will be hard to take this view when you are first admitted to a hospital, but later you may have quite a different view of the experience.

Step 3: Developing a Mania Prevention Contract

Now let's put together everything discussed so far in this chapter into a written contract for relapse prevention. The form on pages 246–247 asks you to summarize what you have concluded about your prodromal phase, the steps you and your significant others can take to prevent a full relapse, and the emergency procedures involving your doctors. Consult with your family members, spouse, doctor, and other trusted persons to make sure that all understand what they are being asked to do.

It is usually best to create this contract when you are feeling stable and have the hindsight to think back on the previous episode and how it developed. Initially, you may feel yourself getting triggered by family members who remember things in a different order than you do or blame you for things that weren't your fault. Try to hang in there during the discussion without getting defensive—your family members may be anxious about what is being expected of them and whether they will be able to follow through.

When filling out this contract, try to include as many options as possible. Some of the options will probably seem more comfortable to you than others, but it's better to write them all down even if you don't end up using them. Encourage your significant others to be open about what they do and don't feel comfortable doing when you're cycling into mania. Write into the contract only those responsibilities you and they are willing to accept. Alternatively, list all of your possible options and rank them from top to bottom in order of preference. Ask everyone to sign the contract.

Contract for Preventing Mania

Your physician's name: _____

Phone number, office: _____ Phone number, emergency: _____

Your therapist's name: _____

Phone number, office: _____ Phone number, emergency: _____

Name of local hospital: _____ Emergency room number: _____

Your insurance carrier: _____ Policy number: _____

Group number (if applicable): _____

1. List your typical early warning (prodromal) signs of a manic episode (from the exercise on page 229).

   _____

   _____

   _____

2. List the circumstances in which these prodromal symptoms are most likely to occur.

   _____

   _____

   _____

3. Ask one or more members of your core circle to add any other early warning signs they've observed and, if relevant, the circumstances in which these signs first appeared.

   _____

   _____

   _____

4. List what behaviors *you* can perform when these symptoms start to appear (*examples:* call your doctor; get your blood level tested; stick closely to your medication regimen; try to get regular sleep; get on a structured daily and nightly routine; avoid alcohol, drugs, or caffeine; give up your credit cards and car keys; avoid major financial or other life decisions; avoid risky sexual situations).

   _____

   _____

   _____

(continued)

5. List what behaviors *your relatives, significant others, or friends* can perform (*examples:* call your physician, talk to you in a supportive way, tell you what you are doing that worries them, tell you how much they care about you, keep you from overscheduling yourself, call the hospital emergency room, remind you to take your medications, accompany you to doctor's appointments, take care of your children, accompany you when you go out at night, help manage your money, help you stay on a regular sleep–wake cycle, help you stay away from alcohol or drugs).

_____

_____

_____

6. List what you would like your *psychiatrist* or your *therapist* to do (*examples:* meet with you on an emergency basis, check your lithium or valproate level, revise your medication regimen as appropriate, call the hospital and arrange for admittance [if needed], explain things to your family members).

_____

_____

_____

Signatures   Date

_____   _____

_____   _____

_____   _____

_____   _____

Troubleshooting Your Contract

Things improved for Robert after his hospital discharge. He found a new psychiatrist, Dr. Barnard, who met with him several times in the weeks after his discharge to help him optimize his medication regimen. Robert and Jessie also met with a psychologist who helped them develop a relapse prevention contract. Together they developed a list of his prodromal symptoms, which included mild irritability, mistrustfulness, standing too close to people and talking too loud, a sudden disinterest in his job, an increase in his sex drive, and a subjective feeling of mental clarity. They made a distinction between these early warning signs and signs of his full-blown manias, such as feeling elated or expansive, socially inappropriate outbursts of anger, spending excessively and impulsively, grandiose beliefs about his musical talents, severe loss of sleep, and a firm denial that anything was wrong. They also agreed on the environmental circumstances associated with his escalations: an excessive workload, family arguments, and financial problems.

Robert and Jessie negotiated a series of prevention steps. One of these involved giving Jessie the freedom to call his psychiatrist if Robert appeared to be escalating. They also agreed that when his symptoms were still mild, Jessie would help get him away from the immediate stressors (for example, encourage him to take a few days off of work with her). They agreed, as a couple, to try to maintain regular sleep–wake routines, especially when one or more of his prodromal signs were observable. Finally, Robert consented to have Jessie accompany him to the hospital emergency room, if it became necessary.

Robert did not stay episode free, however. His next manic episode began about 2 months later, but this time he and Jessie caught it earlier. Once again, he refused to make an appointment with his doctor. He admitted that he was probably escalating but didn't want to take any more medication. He and Jessie began to argue. As Robert later described it, Jessie became "rigid . . . finger-pointing, serious, not loving." Jessie got increasingly desperate when she found that Dr. Barnard was out of town. She called Dr. Barnard's backup, who prescribed an increase in the dosage of Robert's antipsychotic medicine, risperidone. Robert agreed to the medication adjustment, which kept him from going back into the hospital. Nonetheless, more damage was done to their relationship, and Jessie considered leaving. Robert also had more conflicts with his coworkers and other family members during this interval.

A meeting with his psychologist, arranged about a week after Robert changed his medication, focused on troubleshooting the relapse prevention plan. Robert, who was still hypomanic, complained that the plan hadn't worked because of Jessie's emotional stance. He said that he needed her to be "kinder and gentler" in her approach. The psychologist asked him to be more specific, and he said, "I want her to tell me she loves me, and in a more tender way tell me that she thinks I need help and why, even if I'm not receptive." He added that he wished she wouldn't take his irritability so personally and instead see it as part of his disorder. Jessie, in turn, expressed frustration that he hadn't gone to his medication appointments when Dr. Barnard had been in town: "I want him to go for me or for our relationship, if he won't do it for himself." She wasn't sure if she could take a gentler emotional stance when dealing with his escalating mood. "It's hard to smile at a bus that's about to run you over," she said.

The psychologist encouraged Robert and Jessie to practice communicating in the way the other wished: Jessie trying to be more tender in her approach and Robert ceding a degree of control to her. They also discussed the potential involvement of other family members, such as Robert's son, at times of emergencies. Robert decided, however, that he wanted to shield Brian as much as possible from his illness and didn't want his son interacting with his doctors. Jessie agreed.

When she returned from her trip, Dr. Barnard met with Robert and Jessie and told them of a medication plan to undertake if Robert had one or more prodromal signs and could not immediately get in to see her: increase his dosage of risperidone and add a benzodiazepine (Klonopin) for sleep. She wrote a prescription with a plan for increasing the dosage, with the understanding that Robert would come in to see her as soon as possible after initiating the new dosing schedule. These modifications were written into their modified contract (for example, "Robert to increase risperidone dosage; Robert to call his doctor or be willing to let Jessie make the call if he will not; Jessie to try to recognize Robert's irritability as part of the manic syndrome"). Robert and Jessie agreed to reexamine the contract every 3 months and revise it as necessary.

Robert has continued to have mood cycles, but his episodes increasingly resemble hypomanias rather than full-on manias. He feels he has a good relationship with Dr. Barnard and his psychologist, and he and Jessie are still together and working on their problems. He has explained his bipolar disorder to his son, who, with time, has become more understanding.

Think of your mania prevention contract as a work in progress. The prevention steps can be defined, agreed upon, and practiced when you're healthy, but no one can be certain how well they will work until you put them into action. Knowing your prodromal signs, being responsive to the feedback of others, and knowing when to ask for help are all central to making the contract effective in real life.

If you do have a manic episode despite your prevention contract, sit down with your doctor, family, or therapist after the dust has settled and try to decide what did and did not work. Were you unable to reach your physician or a backup physician? If so, ask your doctor to recommend medication adjustments that you can make on your own the next time you start to escalate. Ask him or her to write down your emergency medicine plan in prescription form, with the understanding that you will follow the plan when your early warning signs appear (for example, "increase my risperidone when I feel agitated and unable to sleep") and arrange an in-person meeting as soon as possible thereafter.

> **Effective solution:** If you have a manic episode despite having a prevention contract in place, take time afterward to review with your physician and therapist what went wrong and how the contract should be revised.

Were there other problems that prevented the contract from working? For example, were you hostile to significant others, who then threw up their hands and refused to help any further? Were your relatives unnecessarily controlling? Alternatively, did you ask for help but no one was available? If so, perhaps you can think of other relatives or friends to whom you are less likely to react negatively or who might be available with little notice.

Was the contract ineffective because you found the recommendations made by your significant others unacceptable? If so, how could the contract be modified to make these recommendations more palatable? For example, Gabriel refused to see a certain doctor whom his parents insisted he see. He was, however, willing to see a doctor he had found by himself. Being able to see his preferred doctor was added as a modification to his mania prevention contract. You will find that the contract has a much greater chance of succeeding if you have had input into each step, have listed choices of strategies rather than only one single strategy, and can troubleshoot and revise the contract as you go along.

• • • • • • • • • • • • • •

Because of the influences of your individual neurophysiology, you should not expect to be able to fully prevent manic episodes. *But you have a window of opportunity in the early stages of manic escalation in which you may be able to decrease the severity of your oncoming episode.* Being able to identify your episodes early and receive emergency treatment will give you a greater feeling of autonomy in the long run, even if it means having to give up control to others in the short run. A written contract, especially if it is developed and filled out when you are feeling well, will enhance the likelihood that your and others' prevention efforts are successful.

Depressive episodes have a different quality. They do not come on suddenly and often last longer than manic episodes. But as is true for mania, identifying and combating the early warning signs of depression will help you feel more in control of your disorder. In Chapter 10, you'll see how you can use the support of your core circle, along with certain personal strategies such as behavioral activation and cognitive restructuring, to try to keep your depressions from becoming more serious or debilitating.

Halting the Spiral of Depression

One day you realize that your entire life is just awful, not worth living, a horror and a black blot on the white terrain of human existence. *One morning you wake up afraid you are going to live. . . .* That's the thing I want to make clear about depression: It's got nothing at all to do with life. In the course of life, there is sadness and pain and sorrow, all of which, in their right time and season, are normal—unpleasant, but normal. Depression is in an altogether different zone because it involves a complete absence: absence of affect, absence of feeling, absence of response, absence of interest. The pain you feel in the course of a major clinical depression is an attempt on nature's part (nature, after all, abhors a vacuum) to fill up the empty space.
—ELIZABETH WURTZEL, *Prozac Nation* (1994, p. 22)

In bipolar disorder, depression can occur in "pure" form—in which you feel extremely sad, slowed down, lethargic, fatigued, or numb—or as part of a mixed episode, which means you feel both depressed and manic or hypomanic simultaneously. Many writers have described the despair of depression, both the bipolar and unipolar (major depressive) forms (for example, Jamison, 1995; Jamison, 2000a; Solomon, 2002; Styron, 1992). But most important from the vantage point of managing your own illness is being able to recognize the early warning signs that *your* depression is recurring. ***The central goal of this chapter is to give you psychological self-management techniques that you can use during the early phases of depression, before it becomes incapacitating.*** When self-management techniques improve your mood during these early stages, you may be able to avoid the medical interventions that are usually required when depression reaches its most severe point.

Medical interventions usually include antidepressant agents, higher dosages of mood stabilizers or antipsychotics, ECT, and hospitalization. As discussed in Chapter 6, some of these alternatives carry side effect risks, such as inadvertently eliciting rapid cycling of mood states. Nonetheless, it's essential to consult your physician about the medical alternatives available to you. Self-management and personal psychotherapy have a strong place in the treatment of severe depression, but usually in combination with medical interventions.

In the next chapter, I talk about suicidal episodes and how to combat them. Suicidal thoughts and impulses are a very common component of the bipolar syndrome. They are nothing to be ashamed of—virtually everyone with this disorder has thought about suicide at some point. Fortunately, there are ways to protect yourself from sinking further when you begin to feel hopeless.

Mostly, this chapter is about hope. Depression is a painful aspect of the human condition, and people with bipolar disorder experience it more intensely than virtually anyone else. To make matters worse, the emotional pain may not be obvious to those around you, and they may want you to just snap out of it. You can't do that, but there are some things you *can* do—often with the support of others—to help combat it.

Bipolar Depression: An Illness, Not a Character Flaw

Alexis, a 37-year-old woman with bipolar II disorder, had been dealing with an ongoing depressive state for years—a state that occasionally became worse and incapacitated her. She had tried to alleviate her depression through various antidepressants, medicinal herbs, cognitive therapy, group therapy, and, at times, "exercising to a fault . . . driving myself constantly until my body gave out." Her depressions were usually accompanied by self-accusations about being weak, not having the courage to face up to her problems, and not being able to accomplish her goals. She had heard that depression had a strong biological basis, especially in bipolar disorder, but had never really connected this fact to her situation.

A breakthrough occurred in her therapy when her clinician said to her, "If you had diabetes, would you be blaming yourself for not being able to control your blood sugar levels?" She began to entertain the idea that she needed to "make an end run around my depression" rather than trying to get rid of it and feeling like a failure for not being able to do so. When she started thinking of her depression as a physical illness that was caused by factors not entirely within her control—and something she needed to learn to live with—her mood began to improve, albeit gradually. She learned that accepting the reality of her depression was not the same as giving in to it or becoming immersed in it.

She eventually realized that, when depressed, she needed to slow down, take care of herself (sleep regularly and balance her pleasurable versus work activities), "give myself a break," and not try too hard to drive her depression away with frenetic activity. She has never been entirely free of depression, but now she has a different perspective: "I can now ignore those old tapes in my mind telling me I'm a bad person. I now see that this is the depression talking."

Depression as a Physical Condition

If you had a bad case of the flu, what would you do? Most of us would take time to convalesce and not expect too much of ourselves while recovering. Likewise, if you were suffering from chronic back pain, you would probably give yourself a break in terms of your physical expectations of yourself by declining to lift heavy objects, not sitting in the same position for hours, and selecting a "back-friendly" form of exercise. In all likelihood you would pay close attention to those things that helped alleviate your pain and avoid those that made it worse. Why don't we do the same for ourselves when we're in emotional pain? Emotional and social pain are processed by some of the same brain regions that process physical pain (Eisenberger, 2015).

Try to think of bipolar depression in the same way you would think of a flu, chronic pain, or perhaps a long-term medical illness such as diabetes. No one would think of blaming a person with diabetes for not being able to control the way his or her body processed sugar. No one would blame a person with epilepsy for having seizures, or a person with atherosclerosis for having a stroke. Likewise, you should not blame yourself for having depression. As discussed in Chapter 5, bipolar depression is strongly influenced by biochemical, genetic, and neurological (brain) variables. It is *not* the product of a character flaw, personality defect, or lack of moral fiber.

Even the well-known explanatory concept of depression as the result of low self-esteem is suspect when talking about bipolar depression. Many people think that if you're depressed, you must not think much of yourself. This low estimation might characterize the way you feel when you're depressed, but you may feel quite differently about yourself when you're well. In other words, low self-esteem is not a trait. Rather, it may just be a symptom of your depression. One of the leaders in our field, Dr. Martin Seligman of the University of Pennsylvania, has compared self-esteem to a fuel gauge: It is a measure of how we're doing at any one time—how much fuel is in the tank—which can change depending on what we are able to accomplish (Seligman, Reivich, Jaycox, & Gillham, 1996).

Depression is not due to an unwillingness to accept responsibility, fears of coping with reality, laziness, cowardice, or weakness. It is an illness. To be sure, there are things you can do to make yourself feel better or at least stop your depression from worsening. But the fact that you have depression in the first place, or that you're having a difficult time making it go away, probably says more about your brain and biology than it does about your effort, willpower, or self-esteem. Knowing this basic fact about bipolar depression will not make it disappear, but may make it easier to accept.

Different Styles of Coping with Depression

As you read through this chapter and the next, you'll see that I recommend a diverse set of techniques for coping with bipolar depression. These involve changes in your behavior and thinking as well as in your relationships with others. You'll see that some of the techniques involve distraction. *Distraction* means seeking out and engaging in activities that keep you busy, give you pleasure, draw your attention, and keep your mind off your pain and anguish. A related strategy is *behavioral activation,* in which you become more engaged with your environment, whether through outdoor exercise (for example, hiking, riding a bike), spending time with others whose company you enjoy, listening to music, reading, or visiting places that you haven't been before, even if that is just a local coffee shop. The rewards that come from increased activation can improve your mood such that you want to do these things more often.

Some of the coping strategies involve *emotion-focusing.* That is, you learn to recognize that you're depressed and experiencing pain and teach yourself to look at these emotions, label them, and accept them without becoming overwhelmed, as Alexis learned to do. This is what we refer to as *mindfulness.* Emotion-focused coping can also involve talking about your feelings with people who are supportive and empathic.

A fourth strategy, *cognitive coping,* involves learning to combat and challenge negative thinking patterns about specific situations or events (for example, self-blaming thoughts) and considering alternative ways to view these situations or events. As you'll see, these strategies are not mutually exclusive. In fact, the people who recover most rapidly from bipolar depressive episodes seem able to sample from all four, using different strategies at different times.

Are You Depressed Right Now?

Depression is not just sadness. As you know if you've had a serious depression, it can feel like a blunted, empty, or inhibited state marked by loss of interest in

---

Four Strategies for Combating Depression

- Distraction
- Behavioral activation
- Emotion-focusing/mindfulness
- Cognitive coping

most things, a difficulty or even inability to experience pleasure (anhedonia), and withdrawal from everybody and everything (see the quote by Elizabeth Wurtzel that opened this chapter). Some people don't even feel sad when they're depressed. Instead, they just feel numb or bored. If you've had mixed episodes, you're probably familiar with the feeling of being fatigued and drained but also charged up, irritable, and anxious ("tired but wired"). In the same way that mania is not always a happy state, depression is not only experienced as a sad state; it can be marked by anger and apprehension. Unlike mania, depression is almost never enjoyable or intoxicating.

Try filling out the Quick Inventory of Depressive Symptoms–Self-Report (Rush et al., 2003) on pages 256–258. This scale is intended to measure the severity of your depression as you've experienced it in the past week. Fill it out according to how you've felt most of the time (even if this past week was not typical) and tally your total score, which can range from 0 (not at all depressed) to over 21 (very depressed). The four answers to each item are coded from 0 to 3; you get the total test score by summing the following:

- The highest number (0 to 3) recorded for questions 1–4
- The number from question 5
- The highest number from questions 6–9
- The sum of your ratings for questions 10–14
- The highest number (0 to 3) from questions 15–16

Generally, people who have scores between 0 and 5 are not likely to be depressed. Those in the 6–10 range are mildly depressed; 11–15, moderately; 16–20, severely; and 21 or over, very severely depressed. If you are in the severe or very severe range, you will almost certainly need attention from your doctor or therapist; some people in this range require hospitalization. Scores lower than 20 often warrant treatment as well, both medical and psychological. Also, your score may change from one week to the next. This is the nature of depression, particularly of the bipolar type. Your score should not be influenced by whether you have bipolar I or II disorder.

If you scored in the mild-to-moderate range, the self-management techniques described in this chapter and the next will be particularly relevant to you right now. They may also be helpful if you are not feeling depressed (that is, below 6) but want to develop skills for preventing or alleviating episodes of depression in the future. If your score is in the severe range (over 15), you may want to try medications first; self-management techniques will be hardest to implement in this state.

Quick Inventory of Depressive Symptoms–Self-Report

Please circle the number next to the response to each item (0, 1, 2, or 3) that best describes how you have felt for the past 7 days.

1. Falling asleep:
   0 I never take longer than 30 minutes to fall asleep.
   1 I take at least 30 minutes to fall asleep, less than half the time.
   2 I take at least 30 minutes to fall asleep, more than half the time.
   3 I take at least 60 minutes to fall asleep, more than half the time.

2. Sleep during the night:
   0 I do not wake up at night.
   1 I have a restless, light sleep with a few brief awakenings each night.
   2 I wake up at least once a night, but I go back to sleep easily.
   3 I awaken more than once a night and stay awake for 20 minutes or more, more than half the time.

3. Waking up too early:
   0 Most of the time, I awaken no more than 30 minutes before I need to get up.
   1 More than half the time, I awaken more than 30 minutes before I need to get up.
   2 I almost always awaken at least one hour or so before I need to, but I go back to sleep eventually.
   3 I awaken at least one hour before I need to, and can't go back to sleep.

4. Sleeping too much:
   0 I sleep no longer than 7–8 hours/night, without napping during the day.
   1 I sleep no longer than 10 hours in a 24-hour period including naps.
   2 I sleep no longer than 12 hours in a 24-hour period including naps.
   3 I sleep longer than 12 hours in a 24-hour period including naps.

5. Feeling sad:
   0 I do not feel sad.
   1 I feel sad less than half the time.
   2 I feel sad more than half the time.
   3 I feel sad nearly all the time.

6. Decreased appetite:
   0 My usual appetite has not decreased.
   1 I eat somewhat less often or lesser amounts of food than usual.
   2 I eat much less than usual and only with personal effort.
   3 I rarely eat within a 24-hour period, and only with extreme personal effort or when others persuade me to eat.

(continued)

7. Increased appetite:

   0 My usual appetite has not increased.

   1 I feel a need to eat more frequently than usual.

   2 I regularly eat more often and/or greater amounts of food than usual.

   3 I feel driven to overeat both at mealtime and between meals.

8. Decreased weight (within the last 2 weeks):

   0 My weight has not decreased.

   1 I feel as if I've had a slight weight loss.

   2 I have lost 2 pounds or more.

   3 I have lost 5 pounds or more.

9. Increased weight (within the last 2 weeks):

   0 My weight has not increased.

   1 I feel as if I've had a slight weight gain.

   2 I have gained 2 pounds or more.

   3 I have gained 5 pounds or more.

10. Concentration/decision making:

   0 There is no change in my usual capacity to concentrate or make decisions.

   1 I occasionally feel indecisive or find that my attention wanders.

   2 Most of the time, I struggle to focus my attention or to make decisions.

   3 I cannot concentrate well enough to read or cannot make even minor decisions.

11. View of myself:

   0 I see myself as equally worthwhile and deserving as other people.

   1 I am more self-blaming than usual.

   2 I largely believe that I cause problems for others.

   3 I think almost constantly about major and minor defects in myself.

12. Thoughts of death or suicide:

   0 I do not think of suicide or death.

   1 I feel that life is empty or wonder if it's worth living.

   2 I think of suicide or death several times a week for several minutes.

   3 I think or suicide or death several times a day in some detail, or have actually tried to take my life.

13. General interest:

   0 There is no change from usual in how interested I am in other people or activities.

   1 I notice that I am less interested in people or activities.

   2 I find I have interest in only one or two of my formerly pursued activities.

   3 I have virtually no interest in formerly pursued activities.

(continued)

14. Energy level:

   0 There is no change in my usual level of energy.

   1 I get tired more easily than usual.

   2 I have to make a big effort to start or finish my usual daily activities (for example, shopping, homework, cooking, or going to work).

   3 I really cannot carry out most of my usual daily activities because I just don't have the energy.

15. Feeling slowed down:

   0 I think, speak, and move at my usual rate of speed.

   1 I find that my thinking is slowed down or my voice sounds dull or flat.

   2 It takes me several seconds to respond to most questions and I'm sure my thinking is slowed.

   3 I am often unable to respond to questions without extreme effort.

16. Feeling restless:

   0 I do not feel restless.

   1 I'm often fidgety, wringing my hands, or need to shift how I am sitting.

   2 I have impulses to move about and am quite restless.

   3 At times, I am unable to stay seated and need to pace around.

How Does Your Depression Wax and Wane?

Depression comes and goes in different ways for different people. It is helpful to know that for some people depressive onsets are dramatic, whereas for others the onsets are subtle and slow. If your onsets are gradual, it may not always be clear to you (or your significant others) whether you are having a new episode or the continuation of an existing one. With experience, you may learn to distinguish minor differences over time in the severity of your depressed mood or your energy and activity levels.

In the first type, which I call the *classic recurrent* type, a full-bore depression or mixed disorder develops (1) when you've been functioning at your baseline (your mood when you are between episodes, even if you are not symptom-free), or (2) just after a manic or hypomanic episode, reflecting the downward cycle of the illness. The onset of this depressive episode is usually not as sudden as the onset of a new episode of mania or hypomania. Instead, it involves a gradual winding down of your mood state over a period of days, weeks, or even months, until you reach a state of full clinical depression or mixed disorder. For some people the onset can be tied to specific life events (see Chapter 5).

PERSONALIZED CARE TIP:

Am I in a depressed or a mixed episode?
Is my depression related to bipolar I or II?

Understanding the diagnostic significance of your depressive episodes, such as whether they are mixed, can be an important strategy in treatment planning with your doctor. As I said in Chapter 6, having mixed episodes usually means that you will do better with anticonvulsants and second-generation antipsychotics than with antidepressants. But keep in mind that people mean different things when they use the term *mixed*. In my usage, it refers to a state in which you have a full depressive episode (lasting 2 or more weeks) combined with three or more symptoms of mania or hypomania (for example, depressed and irritable mood with loss of interests, fatigue, suicidal thinking, and poor concentration plus decreased need for sleep, pressured speech, and impulsive spending). It can also mean that you have a full manic or hypomanic episode with three or more co-occurring depressed symptoms. Some health care professionals refer to subthreshold episodes as mixed, such as when you have a depression that lasts only 1 week and is combined with increased activity, grandiose thinking, and distractibility that lasts only 2–3 days.

Another question that people frequently revisit during their depressive states is "Am I bipolar I or II?" Many people with bipolar II wonder if the severity of their depression means that they actually have bipolar I. In fact, it doesn't seem to matter: depressive episodes in bipolar II are just as severe as those in bipolar I, and you can't really tell them apart on the basis of symptoms or duration of episodes. As explained in Chapters 2 and 3, the real difference between bipolar I and II lies in the severity of the manic pole of the illness—people with bipolar II only experience hypomanic episodes, which are shorter and less impairing than bipolar I manic episodes.

In the other type of depressive onset, called *double depression,* you have an ongoing and persistent state of sadness (dysthymia) that may have been present for years and is quite unpleasant but still allows you to function. Then a major depressive episode develops on top of this state of dysthymia. This new episode of bipolar depression is kind of a "slow burn": it develops gradually and perniciously, almost imperceptibly from day to day. When this severe depression remits, you may return to a milder state of depression or dysthymia rather than to a depression-free state. This cycle can be quite frustrating and demoralizing.

Notice that in describing these course patterns, I don't refer to depression as a change from normal mood. In my experience, most people with bipolar disorder do not ever feel like they get to a state of normal mood. In fact, they feel that their moods are always fluctuating. Many say that they are always somewhat depressed. Of course, it's not entirely clear what normal mood means for the typical person—some people seem to feel fine most of the time, whereas others are always somewhat anxious and on edge, angry, bored, or disappointed by things. Having a chronic, low-grade depressed mood can be a personality or temperamental type (remember Eeyore, from *Winnie-the-Pooh*?).

Whether you have classic recurrent or double depression, it is important to be able to recognize your prodromal signs of a new episode—the early indicators that your mood state is changing. If you live in an ongoing state of persistent, low-grade depression, the prodromal signs of a new depressive episode will be more subtle than those experienced by people with classic recurrent depressions and will mainly reflect changes in the *degree* to which you experience depressive symptoms (for example, the seriousness of your suicidal thoughts or the degree to which you feel sapped of energy). Nonetheless, knowing how to cope or ask for help when these changes appear can be central to your recovery and well-being. You may be able to implement the self-care strategies in this chapter to keep the depression from worsening or to make your "rebound" depression more tolerable. Keep these goals in mind—*the fact that your depression doesn't disappear entirely is not a sign that you have failed in your attempts to cope with it* (see the example of Alexis earlier in this chapter).

How Do You Know If You're Getting More Depressed? The Mood Spiral

One symptom of depression seems to feed on others: negative moods like sadness and anxiety, along with the physical symptoms of depression like lethargy or insomnia, produce negative thinking (for example, negative self-statements, the harshly critical, accusatory voice in your head), and this negative thinking fuels low moods. The combination of negative moods, thought patterns, and physical changes can make you feel less motivated to try hard, which can make you withdraw and, in turn, worsen your negative thinking and mood, in a pattern called the mood spiral. Consider the following experiences of two people with bipolar depressions.

Denise, a 27-year-old with bipolar II disorder, was typically mildly depressed and pessimistic in her day-to-day life, despite being loyal to her regimen of lamotrigine (Lamictal) and paroxetine (Paxil, an antidepressant). Her more serious depressions had a gradual but predictable course. Her first sign of a depressive recurrence was ruminating about things that were realistic but blown out of proportion. In the weeks leading up to her most recent episode, she felt slighted by a colleague at work (in the company of others, he had raised his voice and took a tone with her that, she felt, made it sound like he was talking to a child). She was angry at herself for not having responded adequately to the slight. She expanded the significance of this relatively minor event into thinking that no one at work liked her and that her coworkers thought she was incompetent. She became very self-critical, claiming it was her lack of social skills that led others to dislike her. Her depressed mood worsened, and she had more and more difficulty going to work. Her performance started to deteriorate, and she developed insomnia. Sick days followed. Eventually she took a leave from her job and became inactive and withdrawn in her home. At this point she became suicidal.

Denise eventually came out of her depression through a combination of medication changes (for example, an increased dosage of her Lamictal) and regular psychotherapy. In addition to identifying and challenging her negative self-statements concerning her work performance and how others judged her, her therapist assigned her behavioral activation exercises, including spending time with friends and neighbors, various forms of light physical exercise, and activities that involved her young niece, with whom she was close.

Carlos, age 35, had bipolar I disorder with classic recurrent depressions. He'd had numerous episodes and learned to recognize the symptoms that signaled the onset of a depressive episode with mixed features. His prodromal signs took the form of mild fatigue, sleepiness, and poor concentration. These signs were usually intermixed with feelings of anxiety, dread, and a restless "jumping out of my skin" feeling.

Fortunately, when he had been well, Carlos and his therapist had put into place a prevention plan for staving off his worst symptoms. His plan included getting on a regular bedtime/wake-up routine, eating more protein and fewer carbohydrates, avoiding alcohol and marijuana, scheduling at least one contact each day with a person who could give him positive input, and taking breaks from work when he needed to. He also kept a "thought record" (see page 275) in which he recorded examples of self-blaming statements or overgeneralizations about his situation (for example, "My life has never had any joy or fulfillment"). He learned to counter these thoughts with more adaptive ones ("I'm going through a tough time . . . I've dealt with this before and come out of it . . . Depression is going to color the way I feel about things").

The form on page 262 will help you list the prodromal signs of your depression (your mood spiral). The list is not exhaustive, and spaces are left for symptoms that are not included here. In completing the form, try to think back to the last time you became depressed. If you are currently depressed, you may be able to recall the earliest phases of this depression. What were its first signs? If you were already depressed when the new episode developed, how did you know things were getting worse? As you did when listing your prodromal signs of mania (Chapter 9), include the input of your spouse or another family member or friend who observed you during the early phases of your current depression.

Listing Your Prodromal Signs of Depression

List a couple of adjectives describing what your *mood* is like when your depressive episodes first begin (*examples:* sad, anxious, fearful, irritable, grouchy, downhearted, blue, "blah," flat, numb, bored).

Describe changes in your *activity* and *energy* levels as your depressive episodes develop (*examples:* feeling slowed down, withdrawing from people, moving more slowly, talking more slowly, doing fewer things, having little or no sex drive, feeling fatigued, feeling "tired but wired").

_____

_____

_____

_____

Describe changes in your *thinking* and *perception* (*examples:* thoughts go more slowly; can't get interested in things; colors seem drab; people look like they're moving too fast; feel self-doubting, self-critical, or self-blaming; feel guilty; regret past deeds; feel hopeless; concentrate poorly; feel dumb; can't make decisions; think about hurting or killing myself; ruminate and worry about things).

_____

_____

_____

_____

_____

Describe changes in your *sleep* patterns (*examples:* wanting to sleep more or later, waking up repeatedly in the middle of the night, waking up an hour or two earlier than usual and not being able to fall back to sleep).

_____

_____

_____

_____

Describe anything else that seems different when you're getting depressed.

_____

_____

_____

_____

Notice how the prodromal signs of depression differ from the signs of mania discussed in Chapter 9. The depressive warning signals usually involve feeling slowed down, pessimistic, unmotivated, uninterested, mentally sluggish, and hopeless. The mania signals involve feeling sped up, goal driven, energized, mentally swift, and, often, overly optimistic or grandiose. Some people experience the buildup of mania and the descent into depression simultaneously, culminating in a mixed episode.

Keep your list of depression warning signs in a place where you can find it later. If you feel your mood or energy level start to shift, refer back to the list to see if you are experiencing the buildup of a new episode. You can then move on to introducing self-care strategies when one or more of these signs appears. As you did with your mania list, share this list with your close relatives (your spouse or partner, trusted friends, parents) so that they can learn to recognize when you're getting depressed and how they might be able to help (for example, listen supportively, look after your kids, provide a distraction, help you stay active).

Self-Care Strategy No. 1: Behavioral Activation

> *"When I get depressed, it's hard for me to even be out in public. I withdraw, I get tired, I think in very black-and-white terms, I discount anything good that happens. But I've learned not to give up and go back to my lair. I know that 12 in the afternoon is my worst time, so I force myself to go to the gym then. I just pray no one will talk to me. On other days I'll just have coffee with a friend. It's tough, I dread it, I feel like I'm so down and I can't do this, I just can't. But, without a doubt, it helps me."*
> —A 41-year-old woman with bipolar II disorder

Behavioral activation is a treatment used by itself or in combination with cognitive therapy or mindfulness treatment (Martell, Dimidjian, & Herman-Dunn, 2010). There are two assumptions behind behavioral activation. First, depression results in a loss of pleasurable activities or *positive reinforcements*. That is, being depressed makes you less likely to do the sorts of things that will help you get something positive from your environment. Second, the lack of these reinforcements worsens your depression and makes you want to withdraw even more. It is certainly true that being depressed makes it very difficult to get yourself to do anything. But it's equally true that, in combination with your biological predispositions, not engaging with your environment keeps you depressed and eventually makes you feel worse.

Depression has a way of spoiling your experience of things you used to love to do. They just don't seem fun anymore. Sometimes the events that make you depressed (for example, the ending of a relationship) result in limiting your contact with people whose company you used to enjoy and decreasing your access to activities that used to give you pleasure. All of this will make you feel like withdrawing.

When you're depressed, it's certainly understandable that you'll want to stay in bed, sit at home, and avoid people. You may have to from time to time. But if this state of inactivity comes to dominate your life, your depression will only get more severe. As noted psychologist Peter Lewinsohn put it, "The more we do, the less depressed we feel; and the less depressed we feel, the more we will feel encouraged to do things" (Lewinsohn, Muñoz, Youngren, & Zeiss, 1992, p. 74).

The goal behind behavioral activation is to try to increase your contact with your physical and social environment, to the point where you start feeling better about yourself. Of course, you need a regular slate of routines and pleasurable activities even when you're well (Chapter 8), but it's especially important to introduce activating exercises when you recognize a worsening state of depression. In this section, I'll give you a brief set of instructions for implementing the behavioral activation method.

Make a List of Pleasurable Activities

Start by examining the previous week or, if you prefer, take notes on yourself for the forthcoming week. Your mood chart should help you track information about your daily habits. Ask yourself the following:

- "Are my days characterized by a lack of structure?"
- "Are there long periods of time when I have nothing to do?"
- "Are there particular points during the day when I feel down?"
- "Are the mornings long expanses, with nothing to look forward to?"
- "Do I dread the weekend because there is nothing to do?"
- "Do I sleep more than I need to because there is nothing I want to do?"
- [If you are working or going to school] "Is the beginning of the work or school day inviting just because it gets me out of the house?"

Alternatively:

- "Have my days been dominated by too many activities, most of which are required by my work or family life but which I don't find rewarding?"
- "Has there been a good balance between pleasant activities and 'must do' activities?"
- "Am I engaged in enough positive, rewarding activities to keep my mood from spiraling downward?"

Next try to list as many pleasurable or engaging activities as you can in the form on page 265. It can be hard to think of pleasurable things to do when you're depressed, but filling out the form will get you started. At the bottom you'll find a list of examples of activities many people find pleasurable when they're feeling down. List all of the activities that could be pleasurable for you, even if they don't seem feasible (for example, you may really enjoy fishing, but there is nowhere to fish nearby). Some people find self-awareness exercises, such as mindful breathing, to be relaxing and stress relieving (see "A 3-Minute Mindfulness Breathing Exercise," on page 266). You may want to try these as well.

If you'd like to learn more about using mindfulness meditation as a coping strategy, I recommend *The Mindful Way Through Depression* by Williams, Teasdale, Segal, and Kabat-Zinn (2007), which will take you through numerous meditation practices, of which this one is just an example. See also *The Mindful Way Workbook* by Teasdale, Williams, and Segal (2014).

Listing Pleasurable Activities

List as many activities as you can think of that you would find rewarding and pleasurable. Include activities that keep you engaged with other people, activities that increase your sense of competence, and activities that might allow you to experience emotions other than depression.

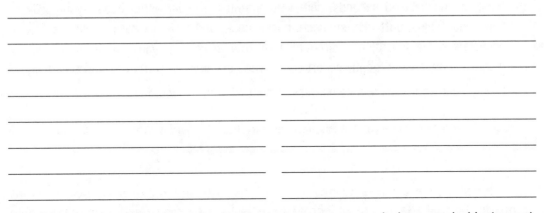

(*Examples:* taking a walk, going to a church or synagogue group, playing a musical instrument, walking the dog, watching a TV program, watching a sports event, going to the library, talking on the phone to a friend, talking to a therapist, playing a sport, watching a comedy movie, having sex, riding a bicycle, visiting the Humane Society, listening to music, practicing a hobby, sitting in a café, going on a social media site, cooking, driving, sewing, dancing, working at a homeless shelter, writing in a journal, taking photographs, taking a class, painting or drawing, soaking in the bathtub, eating at a restaurant, listening to a relaxation tape, shopping, hiking, gardening, praying, meditating, going for a swim, eating lunch outside, attending a lecture, washing your face or hair, lying in the sun, playing with a pet)

Source: Lewinsohn et al. (1992).

A 3-Minute Mindfulness Breathing Exercise

Behavioral activation strategies can be supplemented by exercises that get you in touch with your body, your breathing, and your surroundings within the present moment, or what we call "mindful awareness." Try the following the next time you feel mildly anxious or down:

Find a comfortable chair to sit in: sit with your back upright and your hands on your thighs, not touching the back of the chair. You can also lie on your back.

- Close your eyes or stare at an object in the room. Spend 60 seconds being aware of the noises in your room—the sound of the air conditioner or heating, sounds from the street, music, people's voices. Ask yourself, "What am I experiencing in my thoughts, my emotions, and my body?" Acknowledge to yourself each sensation, thought, or feeling, whether pleasant or unpleasant.

- Now, for the next 60 seconds, focus on your breathing. Keep focusing on your in-breath and out-breath, like you were riding a wave. It's inevitable that your mind will wander. If your attention shifts to thinking of other things, notice what took you away but gently escort your mind back to your breathing.

- Now, for the next 60 seconds, shift your attention to your entire body—your belly, feet, legs, thighs, buttocks, stomach, chest, neck, and facial expression. Notice your posture and the sensation in different parts of your body as you breathe in and out. If your mind wanders, gently escort your awareness back to your body and breathing.

- Slowly open your eyes and come back in contact with the room.

Adapted by permission from Segal, Williams, and Teasdale (2012). Copyright © 2012 by The Guilford Press.

Just because you list a number of activities doesn't mean you should try to do all of them. In fact, the objective here is first to make a list of pleasurable activities and then introduce one at a time, without crowding yourself or feeling stressed by having to do too much. Make a particular effort to list activities that have the potential to (1) keep you engaged with other people and make you feel valued (for example, hiking with a friend), (2) give you a sense of competence and purpose (for example, taking piano lessons or a foreign-language class), and (3) make you likely to experience emotions other than depression (for example, watching a humorous movie, being out in nature, riding a bicycle). Keep in mind that what is pleasurable to other people may not be pleasurable to you, and vice versa (see the extended list provided by Lewinsohn et al. [1992] in *Control Your Depression*). Try to list only activities that you want to do and know you would enjoy.

Scheduling Pleasurable Activities

Next choose one or two activities from this list to do each day of the next week (see the "Scheduling Pleasurable Activities" form on page 268). Pick the day you will do each activity and set a target time in the "Day of the Week" column. If you feel that one activity per day is too much, choose one to do every other day or even one every week and build up from there. If you're feeling very depressed or low in energy, pick easier activities such as putting on a favorite piece of clothing, taking a bath, or spending 5 minutes outside in the sun. It will feel therapeutic to be able to do something small for yourself each day, or every few days, when it feels impossible to do more.

Some activities and events require coordination of your and other people's schedules, extensive travel, money, and reservations made well in advance (for example, concert tickets). You may find it easier to choose activities that do not require such planning. Perhaps activities that require planning can be introduced later.

Try to pick activities that will not disrupt your work (or school) routine or your sleep–wake cycle. For example, if you like to exercise, avoid doing it in the evening because it can keep you awake. If you enjoy conversations with a specific person but feel wired or energized by these talks, avoid them after a certain time of night. If you have discovered interesting connections with people through social media, do not start doing this right before you go to bed. At first, try not to be too ambitious in scheduling activities early in the morning. If you scheduled multiple events for the same time interval and miss the first one, try to forge ahead with the other ones.

> **Effective prevention:** Engaging with your social and physical environment—behavioral activation planning—can help halt the downward spiral of depression. When implementing new rewarding activities, it's good to push yourself, but recognize that you may not be able to do each new activity every day. Give yourself plenty of room to adjust the plan.

Next, record the actual time of day that you completed each activity. Record your mood on the –3 (severely depressed) to +3 (severely manic) scale that you used for your mood chart. Rate your mood before you begin the activity and again as soon as you are finished. For example, if your activity is gardening, record how you felt just prior to going out to the garden and then give yourself another rating for the hour or so after finishing. Make copies of this form (or download and print; see the end of the Contents for information) before filling it out so that you can use it in subsequent weeks.

Notice that I've asked you to keep track of your high as well as your low moods. As you know from previous chapters, certain activities can contribute to manic symptoms. For example, exercise generally improves a person's moods, but some people exercise to excess and become hypomanic. It's important to keep data on yourself so that you can determine whether certain activities improve your mood or "overcorrect."

Scheduling Pleasurable Activities

Day of the week and target time	Pleasurable activities	Actual time of day each activity was done	Mood before and after each activity (−3 to +3)	
			(Before)	(After)
Monday	1. _____ _____	1. _____	_____	_____
	2. _____ _____	2. _____	_____	_____
Tuesday	1. _____ _____	1. _____	_____	_____
	2. _____ _____	2. _____	_____	_____
Wednesday	1. _____ _____	1. _____	_____	_____
	2. _____ _____	2. _____	_____	_____
Thursday	1. _____ _____	1. _____	_____	_____
	2. _____ _____	2. _____	_____	_____
Friday	1. _____ _____	1. _____	_____	_____
	2. _____ _____	2. _____	_____	_____
Saturday	1. _____ _____	1. _____	_____	_____
	2. _____ _____	2. _____	_____	_____
Sunday	1. _____ _____	1. _____	_____	_____
	2. _____ _____	2. _____	_____	_____

Effective treatment: Savoring positive emotions

There are strategies you can use to prolong the good feelings associated with pleasant events. "Savoring" is a meditative practice that refers to attending to, focusing on, and becoming aware of your positive feelings while they are occurring (regardless of what caused them) (Bryant & Veroff, 2007). So, if you are sitting outdoors with someone you like and looking out at the ocean or mountains, be attentive to the positive sensations, thoughts, and feelings that occur in that moment and try to make them last. For example, perhaps your heart is beating faster—experience the feelings of your heart beating and remind yourself that a faster heart rate can mean excitement. If negative thoughts intervene (for example, "Ugh, I have so much to do after this"), simply be aware that your mind went there and gently bring yourself back to the present moment. If you are comfortable, tell your friend about the feelings. Avoid judging yourself on your ability to make this work—savoring is a practice that can take time to learn.

Troubleshooting Your Plan

After scheduling pleasurable activities for a week or more, evaluate whether the plan is working. Are your mood ratings more positive on the days in which you did one or more of the activities? To determine this, complete the "Impact of Your Behavior Activation Plan" form on page 270, in which you rate each day in the last week on the –3 to +3 scale (used in the mood chart) and make a check mark next to the days in which you completed at least one of your activities. If your mood varied considerably during any given day, use the rating that you think best characterizes the whole day, rather than how you felt at a particularly tough moment. Then calculate an average mood rating for the days that you did, and did not, complete your activities. You should be able to tell from this overview whether your activity plan has had a beneficial impact on your mood in the last week. (You can download and print extra copies of the form; see the end of the Contents for information.)

If your plan is not working yet, consider the possibility that you are choosing events that are too hard, that require too much planning, or that you don't really enjoy. For example, if you have included taking a foreign-language class but don't really like the process of learning a language, you may not want to include this activity. Also, consider the balance between activities you must do and those you really want to do. If your depression is related to the absence of pleasurable events as well as the avoidance of unpleasant activities that have to be done (for example, sweeping the garage, preparing your taxes), introduce a combination of pleasurable and required activities into your schedule. Start slowly: if you are severely or even moderately depressed, it may not be possible to schedule a "must-do" activity every day. Work your way up to a reasonable balance, such as two pleasurable activities and one required activity per day.

Impact of Your Behavior Activation Plan

Day of the week	Things you did that day	Mood that day (−3 to +3)	Check (✓) if you followed your activity plan
Monday	_____	_____	_____
Tuesday	_____	_____	_____
Wednesday	_____	_____	_____
Thursday	_____	_____	_____
Friday	_____	_____	_____
Saturday	_____	_____	_____
Sunday	_____	_____	_____

Average mood rating for the days you followed your plan _____

Average mood rating for the days you did not follow your plan _____

PERSONALIZED CARE TIP:
Finding the right balance in a behavioral activation plan

In the midst of a depressive episode it can be quite difficult to initiate a social activity (for example, going to a movie with a friend). Avoid pushing yourself too hard. Start with a couple of nonsocial activities you find easy to do and work up from there. So, you can replace "finding an evening art opening to attend" with "going to a coffee shop and working on my laptop," whether or not you decide to interact with others. If you start to feel overwhelmed by your weekly schedule, adjust your activity level downward: have some regularly unscheduled time, spread tasks out across the week, and cancel social plans if you need to. Use your knowledge of your internal state (hopefully made sharper by mood and sleep charting) to implement a plan that works for you (Suto, Murray, Hale, Amari, & Michalak, 2010).

If things have gone well for you so far, and you've noticed that your mood has improved (or, at minimum, your prodromal depressive symptoms haven't worsened), start introducing more pleasurable activities into various parts of your day. You may find, for example, that you feel better if you have something pleasurable to do during the lunch hour (for example, sitting at an outdoor picnic table) as well as something to look forward to when you get home from work, school, or other activities (for example, playing a musical instrument, taking a walk). If you are not working or going to school, it's especially important to have rewarding activities at the beginning and end of the day so that some structure is introduced into your routines.

The behavioral activation method may seem somewhat superficial or too obvious. You may feel, "Of *course* I should be doing those things—the problem is that I *can't!*" When your depression is gradually worsening, it becomes especially important to reengage with your environment and do the things that give you a different experience of your emotions. The key is not to push yourself too hard with these activities. Don't try to do too many all at once. At first, pick a few you can do easily (for example, taking a short walk, listening to music, taking a bath, drawing,

---

New research: How effective are behavioral activation strategies?

A new study conducted in Goa, a state on the west coast of India, sheds light on the effectiveness of behavioral activation strategies in another cultural setting (Weobong et al., 2017). The investigators randomly assigned 493 people treated in 10 primary health care settings for moderate or severe depression (though not necessarily bipolar disorder) to either a Healthy Activities Program (HAP) or Enhanced Usual Care (EUC). The HAP consisted of six to eight therapy sessions to promote engagement and activation in pleasurable events. The sessions included education about depression and its effects on motivation, activity scheduling, increasing contact with social networks, and problem solving. Importantly, the HAP was delivered by lay counselors who had no formal mental health training. The EUC did not involve any changes to usual patient care, although treating physicians were given instructions on when to refer the patient for additional psychiatric care. Few of the study participants received antidepressants.

Over 12 months, the participants who received the HAP had lower depression ratings and higher frequencies of remission (that is, they became symptom-free) than those in EUC. Those who received the HAP were also less suicidal over time. The program appears to work fast: most of the gains were in the first 3 months of treatment. It appears that becoming engaged with one's environment, particularly one's social network, can have lasting effects on depression. Behavioral activation has not been tested in a randomized trial in bipolar disorder, but we may see such studies in the coming years.

bird-watching, playing cards). Then work on building up to a reasonable number each day, until you find yourself looking forward to the next day because of the pleasant activities you've scheduled. Troubleshoot the plan at the end of each week to determine why it didn't work. On your first few tries, you probably won't be able to complete certain aspects of the plan. Try not to get discouraged; it may take a few weeks to formulate a plan that really works for you.

Even if it sounds simple, you may be surprised at how well your plan helps to prevent your depression from spiraling. In all likelihood, you'll get a feeling of mastery from making your plan work, which will make you want to extend it further.

Self-Care Strategy No. 2: Cognitive Restructuring

You are probably aware that mood states are affected by the things you tell yourself—by what we call *cognitions* or *self-statements*. Many studies have shown that negative thinking is associated with depressed and anxious moods. People with depression may have negative *core beliefs* about themselves (for example, "I'm not a likable person"), about people in general (for example, "People are generally motivated by selfish concerns"), and about their future ("I'm never going to accomplish my goals, be loved, or be healthy"). CBT for depression is based on the assumption that certain events provoke distorted *automatic negative thoughts* that reflect core beliefs about one's unworthiness or unlovability (Beck, Rush, Shaw, & Emery, 1987). These automatic thoughts and core beliefs are important in causing and maintaining depressed mood and behaviors (for example, withdrawing from others). In cognitive restructuring, you hold your assumptions up to the light to see if they are logical and accurate or if there are other ways to make sense of your experiences. You may recall my discussion of CBT in Chapter 6; it is one of the most effective treatments for major depression and anxiety disorders.

The relationship between thoughts and mood states is probably not one-way: depressed moods also generate distorted thoughts and increase a person's access to negative memories or images. Mark Williams and his group at Oxford University (Williams, Russell, & Russell, 2008) have proposed that negative mood states, even when minor, increase access to negative "networks" of information that then worsen our mood, culminating in more serious episodes of depression. In turn, learning to modify negative thoughts and replace them with more adaptive or balanced cognitions—or, at minimum, learning to observe your thoughts and gain some distance from them—can go a long way toward alleviating your negative mood states.

Cognitive restructuring involves a sequence of techniques. First, you identify the automatic thoughts or self-statements associated with certain disturbing situations or life events and link these thoughts with your mood states. You will probably find that certain thoughts or images are more powerful than others in provoking your emotional reactions ("hot" cognitions). Sometimes, hot cognitions take the form of pessimistic predictions about the future (for example, "I will always be isolated and feel lonely"). Second, you evaluate the evidence for and against these automatic thoughts or predictions. Next, based on this for/against evaluation, you learn to replace your original thoughts with self-statements that provide a more balanced interpretation of your experiences. Last, you observe the effects of these new self-statements on your mood.

Cognitive restructuring has been criticized as being superficial or formulaic. (It was lampooned on *Saturday Night Live,* where a self-help guru named Stuart Smalley offered "daily affirmations" such as "I'm good enough, I'm smart enough, and doggone it, people like me"). But CBT is *not* a matter of blithely replacing bad thoughts with good ones. *Instead, it involves thinking up alternative or more balanced ways of understanding the things that have happened to you and looking at your situation from a number of different vantage points.* A simple example: some people automatically blame themselves when someone else treats them badly, without considering the possibility that this other person is having a bad day or behaves in a similar manner with other people.

In this section, I describe the method of cognitive restructuring and outline exercises to help you learn it. Like pleasurable activity scheduling, cognitive restructuring will probably have its greatest power once you have noticed the appearance of one or more depressive prodromal symptoms, before your depression gets really severe. It's much harder to identify or challenge negative thoughts when you are in the midst of a severe depression. If you want to explore this method further, I suggest consulting the workbook *Mind Over Mood* by Dennis Greenberger and Christine Padesky (2015).

Step 1: Identifying Negative Thoughts: Jake

Jake, age 49, struggled with severe bipolar depressive episodes that sometimes took on mixed features such as rapid, ruminative thinking and an agitated, driven feeling. His major episodes were often preceded by several short periods of low mood brought on by seemingly minor events. When he was feeling well, he was a popular coach of a children's soccer team. But when he felt he'd had a bad day of coaching (for example, his concentration had been poor or the kids had not responded to his suggestions), his mood would sink. He became aware of a self-statement that went like this: "I'm just no good with kids. I have major character flaws that they can see in me." Sometimes, just the word character would pop into his mind, and he would feel his mood drop. Character became a hot cognition closely tied to his depressive mood states.

There had been a few minor run-ins with parents that he had exaggerated in his mind, such as when the father of one of the team players had snapped at Jake for not allowing his son more time on the field. Mostly, Jake was quite good with children, and the kids and parents on his team frequently expressed their appreciation of him. Nonetheless, his thinking and resulting mood contributed to his growing desire to quit coaching altogether. When asked to recount why he thought he had a bad character, he tended to focus on one or more mistakes he had made and magnify or overgeneralize these mistakes ("I was impatient with one of my kids. I was too hard on him. I can't work well with people because I can't be patient with myself").

The first step in cognitive restructuring is to become aware of the thoughts, images, or memories that crop up when you have experiences that worsen your mood. Be particularly attuned to experiences involving your work, family, or close relationships. Take a look at the thought record form on page 275, which we'll be completing throughout this section. Pick out three negative (or perhaps annoying) experiences you've had in the past week and record them in the table (column 1). Rate the intensity of your mood (column 2) in reaction to these events on a scale of 0% (not depressed) to 100% (very depressed). (Alternatively, use the –3 to +3 scale if you're more comfortable with that format.) List other moods you may also be feeling (for example, anxiety) and rate their intensity. Try to distinguish how you felt during or immediately after the event, not how you felt that entire day.

Now see if you can recall any negative self-statements that came into your head right before you started feeling bad, or notice and record any that come into your mind now as you review the events. Write these in the "Automatic Thoughts" column. To help you "snag" these statements or automatic thoughts, try to be attuned to questions like these:

- "Why did this event happen?"
- "What was going through my mind just before I started to feel this way?"
- "What does this event say about me or what others think of me?"
- "What does this mean will happen in my future?"
- "What is the worst possible reason this could have happened?"

Don't be surprised if you're not immediately aware of any thoughts or images. You may find that you can't quite remember how you felt or what you thought after a particular event. If you are having trouble remembering, practice by focusing on recent events that caused you to have strong emotional reactions (for example, rejections from a romantic partner, run-ins with people, problems with your boss at work). These events are probably most closely associated with certain identifiable hot thoughts or imagery. Try talking or writing about this experience to see if you can identify *thoughts* as opposed to feelings.

You may find it helpful to carry a note pad or handheld digital recorder to record your thoughts when you experience emotion-provoking events. This kind of in-vivo recording will increase your chances of tracking thoughts accurately, rather than trying to reconstruct them after the fact. With time, as you become more familiar with this thought-tracking method, you will no longer need recording devices.

Thought Record

1. Situation	2. Moods	3. Automatic thoughts (images)	4. Evidence that supports the hot thought	5. Evidence that does not support the hot thought	6. Alternative/balanced thoughts	7. Rate moods now
Whom were you with? What were you doing? When was it? Where were you?	Describe each mood in one word. Rate intensity of mood (0–100%).	Answer some or all of the following questions: • What was going through my mind just before I started to feel this way? • What does this say about me? • What does this mean about me? my life? my future? • What am I afraid might happen? • What is the worst thing that could happen if this is true? • What does this mean about how the other person(s) feel(s)/think(s) about me? • What does this mean about the other person(s) or people in general? • What images or memories do I have in this situation?	Circle hot thought in previous column for which you are looking for evidence. Write factual evidence to support this conclusion. (Try to avoid mind-reading and reinterpretation of facts.)	Ask yourself questions to help discover evidence that does not support your hot thought (e.g., "When I am not feeling down, do I think about this type of situation any differently?")	Ask yourself questions to generate alternative or balanced thoughts (e.g., "Is there an alternative way of thinking about or understanding this situation? If someone else was in this situation, how would I suggest that they understand it?") Write alternative or more balanced thoughts. Rate how much you believe in each one (0–100%).	Copy the feelings from Column 2. Rerate the intensity of each feeling from 0 to 100%.

Adapted by permission from Greenberger and Padesky (2015). Copyright © 2015 The Guilford Press.

275

Some people are more visual, and their hot thoughts come in the form of disturbing images (for example, an image of yourself as a child being picked on by other kids on the playground; your memory of someone's facial expression). For others, specific words are hot thoughts. For Jake, it was the word *character*. For Suzanna, it was the word *crazy*. If single words or images are associated with your mood changes, record them in the "Automatic Thoughts" column, and see if you can expand them into a full sentence (for example, "as long as I act this way, people will always think of me as being crazy").

Let's imagine you had an unpleasant conversation with your father last week and you have been ruminating about it, on and off, since then. Record the event as "Conversation with Dad that didn't go well" in the "Situation" column. Let's also assume your resulting depressed mood was 70% (quite depressed) out of a possible 100% (extremely depressed). For the "Automatic Thoughts" column, you would record the self-statements or images that came up during the conversation or immediately after it. Examples might include "I never will be able to live up to his expectations" or "I let him down again," both of which might fuel your low mood.

Step 2: Challenging Negative Thoughts

Now let's work on modifying your automatic thoughts. Your thoughts can be considered hypotheses, rather than hard facts, about certain events. Complete the next two columns, "Evidence That Supports" and "Evidence That Does Not Support" your hot thoughts. Be a scientist observing your own thought process (Greenberger & Padesky, 2015): Is there any evidence for or against your conclusion that you let your dad down or won't ever be able to live up to his expectations? Did your father say anything that indicated differently? Have you had any experiences with your dad recently that would show that these conclusions are not always true? Are you discounting anything positive that he said? Could your sad mood have made you view the conversation differently from how it really was? Would you have viewed it differently in a different mood state? Was the outcome of the conversation really within your control?

> **Effective treatment:** Think of your thoughts as hypotheses that can be proven or disproven once you collect real-world information about them. Try to design small "experiments" to see if you can evaluate these hypotheses. So, if you believe your immediate supervisor at work has critical attitudes toward you, ask another coworker whether she has seen your supervisor be unnecessarily mean or evaluative to you. Ask whether she thinks the supervisor acts that way with other employees. Tell your supervisor something about yourself that does not pertain to work (for example, "I saw a great movie last weekend") and see how she responds.

The next step is to complete the column titled "Alternative/Balanced Thoughts." This is the chance to consider alternative viewpoints that are more balanced (as opposed to distorted), even if you don't believe them fully. Try writing down all of the other causes, explanations, or conclusions you could have drawn from this event and rate each of them on a 0–100% scale as to how credible you find them (100% means you believe this alternative explanation fully, 0% means not at all). Examples might include: "I think Dad was just in a bad mood that day and I got defensive" (40%); "We got on the touchy subject of money, which always makes us both uncomfortable" (70%); and "Dad expressed disappointment in me, but some important things came to light that we needed to talk about" (50%). Once you have generated and reflected on these alternative thoughts, make new ratings of your moods (depression, anxiety, or any other emotions you listed in column 2) using the same 0–100% (or –3 to +3) scale.

In considering alternative or more adaptive thoughts, consider the following strategies. Write a sentence or two that summarize all of the "for" and "against" evidence for your beliefs about this event. Consider what advice you would give another person who was in the same situation, had the same thoughts and moods, and had given you the same for/against evidence. Consider the best, worst, and most likely (realistic) outcomes if your hot cognition turns out to be true. For example, if the hot cognition "I let Dad down again" turns out to be true, a worst-case outcome might be that he pointedly reminds you of your failings the next time you talk to him and you end up feeling even worse; a best-case outcome might be that he apologizes and admits he was wrong, and you feel great; a realistic outcome might be that you feel tension the next time you talk to him but that you effectively steer the conversation toward more comfortable topics.

> **Effective treatment:** To come up with alternatives to negative self-statements:
>
> - Write lists of evidence for and against the negative statement.
> - Think of how you'd advise someone who had the same negative thought.
> - Consider the best, worst, and most likely outcomes if your negative thought turned out to be true.

Jake, the soccer coach, learned to evaluate the evidence for and against his automatic, self-blaming thought that "I'm no good with kids . . . I have character flaws." There was plenty of evidence to the contrary, given the many positive comments he received on an ongoing basis from his wife, the kids, and their parents. He was able to generate more balanced thoughts: "Sometimes the kids get uncooperative when I'm not feeling my best"; "Coaching can be a difficult task no matter how good you are"; "Sometimes I make mistakes, but that's inevitable when you're working with young kids"; "Today the kids were getting overstimulated and weren't in the mood to learn"; "I'm never going to be able to please all the parents." His mood tended to improve upon introducing and repeatedly restating to himself these countervailing thoughts.

Katrina's Example

Another person with bipolar disorder, Katrina, age 41, had worked as an elementary school teacher in Hungary when she emigrated by herself to the United States. A year after arriving she obtained a job at an inner-city school teaching teenagers who were developmentally disabled. During a particularly difficult day, three of the boys in the class cursed at her and told her she was the worst teacher they'd ever had. They told her she couldn't speak English and that she should go back to wherever she came from. By day's end, she felt quite depressed and anxious and didn't want to go back to work. She took two days off, citing "mental exhaustion." She recounted thoughts in reaction to this event, such as "Maybe I shouldn't be a teacher . . . I don't know if I have the strength and willpower . . . I'm not effective; I can't deal with it by myself . . . I don't belong; I can't make it." She identified "I'm not effective" as the most powerful, emotion-provoking hot thought, along with the prediction "I won't make it here and I'll have to move back to Hungary."

In examining the evidence for and against this thought, Katrina cited the fact that she'd had to call in the school counselor to help mediate the conflict, that the kids liked her only when she was being friendly and casual but not when she was actually teaching, and that she was more powerfully affected by this incident than the other teachers would have been. She was also able to generate evidence against her hot cognition, including the fact that she had received positive evaluations of her teaching from the school administration and that her earlier teaching experiences in Hungary had been quite positive. She admitted that "the kids are troubled and angry at everybody" and "I've seen them curse out other teachers." She also recalled that the incident began after one of the boys had verbally taunted another boy in the class.

She eventually settled on more balanced views that did not rule out her own role in causing the incident but that included the contrary evidence: "I'm a good teacher, but I have a difficult set of students that anyone would have a problem with . . . I sometimes struggle with my own boundaries and how to set limits with people . . . I'm still learning to speak English more colloquially . . . I'm new at this, and it's hard not to get my buttons pushed . . . I'm still making a difference in their lives, and they're teaching me a lot about myself even though they hurt my feelings sometimes." Her mood in reaction to the confrontation improved significantly upon reviewing these balanced thoughts. Over time, as her depression lifted, she focused on the larger question of whether she wanted to teach, which had become confused in her mind with whether she was good at it.

What's Different about Thinking Patterns in Bipolar Depression?

So far, the cognitive restructuring method I've described could apply to almost any form of depression or anxiety. The method applies equally well to bipolar disorder, but bipolar depressions tend to be much more severe than those experienced by people going through life transitions. So, in constructing your alternative or balanced thoughts, consider the role of your disorder—particularly, its biological and genetic underpinnings—in modulating your view of the causes of negative events. Do inherited vulnerabilities of brain activity or circuitry explain your behavior in certain situations better than character flaws? Could your emotional reactions in the heat of the moment have been due to overactivity in certain neural pathways rather than your inability to deal with people?

Jake, for example, recognized that soccer coaching did not go as well when he experienced the physical signs of depression or anxiety (for example, poor concentration, irritability, headaches, low energy). On days in which his coaching and athletic performance were impaired, he introduced balanced thoughts, such as "I can tell that my mood and energy are off kilter today; this is one of those days I can't expect as much from myself . . . This is not about my flawed character; it's about my biology . . . My depression is causing me to view things more pessimistically than I have to—it doesn't follow that I'm not a good person because I can't control my moods." Although he was never happy with himself when coaching didn't go well, these thoughts gave him a sense of self-acceptance when he couldn't live up to his high performance standards.

Katrina worried that "I'm too emotionally unstable to be a consistent figure in their [her students'] eyes." Indeed, negative interactions with her students probably had a more powerful effect on her mood states than might be the case for a person without bipolar disorder, but through no choice of her own. She learned to internally rehearse the self-statements "I'm going to have more severe ups and downs than the ordinary teacher," "Not all of my emotional reactions will be under my control, but that doesn't mean I can't teach," and "I'm good at what I do, and there is a great deal of meaning in it." She also recognized the need to give herself more time to relax and decompress after work than might be required by some of her coworkers.

Consider another example. Say you've had a string of negative interactions with your employer over the last week but generally have had good relations with him or her. Is it possible that your irritability with your boss derives from your depressive or mixed symptoms rather than your "short fuse," "angry nature," "problems getting along with people," or "problems with authority figures"? I am not saying, "Blame everything on your bipolar disorder." I'm recommending that you take a more balanced perspective on the factors influencing events in your life, *including* your disorder.

To sum up, cognitive restructuring has the potential to help you alleviate your depressed mood by identifying and revising the automatic thoughts that trigger low mood states. The role your bipolar disorder may play in stimulating your emotional reactions to persons, situations, and events should not be underestimated. In combination with behavioral activation methods, cognitive restructuring has the potential to help alleviate your depression or, at minimum, keep it in check.

• • • • • • • • • • • • •

This chapter has introduced you to important self-management tools for coping with depression. Implementing these tools—identifying your early warning signs, scheduling pleasurable and/or activating events, and reconsidering the way you think about and respond to the events in your life—can go a long way toward controlling the negative spiral of depression.

Don't be too concerned if you don't take to these methods right away. They require guided practice and skill before they feel natural. If you have access to a cognitive-behavioral therapist, consider doing these exercises with his or her guidance at first.

The next chapter addresses an issue that many—in fact, most—people with bipolar disorder confront at one time or another: suicidal thoughts or actions. This topic is, for many, an uncomfortable one. But as with many other attributes of bipolar disorder, you will put yourself in the driver's seat once you are able to understand suicidal impulses as symptoms of your illness that require management. You will see the special role that psychotherapy, medication, social supports, and self-management tools can play in alleviating feelings of hopelessness and suicidal despair.

CHAPTER 11

Overcoming Suicidal Thoughts and Feelings

> I had been getting more and more depressed and had thought about killing myself, but somewhere in there I decided to finally do it. One night I came home from work to my apartment and went through a whole ritual. I had decided I was going to do it by overdosing on my lithium, since that's the drug I had the most of. I took it, little by little, throughout the evening, pill after pill, and then I got in the shower, but by then I was starting to puke and got the runs really badly . . . I think I lost consciousness at some point, and somewhere in there I had the presence of mind to call Dylan [her boyfriend], who called the paramedics, and they took me to the hospital. I ended up there with a catheter and the oxygen mask and the whole thing. I looked awful and felt awful. Everybody was telling me how fortunate I was to be alive, but that made me feel worse. I sure didn't feel fortunate.
>
> —A 28-year-old woman with bipolar I disorder,
> recounting her first suicide attempt

If you are cycling into a period of depression, it is unfortunately very common to have thoughts of ending your life. You may have been having these thoughts all along, but they can become more severe if your depression is getting worse. You may also find that your suicidal thoughts go along with an increase in your anxiety and worry. Some people with bipolar disorder attempt suicide or even kill themselves accidentally or by impulse when they are psychotic and in the manic phase. Others feel suicidal chronically, not just when they have mood symptoms. One patient said, "I know I'll kill myself someday. It's gonna happen. The only question is when."

By some estimates, people with bipolar disorder are at 15 times more risk for committing suicide than people in the general population. Up to 15% of people with bipolar disorder die by suicide, and as many as one in three attempt suicide at least once in their lives (Novick, Swartz, & Frank, 2010). Although not all studies find rates this high, there is strong agreement that suicidal thoughts and feelings are a common feature of bipolar illness, connected with its biological and genetic mechanisms. For example, we know that abnormalities in certain serotonin genes are associated with an increased risk of suicide across populations (Ghasemi, Seifi, Baybordi, Danaei, & Samadi, 2018). In other words, suicidal impulses are related to the genetics and neurophysiology of your disorder; they are not caused by a moral failing or weakness on your part.

You should not feel alone with or ashamed of having suicidal thoughts. Virtually every person with bipolar disorder has entertained the idea of suicide at one point or another. In fact, many people without the disorder have thought about it, even if just in passing. But among people with bipolar disorder, the thoughts become frequent and intense and are more likely to be transformed into a plan of action (for example, to kill yourself with pills at a specific time). One patient of mine put it like this: "My suicidal thoughts are usually like a radio station that is always on but is never quite tuned in well enough to hear what's being said. When I get really depressed, though, the station comes in loud and clear, almost like someone has turned the dial."

The Desire to Escape

People with bipolar and other depressive disorders often feel hopeless, as if nothing will ever change for the better. They feel a strong need for relief from "psychic pain colored by the fear and anticipation of increasing, uncontrollable, interminable pain" (Fawcett, Golden, & Rosenfeld, 2000, p. 147). Some people honestly want to die. But in my experience, most people with bipolar disorder want relief from the intolerable life circumstances and the emotional, mental, and physical pain that goes along with depression and anxiety. When your depression is spiraling downward and you feel a sense of dread and apprehension, you may desperately want to live, but suicide can feel like the only escape from your intolerable feelings.

Even when severe, however, suicidal thoughts can be managed and controlled medically. There is strong evidence from meta-analyses that long-term treatment with lithium decreases suicide attempts and completions among people with bipolar disorder (Cipriani et al., 2013). Antidepressant, anticonvulsant, and antipsychotic drugs appear to decrease the agitation and aggressiveness that can bring about suicidal actions.

The challenge in dealing with suicidal despair is to find other ways of escaping from your intolerable feelings. As I discuss in this chapter, your options can include various combinations of medications, psychotherapy, the help of supportive friends or family members, and self-management techniques. Your hopelessness, pain, and emptiness are temporary, not permanent states, even though they may not seem that way at the time.

Risk Factors for Suicide

You should know about the factors that increase your probability of actually hurting or killing yourself, so that you and your doctor can determine how imminent the danger to you has become. If you plan on switching doctors, tell your new doctor about your risk factors so that he or she can determine the seriousness of your intent and hopefully be of greater help to you in a crisis.

You are at particularly high risk for committing suicide if you . . .

- Are male
- Have bipolar disorder and are also drinking alcohol or using drugs regularly (in addition to making your illness worse and your suicidal ideation more intense, alcohol and substances make it unlikely that you will take your mood stabilizers regularly or seek help from others)
- Have been ill for a short time and have had only a few mood episodes
- Have panic attacks, agitation, restlessness, or other indicators of severe anxiety
- Are prone to impulsive acts, such as driving recklessly or having violent outbursts
- Have recently been hospitalized
- Have previously tried to kill yourself
- Have one or more relatives in your family tree who committed suicide or committed a violent act
- Have experienced a recent stressful life event involving loss (for example, a divorce or the death of a family member)
- Are isolated from friends and family members
- Do not have ready access to a psychiatrist or psychotherapist
- Have feelings of hopelessness about your future and/or do not feel you have strong reasons to keep living (for example, a commitment to raising children)
- Have thought about a specific plan (for example, to take pills, shoot yourself, jump from a high place) and have the means to do it (access to pills or a gun) (Fawcett et al., 2000; Jamison, 2000b).

If you feel suicidal, you should always inform your psychiatrist, therapist, family members, and other significant people in your core circle. This is especially true if you have one or more of the preceding risk factors. It's best to disclose your suicidal thoughts even if you are afraid of worrying people or hurting their feelings or you are convinced that they can't be of any help. Many people feel this way and then don't get the help they need. Err on the side of informing your doctors and significant others, even if you're not sure how serious you are about suicide. Later in this chapter I discuss what your doctor, therapist, friends, and/or family members can do to help you at these times.

How Can You Protect Yourself from Carrying Out Suicidal Actions?

"Anyone who suggests that coming back from suicidal despair is a straightforward journey has never taken it."

—Jamison (2000b, p. 49)

If you have been spiraling into a depressive or mixed episode from your baseline state, or if your ongoing depression has been getting worse, you may have noticed an increase in your suicidal thoughts. These can be vague at first (for example, "I wonder what it would be like to be dead"), then more serious ("I know that I want to kill myself; I just don't know how"), then even more serious ("I've thought of various suicide plans and have settled on one, as well as a time and a place"). The feelings, thoughts, and behaviors that make up suicidal despair are quite complex and not well understood by behavioral scientists. Nonetheless, we know that there are some things you can do to protect yourself from acting on these impulses. In this chapter, you'll learn how to put together a suicide prevention plan.

Suicide prevention involves decreasing your access to the means to commit suicide and increasing your access to support systems (doctors, therapists, family members, and friends). You might wonder, at what point do these plans work, and at what point is it already too late? Keep a general caveat in mind when you develop your plan: you have more leverage in suicide prevention if you have a plan in place when you're feeling well and begin implementing it at the first emergence of suicidal thoughts or other prodromal signs of depression. Don't wait until you are really feeling desperate—don't let yourself get to that point. When suicidal thoughts and plans accompany the lowest point of a depressive or mixed episode, suicide attempts can occur by impulse.

Self-Harm: Does It Always Mean Suicidality?

"One day, I was so down on myself that I took out a knife and carved 'I hate myself' on my arm. When it was starting to heal, my boyfriend, Ari, saw it and flinched. I tried to explain it to him, but he didn't get it. Good thing I didn't cut myself that deeply—I didn't want it to be permanent. More like a temporary tattoo."

—19-year-old woman with bipolar II disorder recounting self-harm during a depressed phase

Within the category of suicidality are self-harm and nonsuicidal self-injury (NSSI). These terms are sometimes used interchangeably, because both involve self-inflicted damage to your body. However, there is an important difference: self-harm refers to self-inflicted damage with suicidal intent. Self-harm may not be severe enough to kill you (for example, superficial cutting or burning yourself with cigarettes), but it may still be driven by suicidal thoughts or impulses. NSSI refers to self-harm without suicidal intent, such as in the example of the young woman above. In the sections that follow, I am talking mainly about self-injury with suicidal intent, which is the more common case in bipolar disorder. For more information on NSSI in teens and coping strategies to avoid it, I can recommend Michael Hollander's (2017) *Helping Teens Who Cut: Using DBT Skills to End Self-Injury* or Lawrence Shapiro's (2008) *Stopping the Pain: A Workbook for Teens Who Cut and Self-Injure*.

Strategy No. 1: Get Rid of the Means to Hurt Yourself

One practical step you can take right away is to put those items you might use to hurt or kill yourself out of your reach. These include guns, sleeping pills, poisons, ropes, and sharp knives or other weapons. Give them to a trusted friend who lives apart from you, or even your psychiatrist or therapist, or put them in a storage bin you cannot access easily. To avoid overdosing on your psychiatric medications, keep only a couple of days' dosages in your house and have your friend or relative hold on to the rest of the pills, dispensing them as you need them. Although these practical maneuvers may seem like they only scratch the surface (you are, after all, only getting rid of the means, not your intentions), they will greatly decrease the chances that you will actually kill or hurt yourself. In the same manner, limiting your access to guns decreases the chances that you will use them on yourself or

Effective prevention: It has long been known that when guns are locked, unloaded, and stored in a closet that requires keys, and ammunition is kept in a separate locked location, the chances of the gun being used on oneself or one's family members decrease considerably (Grossman et al., 2005). A study of over-the-counter pills demonstrated a similar phenomenon. In the 1990s, drugstores in the United Kingdom changed the way they dispensed Tylenol (paracetamol); instead of selling pill bottles containing large quantities of Tylenol tablets, they dispensed the drug in "blister packets" that required the user to pop out individual pills one at a time from a plastic card. The use of blister packs was associated with a 64% reduction in severe drug overdoses (Turvill, Burroughs, & Moore, 2000). In other words, the greater difficulty of accessing the pills decreased the likelihood of their use in suicide attempts.

someone else. Suicide by firearm is very rare among people who don't already own or have access to guns.

Strategy No. 2: See Your Psychiatrist and Therapist Immediately

If your next appointments with your psychiatrist and therapist are not scheduled for several weeks, call them and let them know you are at risk or ask a member of your core circle to make the contact. It can help to see your doctor and therapist together (assuming they are not the same person) so that they can assist you in developing an integrated plan for managing your suicidal impulses, depression, anxiety, stress, and medications. If it is not logistically possible to arrange a conjoint meeting, ask the clinician you did see to share the plan with the other practitioner.

What will your doctors do to help you when you first start feeling suicidal? In all likelihood, they will start by asking you questions about your suicidal intentions, such as any plans you've been thinking about and your history of suicide attempts (if they don't already know about those). Expect to spend some time on these issues before they get to the reasons you want to kill yourself, which may be foremost in your mind. Be honest about your suicidal intentions, even if these feelings are new to you, foreign, or, in your view, shameful. Tell them how serious you are, that you may not feel safe at home, and that you have access to weapons or other means of hurting yourself.

Some people don't feel comfortable disclosing information to their doctors about their suicidal impulses. In my experience, people with bipolar disorder often fear one of the following: (1) their doctors will immediately hospitalize them and be deeply disappointed that the treatment plan seems to be failing, (2) their doctors will not be comfortable openly discussing suicide with them, or (3) their doctors will take an accusatory stance (such as expressing doubts about whether they are taking their medicines) or suggest that they see another doctor. None of these fears is entirely a distortion. In fact, your doctor may indeed hospitalize you if he or she feels the risk to your life is imminent. Keep in mind that this may be the best thing for you. As I discussed in Chapter 9, hospitalization gives you a chance to get your medications reevaluated and adjusted. It will also get you away from the stimuli that may be provoking your suicidal thoughts (for example, certain family members, noises, or pictures in your home; the computer or gaming equipment; the sound of text messages coming in or telephones ringing). If you do go into the hospital, at least some of your inpatient treatment should involve suicide prevention planning for the interval following your discharge.

Some doctors are indeed more comfortable and effective in dealing with suicide risk than others. If you fear that your doctors (that is, your psychiatrist and/or psychotherapist) will be uncomfortable with your disclosure of suicidal thoughts, tell them so. You may be surprised at how forthcoming they are in expressing their concern for you. Your therapist or medical doctor has probably had experiences with many other people who became suicidal and may work best when he or she knows the truth, even if it does mean reviewing and revising the treatment plan. Your doctors may feel like they haven't done their job right, but it isn't your responsibility to take care of *their* feelings. Rather, it's essential that you can be open with them about your feelings of hopelessness or despair.

Your psychiatrist is likely to reevaluate your medication regimen. Among the options he or she will probably want to discuss with you is adding an antidepressant to your regimen (or switching to a different antidepressant if you are already on one), increasing the dosage of your mood stabilizer or antidepressant, or adding a second mood stabilizer (especially lithium if you aren't on it). In extreme cases your doctor may recommend electroconvulsive therapy (ECT). If you have prominent anxiety symptoms, agitation, or psychosis, your doctor may introduce a second-generation antipsychotic or a benzodiazepine (see Chapter 6). When anxiety or agitation is controlled with drug treatment, suicidal thoughts sometimes diminish correspondingly.

Try to be realistic about the speed with which your medical treatments are likely to take effect. It can be quite frustrating to have to go through a trial-and-error period of adjusting medications and substituting others when you're already feeling hopeless and pessimistic. You may have the impulse to give up when the first modification to your regimen does not immediately achieve the intended result. Your state of suicidal despair will almost certainly improve with the proper medication adjustments, but it may take several weeks before the worst symptoms go away. Nonetheless, I have been continually amazed at the degree to which even minor medication adjustments can positively affect even the most suicidal person. One client with bipolar (mixed) disorder, Gerard (age 48), tried to asphyxiate himself by locking himself in the garage and turning on his car. After a brief hospitalization, his doctor added paroxetine (Paxil), an antidepressant, to his mood stabilizer regimen. His suicidal thoughts and intentions diminished rapidly, and his depression lifted, though somewhat less rapidly.

What will your psychotherapist do? The answer depends on her theoretical orientation and how long she has been working with you. Most will try to provide emotional support and teach you ways to handle your suicidal impulses (for example, using distraction or mindfulness techniques, relaxation techniques, or cognitive restructuring) to alleviate your immediate pain. Your therapist and you may examine the antecedents, behaviors, and consequences of your suicidal thoughts and actions (perhaps using different terms). Many therapists, particularly those with a CBT, dialectical behavior therapy (DBT), or interpersonal orientation, view suicidal thoughts or actions as occurring in a context—as one response in a series of possible responses.

Certain events, situations, images, or memories may stimulate your suicidal thoughts or actions. In turn, these thoughts or actions may be inadvertently rewarded by other people. For Maria, age 39, suicidal thoughts often came up in response to food. When depressed, she would eat voraciously and uncontrollably, and then look in the mirror, thinking she had grown fat and ugly that evening. It was usually then that she felt suicidal. If anyone else was around, she sought reassurances about her appearance, but these reassurances did little to alleviate her suicidal thoughts. Instead, she would become more suicidal and then call more people for reassurance. Maria's therapist assisted her in disrupting this chain of events by working directly with her on binge eating as a means of self-medicating her depression, developing alternative thinking patterns when she felt unattractive, and avoiding the pull to seek reassurance regarding her appearance. Successfully obtaining reassurance from others, he believed, was inadvertently reinforcing her suicidal thoughts rather than alleviating her distress.

Your therapist may also be able to help you frame your suicidal feelings in terms of broader life issues, such as regrets about events in the past or feelings of discouragement about your future. He or she may help you understand your suicidal impulses in terms of how they relate to the cycling of the bipolar syndrome. Your therapist can also help you develop a "safety plan," which can include calling him or her and/or going to the hospital when you experience your next suicidal impulse. Possibly, your therapist will suggest that your family members, spouse/partner, or a close friend come to a session with you to make sure they're aware of your suicidal thoughts and so that they can help you design and implement a suicide prevention plan (discussed later in this chapter, pages 294–297).

> **Effective prevention:** Many interventions and self-care techniques will be most powerful when they are implemented *before* you become actively and dangerously suicidal. Be sure to use your first suicidal thoughts or images as signals that you need to put into effect your suicide prevention plan, usually beginning with seeing your physician and therapist. Although you may overestimate the significance of these stray thoughts, it's better to proceed in a preventive way even if your efforts prove to be unnecessary.

Strategy No. 3: Use Your Core Circle

"When I start thinking about the future, I go into a panic, and that's when I think about killing myself. But somehow when I get with other people, I can fantasize about how things could be, and that injects some energy into me . . . it gives me the feeling of purpose, like I have some effectiveness or competence, like I can channel my energy in a good way. It's not just about getting rid of loneliness, or being needy. It's a feeling of being able to make other people laugh, or affecting other people in some way, that makes me feel alive again."

—A 43-year-old man with bipolar I disorder

As you know, one theme of this book is the value of your core circle of family members, spouse/partner, and friends in helping keep you well. In Chapter 9 I talked about how members of your core circle can help keep you from escalating into a full-blown manic episode. They can also be helpful when you are feeling suicidal. For the man quoted above, contact with other people was like an antidepressant, giving him temporary feelings of relief from painful emotions. When you are becoming suicidal, contact and support from others is absolutely critical to keep you from sinking further.

Be aware that you're more likely to reject help when you're most depressed and suicidal. You will feel vulnerable at those times and expect others to reject you. The thought that "I can't be helped, I'll be disappointed, I might even get worse" will go through your mind, contributing to your sense of hopelessness. You may start to believe that "I'm all alone with this—no one can really help me." It's important to challenge these negative thoughts by making yourself seek support from others, even if doing so feels useless at first. Evaluate the evidence that being with others makes you feel worse. *In all likelihood, your attempts to seek assistance will generate compassion from others, which in turn will help ease your pain. If nothing else, they may provide a distraction from your internal pain.*

Start by reviewing the "Identifying Your Core Circle" form you filled out in Chapter 8 (page 217). Who on your list can help you when you first start feeling suicidal? If you have been depressed or anxious for some time, whom have you relied on when you needed to "vent"? Has this person (or these people) been able to help you clarify important issues and potential solutions without bringing you down further? Have you been able to feel closer to this person as a result of confiding in him or her? Is the relationship bidirectional—does this person also seek you out for help? One of the few positive things about depression is that it can result in your making connections with others in ways you would not typically initiate.

In evaluating your list, try to think of who is likely to be supportive in ways that you would find genuinely helpful. Is there someone on the list who can listen to you talk about wanting to die without freaking out? Some people find they can't discuss these matters with their family members but can do so with a friend, a partner, or a spouse. For others, it's a rabbi, priest, or other religious leader. The important question is whether you trust that person to listen to you calmly and attentively and acknowledge your despair, without judgment. It is also helpful to choose someone whose style is optimistic and hopeful but also realistic (that is, someone aware of the limitations imposed by your disorder and your environment). Don't choose a "Pollyanna." Finally, if you are close to someone who has some understanding of bipolar disorder (see "A Quick Fact Sheet on Bipolar Disorder for Family Members," on pages 330–331), or someone who has personally gone through periods of depression, that person may be able to offer a unique perspective on ways to cope with your despair.

If no one on your list really fits these descriptors, try to choose the person (or persons) who comes closest. It's best to include on your list as many people as possible and not rely too heavily on any one person. Include people in your circle who usually improve your mood (for example, a person with whom you share a pleasurable activity) even if you don't plan on disclosing anything to them. Record their names on the Suicide Prevention Plan on pages 296–297.

Now think about how you can get members of your core circle to assist you. Recall the three coping styles I mentioned at the beginning of Chapter 10 (emotion-focused, cognitive coping, and distraction coping). First, encourage your significant others to *listen to you talk about your thoughts and feelings.* Tell them you don't need them to solve all of your problems or come up with the bromide that will make all the pain go away, but you do need help to focus on what's causing you pain and why. Therapists are usually best at doing this, but if you have a friend or family member who's a good listener, give him or her a chance.

Second, ask your friend or family member to *help you find a way to prevent the immediate danger to yourself.* The objective is to keep you safe. If you haven't been able to get yourself to call your doctor or therapist, ask your friend to do so. Ask him or her to take the weapons or pills off your hands. If you need to go to the hospital, ask your friend to accompany you. If you won't or can't go to the hospital, is he or she willing to stay with you, even overnight if necessary, until you feel you're out of danger? If you feel unable to take care of your kids, can that person do it temporarily or help you make other arrangements with someone who can?

Third, use *distraction.* Many people are concerned that talking about their painful emotions will be a burden to others. If you are concerned about this, consider increasing the amount of low-stress, low-demand social time you spend with your significant others or friends. These activities don't have to involve talking about your struggles. Invite them to see a movie with you, go for a walk, take a drive, have dinner, read together, or do some yoga. Physical or social activities that have a degree of structure and involve other people, such as those on your pleasurable activities list (Chapter 10), are especially important to do right now to take your mind away from suicidal thoughts.

Be Aware of Others' Limitations

You may feel skeptical about the ability of members of your core circle to help you. You are probably correct that if the people you're confiding in do not have bipolar disorder themselves, they will not be able to fully understand the depth of your depression or why your suicidal thoughts are increasing in frequency. People in your core circle will be invaluable to your suicide prevention plan, but it's important to know what each is capable of and willing to do.

You may become distressed by friends or relatives who seem increasingly irritated with you and insist that you pull yourself out of it. Be patient with them.

Their irritation probably derives from anxieties about your fate or their frustration at not being able to help more. Likewise, try not to be frustrated when they give you platitudes (for example, "We've got only one life to live, and we have to live it fully"), which people often issue when they can't think of what else to say. If you're going to have multiple conversations with this person, remind him that what would help most is for him to listen without judgment.

Karen, age 35, complained that no one wanted to hear about her depressive or suicidal feelings, which made her feel even greater despair. Her typical pattern was to spend hours with others talking about her sadness and then to tell them, "Now I feel a whole lot worse." It is not surprising that her friends became burned out and didn't want to help her anymore. It's important to reward or reinforce members of your core circle for their efforts from time to time. Remember, they are trying to help, even if what they do is not always helpful. They need to hear *from you* that talking to them or simply spending time together is helping you. It probably is, even if only minimally, and it's important to tell them so.

Strategy No. 4: Reviewing Your Reasons for Living

There will be times when, alone with your suicidal thoughts and feelings, you will start to become overwhelmed by them. This is because suicide is, in part, a cognitive process. When people feel most desperate, they begin to evaluate the pros and cons of suicide as a means of solving their problems. Suicide feels like a more viable alternative when you believe that nothing you do will yield a positive outcome or that your depression or other life problems will always haunt you.

The flip side is that you will be most protected against suicide if you believe that you will be able to cope effectively with life's problems, view life as having intrinsic value, or feel that others are dependent on your existence (Linehan, 1985; Strosahl, Chiles, & Linehan, 1992). In short, people are protected from suicide when they can access good reasons to live. Marsha Linehan and her associates (Linehan, Goodstein, Nielsen, & Chiles, 1983) developed an inventory of reasons for living (see page 292). The inventory was generated by nonsuicidal people who were asked to write down the reasons they did not kill themselves at a point when they had previously considered it, the reasons they would not do so now, and the reasons they believed other people did not. When people believe they can overcome life's problems, and when they feel a strong sense of responsibility to family and children, they are less likely to make a serious suicide attempt.

While this logic may seem obvious, it has an implication for the things you can do on your own when you start to have suicidal thoughts. When people are suicidal, they usually have a great deal of trouble accessing any positive reasons for being alive. So, when you're feeling well, generate a list of your reasons for living or reasons you would not commit suicide if you were starting to think about it. You can then review these reasons when suicide begins to feel like a viable option.

The Reasons for Living Inventory

Check the statements below that indicate why you would *not* commit suicide if the thought were to occur to you or if someone were to suggest it to you.

___ I have a responsibility and commitment to my family.

___ I believe I can learn to adjust to, or cope with, my problems.

___ I believe I have control over my life and destiny.

___ I believe only God has the right to end a life.

___ I am afraid of death.

___ I want to watch my children as they grow.

___ Life is all we have and is better than nothing.

___ I have future plans I am looking forward to carrying out.

___ No matter how bad I feel, I know that it will not last.

___ I love and enjoy my family too much and could not leave them.

___ I am afraid that my method of killing myself would fail.

___ I want to experience all that life has to offer, and there are many experiences I have not had yet that I want to have.

___ It would not be fair to leave the children for others to take care of.

___ I have a love of life.

___ I am too stable to kill myself.

___ My religious beliefs forbid it.

___ The effect on my children could be harmful.

___ It would hurt my family too much and I would not want them to suffer.

___ I am concerned about what others would think of me.

___ I consider it morally wrong.

___ I still have many things left to do.

___ I have the courage to face life.

___ I am afraid of the actual act of killing myself (the pain, blood, violence).

___ I believe killing myself would not really accomplish or solve anything.

___ Other people would think I am weak and selfish.

___ I would not want people to think I did not have control over my life.

___ I would not want my family to feel guilty afterward.

List other reasons for living:

_____

_____

_____

Adapted by permission from Linehan et al. (1983). Copyright © 1983 the American Psychological Association.

Start by checking the items in the inventory on page 292 that you believe to be true. Then, in the blank spaces, add your own reasons if they are not covered in the other items. Try to do this while you're feeling reasonably stable and not seriously depressed. When you're depressed, your reasons for living may be harder to endorse, even though you might ordinarily believe in them.

You'll see that the items cover a broad spectrum of reasons, including the belief that you can cope with and overcome your troubles, the value you put on life itself, the degree to which you feel optimistic, concerns related to your family and children, fears of disapproval by society, moral beliefs, and fears of the suicidal act itself (Linehan et al., 1983). Some of these reasons may be more relevant to you than others. Reviewing the reasons you do *not* want to kill yourself when the thought crosses your mind may help protect you from acting on a self-destructive impulse later.

Strategy No. 5: "Improving the Moment" Tools

Some people feel that their suicidal despair is always in the background even when they distract themselves from it. Suicide prevention can include learning to tolerate feelings of despair when you can't make them go away (see the personalized care tip on page 294). What follow are some "improving the moment" strategies for tolerating your distress (Linehan & Dexter-Mazza, 2007).

Many people turn to religion when they are alone and feel depressed and suicidal. For some, religion is best practiced in group settings like a church, synagogue, or temple, but others prefer solitary prayer. For some, praying for strength gives them a sense of purpose and belonging. Likewise, some people find spiritual readings helpful because they put suffering into a larger perspective. Readings by the Dalai Lama are quite inspirational to people in pain (*Ethics for the New Millennium* [1999], or *The Art of Happiness,* coauthored by Howard Cutler [1998]).

If your suicidal thoughts or feelings are accompanied by significant anxiety, you may benefit from self-relaxation or mindfulness exercises. Usually, relaxation involves sitting in a comfortable chair; tensing and relaxing each of your muscle groups, starting with your feet and moving up to your face; and imagining relaxing, pleasant scenes (for example, lying on a beach). Relaxation or mindfulness exercises may decrease the anxiety and agitation that accompany suicidal thoughts. Consult books that give you step-by-step instructions or audio files on how to relax and breathe more easily (for example, Davis, Eshelman, & McKay, 2008).

Take another look at the 3-minute mindful breathing exercise in Chapter 10, which gives you a step-by-step method for "decentering" yourself (observing your emotions and physical sensations from a nonjudgmental observer's standpoint, such that you are less motivated to avoid them). Indeed, some people relate better to mindfulness exercises—exercises that make you more aware of your current sensations and experiences—than to relaxation exercises (for example, see Teasdale et al., 2014; Williams et al., 2007).

PERSONALIZED CARE TIP:
The hope kit

Cognitive-behavioral therapists have developed another method to facilitate awareness of reasons to live: the use of a personalized "hope kit" (Berk, Henriques, Warman, Brown, & Beck, 2004; T. R. Goldstein et al., 2015). You can learn to tolerate states of extreme sadness or anxiety by distracting yourself with items that either engage your senses (for example, a perfume, a favorite candy that you never allow yourself to eat) or remind you of happier times (photos of your friends, letters, a favorite song playlist). Some people include things from their childhood, such as photos of pets, a pack of baseball cards, or souvenirs from family vacations. Avoid reminders of former spouses or lovers or events that went awry. The idea is to collect elements from your life that you feel comforted by and that may help you feel hopeful when you are otherwise feeling desperate. The hope kit can be modified as frequently as you wish.

Some people include cards that give responses to their current negative thoughts. For example, if you have just lost your job and are telling yourself, "I'm useless, no one will ever want to hire me," include a card with a counteracting thought (for example, "I've been hired before and know that I have a lot to offer"). Include cards with creative ideas for actions you can take to distract yourself, especially actions that may create a different emotional state. For example, if you are musically inclined, take two or three negative thoughts and make a song out of them. If you are artistically inclined, make a cartoon drawing of yourself attending a job interview.

For many, exercise is helpful. Most people report that their mood improves significantly and suicidal thoughts diminish after they have exercised. Of course, it's hard to work out when you feel low in energy, apathetic, or hopeless. Try some light exercise if you feel especially lethargic, such as walking, stretching, or riding a stationary bicycle for a few minutes. When exercising, focus your attention on your body and the physical sensations that accompany the movement.

If your experience of any of these "improving the moment" tasks is positive, consider adding them to your behavioral activation list (Chapter 10). It's important to try these more than once and to incorporate them into your regular routine.

Developing a Suicide Prevention Plan

Now try to put all of this information together into a suicide prevention plan. The form on pages 296–297 can be used as a template. First, list your prodromal signs of depression (see the exercises in Chapter 10). Be sure to list any suicidal thoughts or impulses, including those that seem fleeting or insignificant (for example, "I start thinking about dying, but I would never do anything about it"). Then examine the list of self-management strategies that have been described in this and the prior chapter. Circle those items that seem like reasonable things for you and others to do when you experience suicidal thoughts or other symptoms of depression.

Next share this exercise with your doctor and/or therapist and the relevant members of your core circle and see if they'd be willing to perform these tasks should you go into a crisis. If a friend or family member is not willing to accept responsibility for a given item (for example, taking care of your kids), consider assigning that task to another person. List each member of your core circle at the end of the exercise and indicate which items on the list can be assigned to him or her. Finally, keep your suicide prevention plan in a place that is readily accessible to members of your core circle.

* * * * * * * * * * * * * * *

Suicide is "a permanent solution to a temporary problem" (Fawcett et al., 2000, p. 147). But the intolerable feelings that go along with suicidal preoccupations can be so painful that they feel permanent. It's important to combat these states with a variety of self-management tools to help activate yourself, view your circumstances from alternate perspectives, and engage with important sources of emotional and practical support. Try to be up front with your doctor and therapist about your suicidal impulses and take into consideration their recommendations for emergency treatment. Most of all, remain hopeful that your most severe depressive symptoms will eventually disappear and that you will return to a more tolerable emotional state. It's hardest to see your way out when you have hit bottom, so try to implement as many of these strategies as possible when you experience the first signs of depression or suicidal despair.

Bipolar disorder is tough to handle for both men and women even in the best of circumstances, but there are complex emotional and health problems related to the illness and its treatment that affect women more than men. In the next chapter, I discuss a number of strategies for women that will make you feel more empowered in dealing with the illness. Some of the topics covered include how to make treatment and health decisions when you are pregnant, are planning pregnancy, have just given birth, or are approaching menopause, as well as how to make the best use of mood-stabilizing medications while minimizing risks to your physical health. You'll see how some of the core strategies discussed throughout this book—educating yourself and others about the illness, communicating with your physician, and learning to manage the effects of stress on your mood and health—apply to the unique challenges faced by women with bipolar disorder.

Suicide Prevention Plan

List your typical early warning signs of a depressive and/or suicidal episode.

_____

_____

_____

_____

Circle the things *you* can do if one or more of these early warning symptoms appear, or if you have suicidal thoughts or impulses.

1. Get rid of all dangerous weapons.

2. Call your psychiatrist and psychotherapist to ask for an emergency appointment.

3. Implement your behavioral activation plan by scheduling rewarding or distracting activities.

4. Challenge negative thoughts through cognitive restructuring.

5. Ask your core circle of friends and family members for support; agree not to hurt yourself if they haven't had a chance to get back to you.

6. Practice meditation or relaxation techniques.

7. Exercise.

8. Rely on input from religious and spiritual sources.

9. Review your Reasons for Living Inventory.

10. Review the items in your hope kit.

Circle the things *your doctor and therapist* can do.

1. See you on an emergency basis.

2. Modify your medication regimen.

3. Arrange a hospitalization (if necessary).

4. Help you understand where your suicidal thoughts are coming from and what effects they are having on you or others.

5. Work with you on behavioral strategies for handling your painful thoughts and emotions.

(continued)

Circle those things that members of *your core circle* can do.

1. Listen to you, validate your feelings, and offer suggestions.

2. Avoid being critical or judgmental.

3. Distract you through mutually enjoyable activities.

4. Help you take care of responsibilities that have become burdensome or difficult to perform (for example, child care).

5. Stay with you until you feel safe.

6. Do a mindfulness exercise with you.

7. Call your doctor to help you arrange an appointment.

8. Take you to the hospital (if necessary).

9. Agree to store your weapons or pills away from you.

List members of your core circle and put numbers after each indicating which of items 1–9 they are willing to perform (list more than one item, if appropriate).

_____ _____

_____ _____

_____ _____

_____ _____

_____ _____

List your doctors' names and phone numbers.

_____   _____

_____   _____

_____   _____

CHAPTER 12

For Women Only

What You Need to Know about Bipolar Disorder and Your Health

> I had always struggled with my periods, which birth control pills to take, and how I felt about my body when I was taking mood stabilizers that made me look fat and feel stupid. But when I think back on my illness, my biggest struggle was when I had to decide whether to stay on medications during my pregnancy. I thought I had it all figured out, but then my psychiatrist told me that if I got pregnant, he wouldn't know how to manage my drugs, so I'd have to see someone else. And at the same time my OB-GYN told me that if I was planning to take medications while I was pregnant, he wouldn't treat me any longer! My husband insisted that I stop taking them. I didn't even know what *I* thought. So I stopped my medications and got pregnant, and then I had another episode and landed in the hospital. Fortunately my baby was born healthy. But I certainly could have used a helping hand or two.
>
> —A 43-year-old woman with bipolar I disorder

> My boyfriend thinks I just have PMS. That doesn't even come close to capturing it. What I have is something much, much worse. It's like bipolar and PMS get multiplied several times over, and the result is an intense, panicky, really angry state, combined with a deep sadness that's weird even for me.
>
> —A 27-year-old woman with bipolar II disorder

> My medications, which were supposed to help my depression when I went through menopause, caused me to gain a ton of weight and messed with my hormones. So I've renamed them: depa-bloat, olanza-pig, and despair-idone.
>
> —A 52-year-old woman with bipolar II disorder

If you're a woman, bipolar disorder presents unique challenges in addition to those you read about in earlier chapters. In particular, various stages and events in a woman's reproductive life can affect and are affected by the disorder. You may face the same problems and decisions that the women quoted above encountered. Mood-stabilizing medications can affect the health of your developing baby during pregnancy (called *teratogenic risk*), but so can an untreated bipolar illness, so the risks must be weighed carefully. At significant events in your reproductive life—puberty (around age 12), pregnancy, and the onset of menopause (usually after 50)—the disorder may change course, requiring you to be alert for the need to modify your treatment. Additionally, the unique nature of the disorder in women sometimes calls for medications that interact with aspects of reproductive functioning.

All of these challenges will be addressed in this chapter. Knowing the facts about bipolar disorder in women will help you find the best available treatment and have the best chance of managing your illness. If you are a spouse or partner of a woman with bipolar disorder, this information should help you understand what she's going through and how you can help her get the treatment and support she needs.

The Course of Bipolar Disorder in Women

Let's start with some well-replicated research findings that will help orient you to how we treat bipolar disorder in women.

■ *Women with bipolar disorder have longer, more frequent, and more treatment-resistant depressions than men.* Early on in your illness, you are more likely to be misdiagnosed with major depressive disorder than a man would be. You may also have to wait several years longer before being treated correctly with medications for bipolar disorder, especially if you have a bipolar II illness course (Baldessarini, Tondo, & Hennen, 1999).

■ *Mixed episodes, rapid cycling, and bipolar II disorder are more common in women.* These conditions are often treated with complex combinations of medications—often mood stabilizers with accompanying second-generation antipsychotics (SGAs) that can pose particular health risks (for example, weight gain).

■ *Women have more manic or hypomanic episodes brought on by antidepressants.* Because you're more prone to depression, you may be more likely to be prescribed an antidepressant without a mood stabilizer. As you know, antidepressants given alone can trigger manic, mixed, or hypomanic episodes.

■ *Women are more likely to have physical disorders and pain conditions than men.* Migraine headaches, thyroid disorders, and other physical or neurological problems can complicate your daily life and decisions about mood-stabilizing medications.

■ *Mood stabilizers are more likely to cause weight gain, insulin resistance, and elevated blood lipids in women than in men.*

■ *The disorder itself—not just the treatments for it—can affect a woman's functioning during pregnancy and the postpartum period, as well as the regularity of her menstrual cycle.* Women with bipolar disorder are at higher risk for postpartum depression and for other pregnancy complications (for example, cesarean section births, preeclampsia, need for labor induction) than women without bipolar disorder (Scrandis, 2017). Bipolar disorder is also associated with weight- and insulin-related disorders like diabetes, polycystic ovarian syndrome, and menstrually related mood changes.

■ *Women are more likely than men to have anxiety, panic attacks, body image problems, and eating disorders.* These comorbid conditions often require separate medications or help through CBT, mutual support groups, or insight-oriented psychotherapy.

The good news is that you can reap the benefits of a wealth of new research findings on the biological and psychological ramifications of being a woman treated for bipolar disorder. (For good reviews of the science in this area, see Haskey & Galbally, 2017; Kenna, Jiang, & Rasgon, 2009; Scrandis, 2017.) We now have a pretty good idea of which medications are safest during pregnancy, as well as the risks associated with stopping them altogether. This knowledge comes to us not just from studies of bipolar disorder but also from studies of conditions like epilepsy, for which anticonvulsants like valproate and lamotrigine have been standard treatments for many years. Likewise, we know more than ever about the effects of mood-stabilizing medications on other reproductive functions, such as the menstrual cycle. Outside of medications, we've learned how crucial family and marital relationships are to a woman's mood stability after an illness episode. We know, too, that various forms of couple- and family-oriented therapy, along with mindfulness-based cognitive therapy (MBCT) classes, can help prevent recurrences and reduce symptoms of bipolar depression (Miklowitz & Gitlin, 2014b).

So, you have a lot of accumulated knowledge on your side. As you tackle the challenges that come with having bipolar disorder and being female, keep in mind the theme of this book: *successfully treating your bipolar disorder involves an ongoing collaboration between you, your doctor, and, in many cases, your family members.* Many of the treatment decisions you make will not have right or wrong answers associated with them, which can be frustrating. Also, you may have to make different decisions at different phases of your life. But knowing what the research literature does and doesn't say about treatment in women will help you make well-informed choices. You'll feel like you have more control over your health and that of your baby should you become pregnant, for example. Pregnancy and the postpartum period are, in fact, issues of considerable concern to women with bipolar disorder, so let's start there.

Pregnancy

"[My doctor] asked me whether or not I planned to have children . . . I told him that I very much wanted to have children, which immediately led to his asking me what I planned to do about taking lithium during pregnancy. I started to tell him that it seemed obvious to me that the dangers of my illness far outweighed any potential problems that lithium might cause a developing fetus and that I therefore would choose to stay on my lithium. Before I finished, however, he broke in to ask me if I knew that manic–depressive illness was a genetic disease . . . I wasn't entirely stupid, I said, 'Yes, of course.' At that point, in an icy and imperious voice that I can hear to this day, he stated—as though he felt it were God's truth, which he no doubt felt it was—'You shouldn't have children.'

"I felt sick, unbelievably and utterly sick, and deeply humiliated. I asked him if his concerns about my having children stemmed from the fact that, because of my illness, I would be an inadequate mother or simply that he thought it was best to avoid bringing another manic–depressive into the world. Ignoring or missing my sarcasm, he replied, 'Both.'"

—Jamison (1995, p. 191)

Many women with bipolar disorder have asked me whether they should have children. I hope I have responded with more empathy and compassion than the doctor that Kay Jamison was unfortunate enough to consult. As I said in Chapter 5, there is every reason to have children if you want them and are in a position, emotionally and practically, to raise them. The chance that a child will develop bipolar disorder if one parent has it averages about 9%. In my opinion, that's not a high enough risk to influence the decision to have a child, as explained in more detail in Chapter 14. Bipolar disorder does not carry the genetic load of conditions like Huntington's disease. When one parent has this neurodegenerative disorder, the chances that his or her children will develop it average 50%. That risk and the fact that Huntington's leads to early death makes many parents with the genetic predisposition to Huntington's decide not to have children.

Bipolar disorder presents a very different picture. It's hardly a death sentence. Even a child who inherits your biological vulnerability may develop only a mild form of the disorder or possibly no disorder at all. There may also be much better treatments available once your child is an adult.

Of course, if you have doubts about whether you want to get pregnant right now, it's important to take the proper precautions to prevent it since people with bipolar disorder are vulnerable to engaging in impulsive sexual activity (see the section on contraception starting on page 313). If and when you do want to become pregnant, it's important to keep in mind several suggestions regarding how to manage your illness and treatments after you conceive.

Pregnancy Caveats

"I have experienced depression on and off since I was in high school. The only thing that has ever really worked for me is the lithium I take. When I found out that I was pregnant, I told my doctor that I didn't want to keep taking it. We stopped it, but then I started feeling down again. My feelings about the pregnancy even changed. I started resenting the baby, the ways in which my life was changing, not to mention my body and all the weight I was gaining. During one appointment with my OB, I started crying and saying I didn't want to be pregnant anymore. I was beyond the first trimester, so he convinced me to start back on my lithium. It definitely helped, and I'm feeling better in general and more positive about the pregnancy, although I worry a lot about how I might be harming my baby with these drugs. I'm between a rock and a hard place."

—A pregnant 33-year-old woman with a history of bipolar I mixed episodes

1. **Pregnancy is a high-risk time for relapses of bipolar disorder. Don't believe the myth that being pregnant will protect you against recurrences of mania or depression.** In fact, you can substantially reduce your risk for relapse during pregnancy by staying on your mood stabilizers or SGAs. A study by Viguera, Whitfield, and colleagues (2007) at Harvard Medical School found that 71% of pregnant women with bipolar disorder had an illness recurrence during their pregnancy. Most of the recurrences were depressive or mixed, and about half occurred during the first trimester. The rate was *twice as high* among those who discontinued, rather than continued, their medications during the pregnancy. The women who stopped their medications also spent *five times* as many weeks in states of depression or mania as those who continued their treatment. If you decide to go off them, do so slowly.

> **New research:** A meta-analysis of 37 studies found that recurrence rates during the postpartum period (generally the first 6 months after the birth) were three times higher in bipolar women who did not take medications during pregnancy compared to those who did take medicines (Wesseloo et al., 2016). In other words, pregnancy and the postpartum period are high-risk intervals for many women, and psychiatric medications used during pregnancy to treat mood symptoms may also help prevent postpartum relapses.

2. *Most psychiatric medications pose at least some risks to the developing baby, but so does not taking medications.* Some women with bipolar disorder have manic episodes during pregnancy, with various forms of high-risk behavior (for example, drinking and smoking heavily, driving erratically, forgetting prenatal obstetric appointments, and not eating regularly or getting enough sleep). When the disorder is complicated by alcohol or substance abuse problems, there is an increased risk of pregnancy and birth complications such as preterm deliveries (Scrandis, 2017).

3. *Beware of "alternative" treatments.* Some doctors—and often friends or family members—will encourage you to replace your prescription medications with herbal supplements, vitamins, or other over-the-counter compounds during pregnancy. Some of these compounds may indeed be beneficial to pregnancy (an example is folic acid to reduce the risk of neural tube defects). But as I said in Chapter 6, there is no evidence that natural compounds like omega-3 fatty acids (fish oil), flaxseed oil, St. John's wort, or valerian root can be substituted for lith-

---

PERSONALIZED CARE TIP:
Maintaining health, mood stability, and fetal health during pregnancy

- Keep in mind the *risk factors for poor fetal health* that all pregnant women should avoid: tobacco, alcohol, drugs, obesity, poor diet, excessive caffeine intake, and dehydration.
- *There are no hard-and-fast rules regarding which medications to take or not take during pregnancy.* The choice—for example, whether to take lithium, lamotrigine, an SGA, or some combination—is often based on which medications have kept you stable previously.
- *The most consistent finding in research is that higher dosages of valproate (divalproex sodium) are related to poorer cognitive abilities in babies compared to the other anticonvulsants.* Current treatment guidelines suggest avoiding valproate during pregnancy (Haskey & Galbally, 2017).
- If your mood is cycling up and down during your pregnancy, *continuing your prepregnancy treatment* may be the safest course of action.
- If you decide to go off your medications, *gradual reduction* is always better than abrupt withdrawal; stopping suddenly can bring on a relapse.
- If you are severely depressed or having a mixed episode, *electroconvulsive therapy* presents less of a risk to the fetus than most drugs (as paradoxical as that may sound). Although there are few studies on it to date, *transcranial magnetic stimulation* (Chapter 6) may be an option for you as well.
- Discuss with your physician the risks and benefits of *breastfeeding* while you are taking medications.
- Always consider *psychotherapy* or *mindfulness-based meditation practices* as additions to your medications, both during pregnancy and during the postpartum period, when you are most vulnerable to recurrences.
- *A relatively structured and predictable daily routine* will help minimize your sleep deprivation and mood instability.
- Keep track of your mood, medications, and, if you are not pregnant, your menstrual cycles using your *mood chart.*

Sources: Cohen (2007); Haskey & Galbally (2017); Kenna et al. (2009); Miklowitz & Gitlin (2014a); Scrandis (2017); Ward & Wisner (2007).

ium, anticonvulsants, or antipsychotics. Be wary of the common assumption that medications bought over the counter in health food stores are safer than prescription medications.

"What Can I Expect from My Doctor If I Want to Get Pregnant?"

Once you've decided you want to conceive (regardless of whether you've been pregnant before), see your psychiatrist and your obstetrician to discuss your conception plans. Make sure the following topics are covered:

- Your current method of contraception
- The reproductive risks of your current medications
- Your prior history of mood cycling when you've been off medications (especially during prior pregnancies)
- How well you are responding to your current medications
- Your physical health
- The current regularity of your menstrual cycles and your reproductive and menstrual history
- The risks of conceiving on your current medication regimen

If you have severe bipolar disorder (that is, you have recently had a full manic or mixed episode, and you have a history of severe recurrences when going off your medications), you may require treatment throughout your pregnancy. Lithium alone or in combination with an antipsychotic medication is generally safer than valproate or carbamazepine (Haskey & Galbally, 2017; Scrandis, 2017). If you have mild to moderate bipolar disorder and are currently stable (for example, you have gone a full year without an episode of major depression; you have hypomanias but not full manias), you may be able to slowly discontinue your medications before you conceive.

Most obstetricians will recommend a regular schedule of prenatal visits, a healthy diet, and childbirth classes (especially if this is your first pregnancy). They may also recommend prenatal vitamins or supplements. If you are not already in psychotherapy, consider starting therapy before you get pregnant, particularly if you are having significant stress in your life (for example, marital or couple problems) or are ambivalent about having a child (see Chapter 6 for a discussion of effective therapies). These kinds of issues are very common among women planning pregnancy, whether they are bipolar or not.

"What If I'm Already Pregnant?"

As many as 50% of all pregnancies are unplanned. The risk of unplanned pregnancy is even higher among women with bipolar disorder, because mania and hypomania can lead to impulsive sexual choices and because mood-stabilizing medications can influence the effectiveness of contraceptive pills (see pages 313–314). Take a look at Chapter 9, especially the section titled "Avoiding Risky Sexual Situations," starting on page 235, when your mood is escalating. Working with an OB-GYN who is familiar with mood disorders and the effects of different contraceptives on mood can be quite helpful.

Whether your pregnancy is planned or not, you may not know you're pregnant until you're well into your first trimester, when many of the medications for bipolar illness have already had their effects on the developing fetus. Here are a few risks that you may want to discuss with your doctor.

- The risk of neural tube defects (for example, spina bifida, an incomplete closure of the vertebrae over the spinal cord) increases if you're taking valproate or carbamazepine (Tegretol) between 17 and 30 days after conception.

- The risk of cardiovascular (heart) anomalies is influenced most by medications taken between 21 and 56 days after conception. Lithium poses risks for cardiovascular abnormalities (4.1% vs. 0.6% of women who did not take lithium during pregnancy) (Diav-Citrin et al., 2014).

- In rare cases, lithium use throughout pregnancy can be associated with "floppy baby" syndrome: lethargy, blue coloration of the skin, abnormal muscle tension, and hypothyroidism. Fortunately, this syndrome is temporary.

- Fetal lip and palate abnormalities are associated with medications (particularly anticonvulsants, including lamotrigine) taken between 8 and 11 weeks (8 to 20 weeks for craniofacial abnormalities).

- The alarming rates of major fetal malformations (for example, heart defects, spina bifida) reported for some mood-stabilizing medications (see the next section) have to be compared to the usual base rate of 2–4% in the infants of healthy mothers who aren't taking psychiatric medications (Stewart, 2011).

Weighing the Medication Risks

The risks listed in the previous section are enough to convince some women to discontinue medications when they discover they're pregnant. Before you make a decision, weigh the risks of discontinuing your medications against the risks of experiencing mania or depression while pregnant. Depression during pregnancy has been correlated with low birth weight and premature delivery, possibly because depressed women often have a decrease in appetite and are less likely to get adequate prenatal care. Depression late in pregnancy is associated with more C-sections and a greater need for neonatal intensive care (Chung, Lau, Yip, Chiu, & Lee, 2001). Indeed, women who are depressed often have less emotional energy to prepare for a vaginal delivery. To get an idea of whether you are depressed while pregnant, see the box on this page.

When manic and pregnant, some women impulsively stop their medications and endanger themselves or their baby through risky behavior like abusing substances, driving recklessly, or having multiple sexual partners. If untreated, pregnant women with bipolar illness are also at high risk for suicide.

"How Will I Know If I'm Depressed While I'm Pregnant?"

It can be difficult to tell whether you are depressed or just experiencing the fatigue, weight gain, sluggishness, appetite changes, and sleep disturbance that often go along with pregnancy or the postdelivery period. In fact, doctors often miss the diagnosis of depression in their pregnant patients. Nonetheless, there are important differences between the fatigue states of pregnancy and clinical depression.

Lori Altshuler and colleagues (2008) have identified seven symptoms that indicate major depression during pregnancy. These symptoms can occur during any of the three trimesters and can extend into the postpartum period. Take a look at the list and circle any that you have had *most of the time* in the *past week*.

- Depressed mood
- Feelings of guilt
- Reduced time and interest in work/activities
- Slowness of speech and movement
- Feeling much worse in the morning or the evening
- Feeling more tired than usual
- Withdrawing from others

If you have several of these symptoms, consider seeing your psychiatrist or OB to determine whether you should restart the medications you stopped before your pregnancy or need higher dosages. If you have a therapist, you may also want to step up the frequency of sessions.

During the postpartum period, try filling out the Edinburgh Postnatal Depression Scale, which can be found at *www.fresno.ucsf.edu/pediatrics/downloads/edinburghscale.pdf*. The scale has items that are most characteristic of depression during the postpartum interval (e.g, feeling panicked, feeling like one can't cope).

As you see, deciding whether to stop or take medications when pregnant is a difficult choice and often a very emotional one: it may feel like your baby's health is being pitted against your own. On balance, most doctors will tell you it's safer to continue your medications if your mood has been unstable prior to conceiving. But some medications are safer than others.

"Which Medications Are Safe to Take?"

No mood stabilizer or atypical antipsychotic is approved by the FDA for use during pregnancy (Grover & Avasthi, 2015). Not surprisingly, exposure to only one medication is safer for the fetus than exposure to several different ones. Here are some comparisons:

■ If you are choosing between lithium and valproate, lithium is generally considered the safer of the two alternatives. Because valproate has the highest teratogenic risk in the first trimester, it is usually best to switch to something else. You should discuss with your doctor medications other than these as well. Lamotrigine appears to be somewhat better than valproate in terms of fetal risks but has its own complications (see above).

■ As discussed in prior chapters, it's generally better to stay away from antidepressants if you have bipolar disorder because of the risks of rapid cycling or mixed episodes. But some women with bipolar disorder do well with antidepressants in conjunction with mood stabilizers. It may be better to stick with them if you were taking antidepressants before the pregnancy and they helped you recover from periods of depression. The SSRIs (for example, Prozac) do not appear to cause fetal malformations, although there are few studies of this issue.

■ Consider the option of switching from an anticonvulsant (like valproate) to an SGA such as quetiapine (Seroquel). SGAs appear to have lower teratogenic risk than the anticonvulsants, although there are few comparison studies (Einarson & Boskovic, 2009). The problem with some of the SGAs (for example, Risperdal) is that they can elevate your prolactin levels (discussed below) or cause weight gain.

"Can Any Fetal Testing Be Done during the Early Phases of Pregnancy?"

Some fetal abnormalities can be detected prenatally. One option includes *high-resolution ultrasonography* (ultrasound), which can be done at 10–13 weeks to look at the nuchal fold and nasal bone (markers of Down syndrome) and at 16–18 weeks to assess heart formation, vertebral development, facial/palate abnormalities, and the status of other anatomical structures. In addition, evidence of neural tube defects in your baby is usually suggested by high levels of *alpha-fetoprotein* in your blood, usually tested first at 10–13 weeks and again at 15–21 weeks. Your doctor may also recommend *amniocentesis* (testing of the amniotic fluid for chromosomal abnormalities or fetal infections) between 16 and 21 weeks. Between weeks 18 and 24 your doctor may recommend a *fetal echocardiogram*, which is like an ultrasound but gives more direct information about the structure and function of the baby's heart. Discuss the recommended testing regimen with your OB, ideally as soon as you start prenatal care.

"What Do I Need to Consider Later in Pregnancy and during Delivery?"

Again, weigh the medication risks against the risks of relapse if you are doing well. Consider the following issues and discuss them with your doctor when you're entering your second trimester:

■ The teratogenic risks of some medications continue into the second and third trimesters and can include minor physical malformations (for example, abnormalities in late stages of lung development), low birth weight, premature delivery, hypothyroidism, or later behavioral problems. Many doctors, however, will recommend you stay on your medications if you were taking them during the first trimester and your mood has been stable.

■ Because your body will metabolize medications differently when you are pregnant and when you deliver, you have to be alert to the signs of drug toxicity in yourself and your newborn. Drug toxicity can occur when you have abnormally high blood levels of a medication. Signs that you may have developed lithium toxicity include disorientation, vomiting, or dizziness; your infant's signs could include restlessness, muscle twitching, vomiting, and fever. Your doctor should take a lithium level as soon as possible after you deliver and may recommend that you adjust your dosage.

■ More lithium is excreted by the kidneys as a pregnancy progresses, meaning that lithium levels decrease. In other words, you may need to have a higher dose in the late second or third trimester. Then the dose needs to come down significantly as you go into labor. This balancing act can be quite confusing, and it's important to discuss what your physician's approach is to monitoring your blood levels.

■ Discuss fluid intake with your doctor. Lithium can cause dehydration.

■ Are you are planning to breastfeed? (See pages 310–312.)

■ Are family members or a current partner available to spell you and enable you to get enough sleep during the exhausting first few weeks following delivery? If not, what are your options to ensure regular sleep (as much as is realistic with a newborn)?

Treatment after Delivery

"When we first started to talk about having another child, my tendency toward post-partum depression was a big factor. Being depressed had been hard not only on me; it had been really hard on my husband too, seeing me go through it, worrying about me, having to do a lot of the child care, and dealing with the ways in which I treat him when I'm depressed. I knew I was at risk for getting depressed again if I had another baby—I wasn't sure if I should even try to get pregnant. I wanted to be a mother again, but I was afraid of what it would do to the people around me. I cried a lot. I'm glad we went ahead, because we had a healthy son, but it was a hard decision."

—A 39-year-old mother with bipolar I disorder

For many women with bipolar disorder, the highest-risk time for an episode of depression or mania is during the postpartum period, usually defined as the 6 months following delivery. About 15% of women in the general population have episodes of depression at this time, but the risk is as much as three times higher among women with bipolar disorder (Viguera et al., 2000; Wesseloo et al., 2016). Some women with bipolar disorder go on to develop postpartum psychosis (delusions or hallucinations) within 4 weeks after they give birth, especially those who have had a manic episode triggered by sleep loss (Lewis et al., 2018). Postpartum psychosis can include homicidal fantasies about the infant. Women with postpartum psychosis need immediate treatment and often hospitalization.

"What Is Postpartum Depression?"

Not surprisingly, women who were depressed during their pregnancy are highly likely to develop postpartum depression as well. This is another reason that receiving effective treatment for depression during pregnancy is so important.

Postpartum depressive episodes are not the same as the "baby blues," a 3- to 5-day period of hormonal readjustment following delivery. During those days you may cry frequently, feel intensely sad, feel inadequate as a mother and like you made a big mistake, and find it difficult to concentrate or sleep. Typically, this period lifts within 10 days after delivery. A postpartum depressive episode, in contrast, lasts for at least 2 weeks (usually much longer if untreated) and is characterized by the full depressive syndrome, with difficulty in carrying out day-to-day tasks. Fathers are at risk for depression and anxiety during the postpartum period also (Hoffman, Dunn, & Njoroge, 2017; Singley & Edwards, 2015). Babies born to parents with postpartum depression may develop emotional, cognitive, and language or motor problems, some of which can be detected even in the first few months (Forman et al., 2007).

The good news is that starting or restarting lithium just before or around the time of delivery, or within a day or two after delivery, reduces the rate of postpartum episodes of mania or depression from as much as 50% to 10% (Cohen, 2007; Rosso et al., 2016). In turn, babies born to women with postpartum depression often "catch up" in terms of developmental delays once the mother's depression lifts (Hoffman et al., 2017; Weissman et al., 2015).

Some mothers experience reductions in their levels of thyroid hormone during the postpartum period. The signs of hypothyroidism include hair loss, extreme fatigue, sadness, and a low milk supply. Check with your doctor to see if a thyroid supplement would help you during the postpartum period (see below).

"What If I Want to Breastfeed?"

The health benefits of breastfeeding for the mother and infant are well known, but you may be understandably concerned about the effects of your medications on your baby. A review in the journal *Pediatrics* (Fortinguerra, Clavenna, & Bonati, 2009) concluded that most psychiatric medications are secreted in breast milk, but they differ considerably in their adverse effects on the infant.

Lithium and the anticonvulsants can both be detected in the blood of newborns. Right after birth, the liver, kidney, and blood–brain barrier of an infant are still maturing, which means the baby can have higher blood concentrations of any medication that the mother takes. But there is disagreement about whether these medications should be taken during breastfeeding. The American Academy of Pediatrics has said that lithium should not be taken at all when breastfeeding, but this recommendation is based on very limited data. In fact, Viguera, Newport, and colleagues (2007) found that blood concentrations of lithium in breast-fed infants were only about 25% of those in the mother who was taking lithium, much lower than expected. Moreover, no serious growth or developmental delays or other serious adverse effects were found, and minor changes in the infant's laboratory tests were not clinically significant.

PERSONALIZED CARE TIP:
Discontinuing medications when pregnant

If you opt to go off your medications for your pregnancy and/or when breastfeeding, discuss the proper method of titration with your physician. Go off gradually, not all at once. Make sure you have other protective influences in place such as therapy or mindfulness groups (see below) and regular prenatal visits with your OB-GYN and psychiatrist. Consider going back on your medications once you have stopped breastfeeding, which may require some time to escalate your doses to where they were before.

Although the actual risks of lithium or valproate to breast-fed infants (for lithium: sedation, poor feeding, dehydration, muscle twitching; for valproate: lethargy, sedation) appear to be low, you will feel more confident if you take a few precautions:

- Make sure you and your baby are adequately hydrated; rapid dehydration is a side effect of lithium and can cause a sudden fever in you or your infant.

- Take your medications *after* you have finished breastfeeding or when your infant starts a long nap, so that there will be less in your breast milk the next time you feed. You can also pump your breast milk before you take your next medication doses.

- Talk to your doctor about simplifying your medication regimen so that you take fewer medications or take them in single daily doses.

- Make sure your obstetrician is monitoring your and your baby's blood levels of lithium or valproate at least monthly to avoid any risks of toxicity, especially if your infant is under 10 weeks old.

Of course, you may not be taking lithium or valproate. Here are some additional suggestions:

- If you are taking carbamazepine (Tegretol or Equetro), be on the lookout for decreased feeding, sedation, or spasms in your newborn. A small number of infants develop a temporary liver dysfunction on carbamazepine.

- If you are taking lamotrigine, and especially if you started it recently, make sure to check yourself and your baby for skin rashes (see Chapter 6). The postpartum period is a high-risk time for developing rashes on lamotrigine, and you will almost certainly need to stop taking it if severe itching begins.

- Antipsychotics appear to be among the safest compounds to take when breastfeeding, especially at low dosages. However, as you know from prior chapters, some of these medications (notably olanzapine [Zyprexa]) can cause you to gain a significant amount of weight, which puts you at risk for diabetes and other metabolic syndromes. Some breast-fed infants develop sedation and lethargy when their mothers take antipsychotics.

Breastfeeding and Sleep Regularity

Women who breastfeed have more chaotic sleep–wake cycles than women who bottle-feed, which can put you at risk for a manic recurrence. The postpartum period is a particularly important time for you to get regular sleep, but also one of the hardest times to make it happen.

Of course, the decision to breastfeed is a very personal and often a very emotional one, and the effects on your sleep cycles will probably not be at the forefront of your mind after you deliver. But try to weigh the benefits of breast-feeding against the risks. If you decide to breastfeed, enlist your family members (husband/partner, in-laws, siblings) and others in your support system to help you with other nighttime child care tasks that can interfere with your sleep.

"What Other Treatments Are Available during the Postpartum Period?"

The postpartum period is a very stressful and chaotic time for anyone. Although you are most likely enjoying the excitement and joy of having a new baby, you may also be dealing with your baby's illnesses (or those of your other children), long and sometimes conflictual visits from in-laws, and unpredictable routines. You may feel closer to your husband or partner than ever before, but, understandably, you may also be arguing more. If you had a job during or before your pregnancy, you may not feel like going back, but your employer may be pressuring you to return. These stressors, along with your biological vulnerabilities, can contribute to postpartum depressive episodes.

Some women with bipolar disorder elect to take antidepressants (in addition to their mood stabilizers) during the postpartum months to help deal with their anxiety and depression. If you have done well on them before, and they have not brought on mixed episodes or rapid cycling, adjunctive antidepressants are one treatment option to consider for postpartum depression. The antidepressants vary in their milk transfer rate, so discuss with your doctor which one is best for you. Some doctors recommend sertraline (Zoloft), paroxetine (Paxil), or fluvoxamine (Luvox) over other agents (Fortinguerra et al., 2009), but few studies on bipolar disorder have been done.

The risks of SSRI antidepressants to your infant include sedation, nausea, and reduced feeding. There are a few studies that indicate a higher risk of "primary pulmonary hypertension" (difficulty breathing) and "neonatal adaptation syndrome" (irritability, alterations in muscle tone, temperature instability) in infants of women who took SSRIs in the third trimester of pregnancy (for example, see Occhiogrosso, Omran, & Altemus, 2012; Salisbury et al., 2016). It is unclear how long these symptoms last; 2–4 weeks is the current estimate. They can be a source of considerable anxiety for parents in the meantime.

Many women resist psychotherapy during the postpartum months, believing that their emotional ups and downs can be explained by hormones, sleep disturbance, or simple exhaustion. Certainly these factors will contribute to your mood states. But you may also be cycling into a depressive episode, your prior depression symptoms from the prepartum period may be getting worse, or you may be developing a mixed state (depression with agitation, hypomania, or even full mania). If you have had a therapist before, now is a good time to reconnect and, if possible,

New research: Mindfulness classes during pregnancy

If you don't have the time or financial resources for individual psychotherapy, consider meditation practices such as MBCT (see Chapter 10) or mindfulness-based stress reduction, usually done in groups that meet once a week for about 2 hours. These groups are generally inexpensive or even free and can often be found at community mental health centers or recreation centers.

Mindfulness aims to interrupt our natural tendency to respond with strong emotions to negative thoughts or bodily sensations that are associated with stress and sad mood. In MBCT, one learns to become present, focused, and nonjudgmental when observing one's internal emotional and thought processes.

There is research supporting the use of MBCT for pregnant women with depression. In a recent study, 86 pregnant women who had a history of depressive episodes (and who were therefore at high risk for depressive recurrences) were randomly assigned to a series of eight MBCT classes or usual treatment (access to mental health care within the Kaiser Permanente system). The group that got MBCT reported significantly lower levels of depressive symptoms and lower rates of depressive relapse for up to 6 months postpartum compared to the group that got usual treatment (Dimidjian et al., 2016).

Given how many changes occur when a baby is born, and how different your body may feel, a meditative approach to looking at one's world may be an important strategy for reducing the impact of your mood symptoms. Developing a daily meditation practice is time consuming, and the rewards may not be immediately apparent, but the long-term effects can be quite powerful.

resume sessions. You can ask for help in developing daily and nightly routines, making sense of the changes in lifestyles and family relationships you are now facing, and dealing with distress in your primary relationship. Additionally, some of the cognitive-behavioral techniques outlined in Chapter 10 can be done on your own during the postpartum period (for example, scheduling pleasurable activities).

Contraceptive Choices

Planning pregnancy obviously gives you more control over the management of your disorder and the healthy development of your baby. That's one reason that effective contraception is important. But even if you never intend to become pregnant, you should know about the interactions between the psychiatric medications you're taking and oral contraceptives (birth control pills). Some of the anticonvulsants, including carbamazepine, oxcarbazepine (Trileptal), and topiramate

(Topamax) increase the metabolism of sex hormones like estrogen and progesterone and may make your contraceptive less effective. As a result, you may need to use a different form of contraception (for example, a diaphragm, condoms, or a birth control pill with a higher estrogen dose) if you're taking these medications (Joffe, 2007).

Birth control pills can also make certain medications—lamotrigine and valproate in particular—less effective by reducing the blood concentrations of the medication. So, if you are taking birth control pills, you may need to increase your dosage of lamotrigine or use another contraceptive to get the full mood-stabilizing benefit (Scrandis, 2017). Additionally, if you suddenly stop your birth control pills, your estrogen will drop and you may have a sudden increase in lamotrigine levels, which puts you at greater risk of rashes or Stevens–Johnson syndrome (see Chapter 6). So, make sure your doctor is aware of when you are starting or stopping oral contraceptives.

Bipolar Disorder and the Menstrual Cycle

You may find that your menstrual cycle is affected by bipolar disorder—both the biology of the illness and the medications you take to manage it. Typical menstrual abnormalities include absence of a period (amenorrhea), cycles longer than 35 days (oligomenorrhea), and cycles that are irregular from month to month. Irregular menstrual cycles, usually defined as cycles shorter than 25 days or longer than 35 days, occur in 15–20% of all women. In one of the few studies of women with mood disorders, menstrual cycle dysfunction was reported in 34.2% of women with bipolar disorder compared to 24.5% women with major depression and 21.7% of healthy, nondepressed women (Joffe, Kim, et al., 2006).

Normal or Abnormal Irregularities?

Your doctor should be taking a detailed menstrual cycle history from you, especially if you're gaining weight on medications (see pages 317–318) or you develop menstrual irregularities. There are both normal and abnormal reasons for irregular cycles. Typical reasons include having just reached puberty (younger females), breastfeeding an infant, or being close to menopause. More troubling reasons can include polycystic ovarian syndrome (see pages 316–317), elevated prolactin levels or hyperprolactinemia (often caused by antipsychotic medications; see page 317), hypothyroidism (see page 319), benign growths on the anterior pituitary gland, excessive exercise or weight loss, and severe psychological stress.

What Does Medication Have to Do with It?

If you've had recent irregularities in your menstrual cycle, it's important to know whether these irregularities *predated* taking medications like lithium, valproate, or SGAs. In a study by Natalie Rasgon and colleagues (2005), about 50% of women with bipolar disorder who had menstrual abnormalities reported that these abnormalities started before their first medication use. But even if your menstrual problems did occur early on, your medications can worsen them because of the effects of mood stabilizers on the hypothalamic–pituitary–gonadal (HPG) axis and their peripheral effects on testosterone metabolites. Valproate seems to have a greater effect on menstrual cycles than lithium or other mood stabilizers (Rasgon et al., 2005). Discuss these issues with your doctor: disrupted menstrual cycles can reduce fertility and contribute to longer-term illnesses such as osteoporosis, non-insulin-dependent diabetes, and cardiovascular disease (Kenna et al., 2009).

PERSONALIZED CARE TIP:
Tracking menstrual irregularities

Most women report that their mood symptoms—notably their depression and anxiety—get worse prior to and during their periods. But women with bipolar disorder have more extreme mood variations related to their cycles (Rasgon, Bauer, Glenn, Elman, & Whybrow, 2003). It can be very difficult to tell whether your mood changes worsen your menstrual periods or whether your periods worsen your moods. Do your medications make your cycles worse or better? Do birth control pills reduce your menstrually related mood changes?

Your mood chart (page 191) can help you figure out whether your menstrual irregularities and mood changes are due to your disorder, your medications, or other factors. Start by circling the days on which your periods started and ended. Over several months of keeping the chart, patterns may emerge. You may find, for example, that mood changes associated with your period are less common since you started antidepressants or that increases in your work demands are related to your menstrual irregularities. You may also find that the menstrual irregularities you have been attributing to your medications actually have a life of their own.

Take your completed mood charts to your psychiatry or obstetric appointments and discuss your options. Your doctor may recommend that you stop certain medications or alter the dosages to see whether your menstrual cycles (and any associated hormonal imbalances) go back to normal. Of course, you may decide that you don't want to risk stopping or changing your medications, but you'll have one more piece of information that may be valuable in the future.

Other Physical Conditions Related to Bipolar Disorder and Its Treatments

Several endocrine (hormonal) conditions can be brought on or worsened by the medications you take for bipolar disorder. Other endocrine conditions may be part of the biology of the illness. In some cases, your medications and individual neurochemistry combine to cause the problem. What you do to address the conditions varies depending on what the main cause is likely to be.

Polycystic Ovarian Syndrome (PCOS)

PCOS is an endocrine disorder that increases your risk for type 2 diabetes, endometrial hyperplasia (which can presage endometrial cancer), lowered fertility, and heart disease (Kenna et al., 2009). About half of women who develop PCOS have significant weight problems (some of which are caused by the mood-stabilizing drugs they take). As the name implies, the signs of PCOS include abnormal cysts on the ovaries, but also facial acne, male pattern balding, growth of excessive facial hair, weight gain, and high levels of testosterone (Barthelmess & Naz, 2014). The condition is diagnosed by infrequent ovulation, hyperandrogenism (an elevated level of or an increased sensitivity to the androgen steroid hormones, such as testosterone), insulin resistance, and infertility. The abnormal cysts are detected through ultrasound, and the hyperandrogenism is usually detected through blood tests of sex steroids (for example, testosterone) and reproductive hormones (for example, estrogen or progesterone).

> **Effective prevention of PCOS and other reproductive disorders:** Watch for the development of menstrual irregularities or significant weight gain after you start any new mood-stabilizing medication.

PCOS affects about 1 in 20 women in the general population, but you are at a higher risk if you take valproate. PCOS and bipolar disorder probably have some common genetic underpinnings (Jiang, Kenna, & Rasgon, 2009), but valproate, carbamazepine, and oxcarbazepine (Trileptal) increase your risk substantially. The STEP-BD study (see Chapter 6) found that 10.5% of women with bipolar disorder developed irregular menstrual cycles and hyperandrogenism in their first year of taking valproate, compared to 1.4% taking lithium or other anticonvulsants like lamotrigine (Joffe, Cohen, et al., 2006). Among women who then stopped taking valproate, there was an improvement in menstrual cycles and lower levels of testosterone.

If you're taking an anticonvulsant and you experience menstrual irregularities, don't assume you have PCOS. Irregularities can also signal the impact of stressors, unexpected pregnancy, elevated prolactin levels (see the next page), or the onset of menopause (all covered elsewhere in this chapter).

At minimum, if you are on valproate, carbamazepine, or oxcarbazepine and have developed menstrual irregularities, gained a significant amount of weight, developed facial hair, or had any of the other reproductive signs listed on the previous page, you should get your testosterone levels checked and, possibly, have an ultrasound to see if your ovaries show any polycystic changes (Isojärvi, Taubøll, & Herzog, 2005). If they do, in all likelihood you'll need to stop taking these anticonvulsants and switch to a different mood stabilizer (for example, lamotrigine).

Prolactin Elevation

Elevated levels of the hormone prolactin (hyperprolactinemia) are dangerous because they can increase your risk of breast cancer and, when you also have infrequent menstrual cycles, lead to reductions in the production of estrogen. Low levels of estrogen can in turn lead to infertility and reduce bone density, which puts you at risk for osteoporosis (Joffe, 2007). When elevated, prolactin can cause infrequent menstrual cycles, galactorrhea (breast leaking), breast enlargement, amenorrhea, migraine headaches, or decreased sex drive (Ali & Khemka, 2008).

You are at greater risk of hyperprolactinemia if your treatment includes certain antipsychotic drugs. Between 48 and 88% of people taking risperidone develop hyperprolactinemia. The risk is also high with some of the other SGAs (Kishi et al., 2017). So, if you have a family history of breast cancer, it's particularly important to have your prolactin levels checked while taking SGAs.

If you have prolactin elevation but no evidence of menstrual irregularities, you may not have to be treated for it. But if you're having active symptoms of hyperprolactinemia, you may need to stop taking your antipsychotic medication and switch to an agent less likely to cause prolactin elevation. If your doctor detects low estrogen levels as well as high prolactin, a hormonal contraceptive that increases estrogen may also be recommended.

Weight Gain and the Metabolic Syndrome

Both men and women with bipolar disorder are at increased risk for developing obesity, but the risk is higher among women. *Obesity* is usually defined as a body mass index of 30 kg/m² or more; being overweight is usually defined as at least 25 kg/m² (to calculate your body mass index using pounds and inches, use the online calculator at *http://smartbmicalculator.com*). You may have struggled with weight problems before you started taking psychiatric medications; these symptoms are suspected to be part of the illness. Nonetheless, medications can worsen preexisting weight problems.

A particularly worrisome effect of weight gain and obesity is the *metabolic syndrome*, which consists of insulin resistance or glucose intolerance (in which the body does not properly use insulin or blood sugar), hyperglycemia (excessive blood glucose), excessive fat tissue around the stomach, dyslipidemia (usually indicated by high triglycerides and low HDL and high LDL cholesterol), high blood pressure, and other symptoms. The metabolic syndrome affects 17–49% of people with bipolar disorder and, like weight gain generally, affects more women than men (Kenna et al., 2009). Obesity and the metabolic syndrome are risk factors for serious health problems, including diabetes, hypertension, and cardiovascular problems.

The first thing you can do to protect yourself against developing the metabolic syndrome is to be aware of any weight gain on a certain medication. Whether it be an SGA, valproate, or lithium, ask your doctor to check you for evidence of metabolic disturbances (for example, by testing your cholesterol and triglycerides, conducting a fasting insulin or glucose tolerance test, and doing a blood lipids profile). If there is evidence that your body is reacting poorly to your prescribed medications, discuss your other treatment options with your physician (see the personalized care tip at the bottom of this page). Some medications for bipolar disorder are better than others: for example, people with bipolar disorder generally gain more weight on the SGA olanzapine (Zyprexa) than on valproate (Novick et al., 2009). Among the SGAs, ziprasidone (Geodon) and aripiprazole (Abilify) appear to be more "weight neutral" than olanzapine. Quetiapine (Seroquel) and risperidone (Risperdal) are both associated with weight gain, but not as much as olanzapine. Most of the SGAs and valproate are associated with risk of insulin resistance or hyperlipidemia.

Among the mood stabilizers, lamotrigine appears to be better than lithium or valproate in terms of weight gain. Although topiramate has weight-loss properties, there is poor evidence for its efficacy as a mood stabilizer; avoid taking this medication just to lose weight. If you are gaining weight, your doctor may recommend you add a drug called metformin (Glucophage), an antidiabetic agent that appears to cause weight loss with relatively few side effects.

Of course, if you have gained weight, most doctors will recommend you get regular exercise and maintain a healthy diet. We all know the importance of these lifestyle adaptations, but they can be extraordinarily difficult to implement when you are depressed, which can make you feel even more down on yourself. Try not to be critical of yourself if you can't stick to a diet or exercise plan: you may be able to return to these lifestyle habits when your mood improves.

PERSONALIZED CARE TIP:
Protecting yourself from metabolic problems

If you start gaining weight, talk to your doctor about changing your medication dosage, taking your medication at a different time of day, switching to medications that have less risk of weight gain (for example, aripiprazole, lamotrigine), or, if you do not have liver or kidney disease, adding the drug metformin to promote weight loss.

Thyroid Disorders

Thyroid disturbances appear more often with depression than with other types of psychiatric disorders. Be alert for such conditions, particularly low production of thyroid hormones, or *hypothyroidism,* which is more common in women than men. Some women first develop thyroid problems around the time of menarche, others after giving birth, and still others as a normal part of aging. A variety of factors—autoimmune disease, iodine deficiency, genetic predisposition, and certain medications—can cause thyroid disorders.

There is some evidence that rapid cycling and hypothyroidism (both of which are more common among women) are linked, but not all studies find this (Buoli, Serati, & Altamura, 2017). Lithium suppresses thyroid hormone and causes hypothyroidism in some people. Therefore your doctor should be checking your thyroid levels as part of your regular blood work, especially when you start a new medication.

If you have a low thyroid level you might need a supplement such as levothyroxine (Synthroid). Because it has been found to reduce the frequency of depressive episodes, you don't necessarily have to have an underactive thyroid to benefit from thyroid supplementation. But if you do start thyroid supplementation, be aware of the symptoms of becoming *hyperthyroid,* which can put you at risk for atrial fibrillation or osteoporosis. The symptoms of an overactive thyroid are fairly recognizable: changes in your menstrual cycle, feeling hot and sweaty, heart palpitations, having "salty skin," bulging eyes, changes in weight or appetite, anxiety, and frequent diarrhea or bowel movements. Your doctor can measure whether you are hyperthyroid using standard blood tests. If you are, you will probably have to stop taking the supplement, reduce your dose, or change to a different form of supplementation. Taking a thyroid supplement can be a balancing act, but when you are experiencing depression that is not responding to treatments, it can be simpler and more effective to take the supplement than to add another mood stabilizer or atypical antipsychotic into the mix.

Migraine Headaches

There is a clear link between migraine headaches and mood or anxiety disorders. One recent study found that the rate of bipolar disorder among women with migraines was four times higher than among women without migraines (Jette, Patten, Williams, Becker, & Wiebe, 2008). Of people receiving treatment for migraines, as many as 19% may have bipolar disorder (Kivilcim, Altintas, Domac, Erzincan, & Gülec, 2017). Although men also develop migraines, the rate is at least twice as high among women. Girls often develop migraines around the time of their first menstrual period and then go on to have them repeatedly in the premenstrual or menstrual phases of their cycles.

Migraines are far worse than ordinary headaches: they usually begin in the morning and last for at least 4 hours, occur on only one side of the head, create a throbbing sensation, are worsened by physical activity, and often require bed rest. To treat them, you can use "triptan" medications intended specifically for migraines, such as sumatriptan (Imitrex) or zolmitriptan (Zomig). But migraines can also be treated successfully with valproate or other anticonvulsants. If you are prone to migraines, avoid drugs (for example, risperidone) that elevate prolactin levels.

Lithium may improve migraines but is not considered a primary treatment for them. One of the older antidepressants, amitriptyline (Elavil), has been shown experimentally to reduce the frequency of migraines, but the difficulties of taking tricyclic antidepressants when you have bipolar disorder make this a risky option. The Mayo Clinic has an informative website on new treatments for migraines (*www.mayoclinic.org/diseases-conditions/migraine-headache/diagnosis-treatment/drc-20360207*). More generally, make sure the doctor who is treating your migraines is talking to your psychiatrist about the effects of the migraine medications on your mood and potential drug interactions with your mood stabilizers.

Menopause

> *"Going through menopause was absolute hell. I finally got stabilized on estrogen supplements, and then after all those years my doctor wanted to take my estrogen away. Why didn't he understand that without it I'd be a complete mess?"*
>
> —A 52-year-old woman with bipolar II disorder

Not much is known about bipolar disorder and menopause, except that menopause is a time of heightened risk for mood swings and recurrences. A synthesis of nine studies found that 46–91% of bipolar women reported a worsening of their depressive symptoms during menopause and, less frequently, their mania or hypomania symptoms (Perich, Ussher, & Meade, 2017).

Women with bipolar disorder may be more sensitive to the reductions in estrogen that occur during menopause. Of course, just because your moods worsen near, during, or after menopause doesn't mean that hormones explain everything. Many women have other life changes in their late 40s and 50s, including kids moving away from home, divorces, remarriages, illnesses, deaths of parents, and other transitions. So, if you are of perimenopausal age and start experiencing a destabilization or worsening of your mood, ask your OB-GYN for an endocrinological workup (for example, levels of follicle-stimulating hormone, estradiol, luteinizing hormone, thyroid hormone) and talk to your psychiatrist about whether you need to adjust your medications (for example, you may need to lower your dose of lamotrigine because of its effects on estrogen levels). You can also use psychotherapy or group therapy sessions to explore the effects of aging and recent life transitions on your emotional and physical health.

Some women with bipolar disorder decide to start hormone replacement therapy, or HRT (usually estrogen and progesterone, although some women take only estrogen). There is some evidence that HRT can help stabilize moods around the time of the perimenopausal transition (the time immediately before menopause; Freeman et al., 2002), and it also reduces symptoms such as hot flashes. HRT also has other health benefits, such as increasing bone density, but there are case reports of women on HRT getting manic or beginning to cycle rapidly. Plus, HRT puts you at higher risk for breast cancer and heart disease. Discuss the HRT option with both your OB-GYN and your psychiatrist and consult *http://womensmental-health.org* for updates in this rapidly changing area.

If menopause affects depression, is the reverse also true? The Harvard Study of Moods and Cycles, which involved 976 depressed and nondepressed women between the ages of 36 and 45, investigated whether depression has an effect on the *perimenopausal transition,* during which a number of biological and hormonal changes occur (Harlow, Wise, Otto, Soares, & Cohen, 2003). Perimenopause starts at an average age of 47.5 years and can last from 4 to 8 years. It is marked by a decline in ovarian function and is a time of increased risk for recurrences of depression.

Compared with women who did not have a history of depression, women with depression reported having their first menstrual period at a younger age. In a 3-year follow-up, women with a history of depression reached perimenopause sooner than women who had no depression history, particularly if their depression was severe and they were taking antidepressants for it. Women with depression also had higher follicle-stimulating hormone and luteinizing hormone levels and lower estrogen levels than their nondepressed peers (Harlow et al., 2003).

Although no women with bipolar disorder participated, the results may have implications for you if you are approaching the age of menopause: you may develop perimenopausal symptoms earlier than your age-mates, especially if you are taking antidepressants as well as mood stabilizers. If your periods start to become irregular, shorter, involve mid-cycle spotting, or stop altogether, see your OB-GYN to have your hormone levels checked and determine whether you might be starting menopause. Some women opt for HRT at this time (see *http://medlineplus.gov/hormonereplacementtherapy.html*).

• • • • • • • • • • • • • •

Some of what you've learned in this chapter may discourage you and make you feel like you're "damned if you do, damned if you don't." Indeed, for women, coping with bipolar disorder can be a much more difficult balancing act than for men, and the choices you will be asked to make will often seem quite unfair.

Fortunately, you can adjust your treatment to minimize teratogenic effects during pregnancy, the effects on your menstrual cycle, and the likelihood of developing polycystic ovaries, metabolic conditions, thyroid conditions, or hyperprolactinemia. Before starting any new medication, discuss with your doctor the ways that adverse effects can be reduced. Remember that all medications, even aspirin, have long-term side effects. (For more information on bipolar disorder in your children or any children you plan to have, see Chapter 14.)

Chapter 13 offers a different window on the question of self-management: how to cope effectively in your family and work environments after an illness episode. People with bipolar disorder often experience trouble in both settings—trouble not entirely due to their own behavior. Many of their problems derive from others having an inadequate understanding of the disorder (see Martha's story in Chapter 1). I will discuss several strategies that may empower you in negotiating your family, social, and work relationships. As you've seen throughout this book, managing your disorder involves acquainting others with the facts about it and being clear yourself on what will, and will not, be helpful to your recovery.

CHAPTER 13

Succeeding at Home and at Work

Communication, Problem-Solving Skills, and Dealing Effectively with Stigma

Bipolar disorder poses significant challenges for your daily life with your family, at work, and in your friendships and other relationships. When your family members first learned about your disorder, they may have been supportive, intrusive, anxious, or angry. Some may have been eager to help, while others subjected you to overt rejection. But even after everyone has seemed to adjust to your life with bipolar disorder, difficulties often reappear with the next mood episode.

Likewise, you may experience frustration in the work setting. You probably want to work and be productive, but you may not know how to deal with the stigma of the disorder, the lack of understanding by employers or coworkers, or workplace demands that are incompatible with your attempts to manage your illness. We know that the symptoms of bipolar disorder affect a person's ability to function in the family or work setting. The good news is that you can learn to negotiate the conflicts and demands of your family and work life through a variety of communication skills and self-care strategies.

If you have time, go back to Chapter 1 and reread the case illustration of Martha. After her manic episode and hospitalization, her children became suspicious, withdrawn, and fearful. Her husband was rejecting at some points and overprotective at others before he came to a better understanding of the disorder through their couple therapy. Back at her computer programming job, Martha had problems concentrating. She found the computer screen newly confusing and forgot how to use the programs she had been so expert at using before. Her boss quickly became impatient with her low performance. Her coworkers avoided her and even seemed nervous in her presence after learning of her diagnosis.

If you've recently recovered from a manic, mixed, or depressive episode, you may feel ready to reintegrate yourself into the family and the workplace, only to find that those you live and work with don't treat you the way they used to. Your loved ones may become angry and critical or overprotective. Your partner may seem hesitant to reestablish intimacy with you. At work you may feel like "It's the same old me" but get the impression that your colleagues don't see it that way. And if you really do need to adjust your work setting and work routines to help maintain mood stability, how much can you tell them about your disorder and still get them to treat you as the confident, competent person you were before?

These issues pose undeniable challenges, but I have been continually impressed with how effectively people with bipolar disorder learn to deal with them. Establishing close family or couple relationships is possible even after the most severe of mood disorder episodes. So is reclaiming successful work lives and reaching career aspirations. As you'll soon see, maintaining successful family and work relationships has a lot to do with how you communicate and solve problems with others and educate them as they go through their inevitable ups and downs in reacting to your disorder.

"What Family Problems Might I Encounter after an Illness Episode?"

During the period after an acute episode—when you are on the road to recovery—your close relatives (parents, spouse, siblings, kids) will usually try to be helpful. Some succeed in being valuable allies. For example, after a manic episode, they may let you know that you are overscheduling yourself or that your level of daily activity is escalating. However, relatives and partners often have confusing feelings about your illness and confusing thoughts about how to help you, especially if you are having your first or second episode. In the following sections I explore the most common problems that arise in families and couples.

Negative Emotional Reactions from Your Relatives

Randy, a 45-year-old plumber, had two episodes of major depression and several hypomanic episodes. His most recent episode, a severe depression, led to the loss of his job. His wife, Cindy, had a rudimentary understanding of bipolar disorder from her readings and Internet searches but was fairly intolerant of his apparent inability to function. She made the mistake many relatives make—overpathologizing her husband's behavior and using newly learned psychiatric terms in a derogatory manner: "That's your mania talking"; "Last night when we got into that argument, you were totally rapid cycling"; "You're doing your ADD [attention deficit disorder] thing again." In couple sessions, Cindy revealed that she really didn't believe his mood problems had a biological origin. She blamed them on his "crazy, dysfunctional family," his "temperamental nature," and "unconscious, unresolved stuff with me." She also wasn't convinced by the genetic evidence that Randy's father had had bipolar disorder.

Their debates about the causes of Randy's behavior tended to degenerate into escalating interchanges in which Cindy would berate Randy and he would try to defend himself. He typically ended up agreeing with her, just to stop the argument, but then would feel resentful and withdraw to punish her. Annoyed at his withdrawal, she would continue her attack later with the accusation that "You've never been able to deal with things directly." He began to consider going off his medications just to prove "that I can deal with all of this without anyone or anything's help."

Why is Cindy so angry? Most of the family members I have worked with are well-intentioned, caring people who honestly want to do what's best for their relative with bipolar disorder. But they don't always know what to do when their family member reacts negatively to their attempts to help. They end up feeling frustrated and burdened by the effort required of them to adapt to the disorder and then often say and do things that are critical or unhelpful.

Your relatives' reactions to your disorder, particularly during the period when you are recovering, often reflect the same styles of coping or *causal attribution* that you used at various stages of adjusting to your illness (see Chapter 4): *underidentifying* with the disorder (attributing your behavior changes—those that are likely part of the illness—to your personality or habits) or *overidentifying* with it (attributing all or most of your behaviors, even normal ones, to your illness). Highly critical relatives are often underidentifying you with the disorder, as Cindy was doing. They may believe that your biologically based, illness-related changes in behavior—including any residual mood swings from your last episode that haven't cleared up yet—are really caused by your character or morals, your unconscious motivations, or your lack of effort. A family member who believes that these factors play a causal role will also believe that you have more control over your mood swings than you really do. Your relative may then become angry and critical or even hostile.

Overprotectiveness

Alternatively, you may find that your relatives want to watch you very carefully and micromanage your disorder to the point where you feel you're being treated like a child. This is often called "emotional overinvolvement." Relatives who are overinvolved (most typically a parent or a spouse) often tend to overidentify you with the disorder or label your everyday reactions as signs of your illness. For example, they say that your illness is reflected in your getting angry about things you might very well have gotten angry about before you became ill. Sometimes you and they are both right—your anger may be stimulated by real things, but your disorder makes you react with a level of emotional intensity that is out of proportion to the circumstances. Nonetheless, you may begin to register that their labeling of your behavior is making you feel worse. Relatives may remind you repeatedly to take your medications, tell you to talk to your doctor or therapist about minor problems you have at home or at work, or even go behind your back to talk with your physician.

You may even find, as some of my patients have found, that when you confront your relatives about their overprotectiveness they use your bipolar diagnosis as a weapon against you. For example, you might express annoyance at a relative for asking you too many questions about your medications, only to have the relative tell you that your reaction is a sign of your illness. You can get into a vicious cycle in which you complain about their intrusiveness, your relatives react as if you are cycling into an episode, you get more annoyed with their labeling of you as mentally ill, their beliefs about your cycling become more confirmed, and then they become increasingly critical or overprotective. This is known as a "high expressed emotion" interaction pattern, which can put you at higher risk for recurrences (Miklowitz, Biuckians, & Richards, 2006; Miklowitz & Chung, 2016).

Problems with Intimacy

Now let's consider a different kind of emotional reaction that often arises between spouses or partners during the recovery period: a discomfort with physical intimacy. Your partner's discomfort may not be associated with criticism or overprotectiveness; instead, you may experience him or her as emotionally distant and withdrawn. Physical intimacy may have stopped altogether during, or shortly after, your last episode (as Martha experienced with her husband after her hospitalization), or it may have gradually diminished over time after multiple episodes.

It is quite common for relationships to be at a vulnerable point during the recovery period, even if the episode was only a minor one. Many spouses feel angry about events that occurred during the episode and don't feel comfortable being close. This is particularly likely to happen if you went off your medications (against your spouse's wishes) prior to your most recent episode.

If you are currently hypomanic, you may have an increased sex drive, but your spouse may have pulled away because of mistrust related to your disorder. For example, she may be cautious because of your recent bouts of irritability. The opposite can also occur: You may be depressed, and your spouse may want to reestablish physical contact, but you may feel under pressure, uncomfortable with your body, or bad about yourself as a sexual partner. It is not unusual for people to lose their sex drive during and after a depressed episode.

If you've been well for some time, you may have an easier time negotiating intimacy with your partner. But even clients of mine who have remained well complain that basic issues of trust between them and their partners were violated by their earlier illness states and that emotional and physical intimacy has been hard to reestablish. If you are experiencing one or more of these problems, you are certainly not alone. Fortunately, these couple problems can be addressed using a number of relationship-rebuilding skills, outlined in the next few sections.

> **Effective solution:** The first step in dealing effectively with family members after an illness episode is to educate them about your disorder. This is generally a good idea even if your family is functioning well, but it is especially important during the period after an episode, when negative emotions are often at their peak.

Tools for Improving Family Relationships after an Episode

Educating Your Family

Your relatives or spouse/partner may harbor many misconceptions about the illness, its treatments, or what the future holds for all of you. This can happen even if they have interacted with your doctors, read any of the popular books or seen movies on the subject, and listened to your explanations.

Flawed or incomplete information about bipolar disorder can cause your loved ones to be critical or overprotective of you. Make copies of the box on pages 330–331, which summarizes the basic facts about bipolar disorder (you can also download and print it; see the information at the end of the Contents). Make this fact sheet available for all family members (whether or not they have been with you during your episodes), including your adult or teenage children, parents, spouse/partner, siblings, and other extended relatives.

It is important to have a common language when communicating with close relatives about your symptoms or changes in functioning. Hidden within the different terms your family members use in discussing your behavior are often subtle differences in beliefs about what causes you to behave in these ways. Acquainting your relatives with the facts about the disorder may make them think twice about what causes your mood swings. For example, your family members will be more supportive of you if they understand that increases in your irritability are a sign of the disorder's cycling rather than evidence that "you've gotten mean" or "you're more hostile than you used to be" or "you've got a temper problem." Likewise, they should come to understand that you are suffering from "depressed mood" or "fatigue" or "concentration problems" rather than "mental laziness" or "a pessimistic outlook on life." Family members who become highly critical toward an individual with a psychiatric disorder are often harboring the belief that the individual's symptoms are due to personality or lack of effort (Hooley, 2007).

Family members who know the basic facts about bipolar disorder will also be more supportive of your efforts to maintain consistency in your treatment. Well-meaning relatives who do not understand the disorder may view drug treatment or psychotherapy as crutches, or believe that you're being too watchful over your health and moods. They may give you direct or indirect messages about how they liked you better before you began your medicines or therapy. Alternatively, they may repeatedly plague you with reminders to take your medicines, to the point where you don't want to take them for revenge. In either case, these reactions may make you feel even more ambivalent than you already feel about your treatments. Your family members need to know why you are taking medications, attending psychotherapy, engaging in self-management tasks like sleep–wake regulation, and most important, where you do or don't need their help.

Spend some time answering their questions after they have read the fact sheet. Depending on their age or education level, they may have trouble understanding how you have experienced certain symptoms, where in the family tree the illness may have originated, or why you are taking a certain combination of medications (for example, a mood stabilizer *and* an antidepressant). If you are sharing information about your disorder with your school-age children, try to see if you can simplify it to fit their developmental level. One man explained to his 6-year-old son, "You know how happy you get during your birthday parties? I get that way sometimes for a whole week, and then it gets hard for me to do my work." One woman explained to her 7-year-old, "You know how when you get excited, you can usually calm yourself down? When Daddy gets excited, he gets going really fast and he can't calm down right away." Another woman explained to her daughters that when she became sad she couldn't turn off her feelings like they could. "You know how when you're upset and someone tells you a joke, you feel better? Mommy gets upset, but things like jokes won't get her over it right away—she needs more time." She also made it clear to them that they should not blame themselves when she became depressed or withdrawn.

Use age-appropriate terms when describing your disorder. Kids and adolescents relate better to terms such as "down," "crashed," "stressed out," "amped," "wired," "sad," or "bummed" than to "manic" or "depressed." You may have to explain the disorder to them in several different ways and at different times. Be attuned to what they do and don't understand. Following a lengthy discussion of the disorder and its biological bases, one parent reported hearing her 9-year-old son say to one of his friends, "My mother has a bipolar in her head!"

Helping Your Relatives Understand the Medical Bases of Your Disorder

It's important that your close relatives understand that at least a portion of your behavior is biologically determined. Whereas it is not critical that they understand the disorder's mechanisms involving cellular communication, they will benefit from knowing that the disorder is not fully under your control. When they finally come to accept this, they will probably become less angry or hostile, as Rebecca did:

"I had bought concert tickets and was looking forward to the event for weeks. The night we were supposed to go, my husband said he wasn't going to go, that he was too tired and depressed. I was enraged—it just seemed like something he should've known before. It felt like he was doing it to hurt me and disappoint me. I had really wanted us to do this together. I called to cancel the babysitter and the next day went to the ticket office for a refund, feeling like I was arguing from a position of weakness. To my surprise, I told them, 'My husband has a medical illness.' Somehow, that cut through my anger. It helped me do away with the feeling that he was doing something to hurt me. That was how I decided to explain it to myself and to the outside world."

Rebecca's realization that her husband skipped the concert not because he didn't *want to go* but because he *couldn't make himself go* made her feel less resentful of the limitations his illness placed on their lives. Understand, however, that your relatives' frustration and dissatisfaction over your difficulties or limitations will not evaporate overnight. Family members need time and practice to come to grips with the changes in their lives. Consider the way that Evan's relationship with his father evolved:

"For years, he didn't understand, and we could barely talk to each other. I'd shout and scream and spread my self-loathing all over him, and of course he'd get pissed off. Then I'd get depressed and even less able to deal with him. But after my second wife and I split and then I lost my job, I finally told him I had bipolar disorder, and we were really open about it. I just told him, 'Dad, this is one of the main reasons we've had so many problems between us.' I explained how it's a chemical thing and that it wasn't about how he raised me, and he didn't believe me at first. But in another way it made sense to him—he's got a scientific mind and it put so many different things into place . . . my temper, my job stuff, my problems when I was a teenager. When he came to accept it and we could talk about it, he was able to pull back and think about his own responses to me. And I've gotten a lot calmer and less reactive to him . . . we get along much better now."

A Quick Fact Sheet on Bipolar Disorder for Family Members

What Is Bipolar Disorder?

Having bipolar disorder means that I have severe mood swings, in which I go from a very highly energized state (mania, or a milder form called hypomania) to a very low, unmotivated, and lethargic state (depression). My high periods may last from a few days to a month or more. My low periods may last much longer, from several weeks to several months. About 1 in every 50 people has bipolar disorder. It most often affects a person for the first time in adolescence or young adulthood.

What Are the Symptoms?

My main symptoms during a high period may include feeling *overly happy* and *excited* or *overly irritable* and *angry.* I may also feel like I can do things that no one else can do (*grandiosity*). I may sleep less than usual or not at all, do many things at once (some of which seem goal driven and some not), have more energy, talk faster and express many ideas (some realistic and some unrealistic), and be easily distracted. I may do things that are impulsive when manic, like spend a great deal of money unwisely or drive recklessly.

I may experience the symptoms of depression at other times, which can include feeling very sad, down, irritable, or anxious, losing interest in people or things, sleeping too much or being unable to sleep, having little or no appetite, having trouble concentrating or making decisions, feeling fatigued or low in energy, moving or talking slowly, feeling very bad or guilty about myself, or contemplating suicide or actually carrying out suicide attempts.

How Does Bipolar Disorder Affect the Family?

My bipolar disorder may affect my ability to relate to others in our family or in the work setting, especially when I become ill. Our family or relationship problems may be most apparent during or just after my episode of mania or depression, but then will probably improve as I get better. We can resolve our family conflicts through good communication and problem solving, emotional support for each other, and encouragement. We may want to get the additional help of a family or couple therapist or a family support group.

(continued)

A Quick Fact Sheet on Bipolar Disorder
for Family Members *(continued)*

What Causes Bipolar Disorder?

Having bipolar disorder means that I may have dysregulations in the emotional circuitry of the brain, especially the amygdala and the prefrontal cortex. It's possible that I inherited these dysregulations from my blood relatives, even if I can't pinpoint who else in my family tree had it. My mood swings may also be affected by life stress or sudden changes in my sleep–wake habits. Nobody chooses to become bipolar.

How Is Bipolar Disorder Treated?

My treatment will probably include mood-stabilizing medications such as lithium, valproate (Depakote), or lamotrigine (Lamictal), or second-generation antipsychotic medications like risperidone (Risperdal), quetiapine (Seroquel), aripiprazole (Abilify), ziprasidone (Geodon), olanzapine (Zyprexa), lurasidone (Latuda), paliperidone (Invega), or asenapine (Saphris). I may also take antidepressant medications (for example, sertraline (Zoloft) or escitalopram (Lexapro) or drugs to control my anxiety or problems with sleep. These medications require that I see a psychiatrist regularly to make sure my side effects don't get out of hand and, for some medications, to get my blood levels tested. I may also benefit from individual therapy, family or couple therapy sessions, or support groups. Therapy may help me learn how best to manage my moods, identify new episodes early on, monitor moods and sleep–wake cycles, and function better in the family and workplace. If I am one of the many people with bipolar disorder who have problems with drugs or alcohol, mutual support programs like Alcoholics Anonymous may also help me and our family.

What Does the Future Hold?

It is likely that I will have high and low mood episodes in the future. But there is every reason to be hopeful. With the help of a regular program of medications, therapy, exercise, and support from others, my mood disorder episodes can become less frequent, less extreme, and less disruptive. With help and support, I can accomplish many of my goals for my family and work life.

It's unlikely that your relatives will immediately adopt a medical view of your disorder—it took Evan's father quite some time. But with repeated exposure to educational information, your relatives may begin to reevaluate their belief that you are behaving out of ill will or negative intentions. This was the case for Gray, who, with his wife, Arlene, was getting marital therapy to help him adapt to Arlene's bipolar disorder.

> *Arlene:* When I get depressed, it's like a veil just comes over me. It's not at all like when you get tired after work. It's like being numb, like a ton of cement sitting on my heart.
>
> *Gray:* I know, honey, but I just don't think the answer is to mope. You've gotta get out there and deal with things.
>
> *Therapist:* Arlene, can you say more about what that depression is like, and what you think causes it?
>
> *Arlene:* It's probably something in my brain that goes haywire. It feels physical; it doesn't feel like I'm not trying. I know how frustrated you get, Gray, but you have to realize it's not something I want either. If I could pull myself out, I would—in a minute.

Communication Skills for Reducing Criticism and Conflict

In the interchange between Arlene and Gray, Arlene made an effort to validate her husband's point of view. *Effective communication is a very important component of managing your family or marital relationships and can even help facilitate your recovery from an illness episode.* In one of our studies of family-focused therapy, one of the most consistent changes over time among patients whose bipolar disorder improved was an enhanced ability to communicate with their spouse or parents (Miklowitz et al., 2003). The following is a selection of communication skills you can try out when dealing with criticism, tension, or conflict in your close relationships.

Although the skills look easy on the surface, they can be difficult to apply under stress and require regular practice. Certainly, couples and families not affected by bipolar disorder have to work to use effective communication on a day-to-day basis. Yet the stress of family life after a mood episode requires you to be even more skillful in your communication than you would ordinarily have to be. And when your mood is swinging up and down and you feel that your relatives are unfairly jumping on you, using new communication skills can be doubly hard. These skills require that you step back when you feel the heat rising and put yourself in another person's place. As with many self-management strategies, familiarizing yourself with these skills when you are well makes them easier to use when you are ill.

Skill No. 1: Active Listening

After dealing with an episode of bipolar disorder or any other kind of significant stressor, you may have trouble listening to the feelings, objections, or troubles of your spouse, parents, or other family members. This difficulty is quite understandable; you have just gone through a period of intense emotional upheaval and are not in the mood to empathize with others' pain, especially if they imply that you caused it. But if your family members don't feel that you or others in the family care enough to listen, they will probably be unwilling to perform some of the other tasks that are essential to your recovery (for example, helping keep the home environment as low in stress as possible). So, if your parents, spouse, or kids are responding to you negatively or with criticism, consider helping them modulate their anger by listening and expressing an understanding of their position, even if you do not agree with it. This is a technique called active listening, and attempts to use it will almost certainly change the outcome of what would otherwise be unproductive interchanges. The box at the bottom of this page lists the steps.

In active listening, you become less active in the speaking part of communication than you might be used to, and you become more active on the listening end. You maintain eye contact with the person speaking to you, offer nonverbal acknowledgments like a nod of the head, paraphrase or otherwise check out what you've heard (otherwise known as *reflective listening*), and ask questions to get the speaker to clarify his or her point of view. This is a good skill to use whenever you talk with your family members, but it will be especially helpful when arguments start to escalate. There is nothing like validating someone else's point of view in the middle of an argument to reduce her anger—it's hard to be mad at someone who is making a genuine attempt to understand you.

Active listening requires that you avoid any implication of blaming the other person. That is, stay away from any reflective statements or questions that imply the other person is at fault for his or her reactions, or that involve name-calling. For example, the statement "So you feel that if you're mean to me, I'll change for

---

Steps of Active Listening

- Look at the speaker.
- Attend to what is said.
- Nod your head or say "uh-huh."
- Ask clarifying questions.
- Check out what you heard (paraphrase).

Adapted by permission from Miklowitz (2010). Copyright © 2010 by The Guilford Press.

the better" is not really a reflective statement but more of an accusation. The question "Why would you want to be a nag if you are trying to get me to do something on my own?" may feel like a reasonable question, but it will not help resolve the disagreement. It's hard to avoid saying things like that when you're angry or irritable. But if you stay at the level of asking simple, straightforward questions and paraphrasing exactly what you have heard from your relative (even word for word, if necessary), you will be less likely to say something that escalates the conflict.

Consider the following interchange between Randy and Cindy. Randy is practicing the skill of active listening.

> *Randy:* You were pretty mad at me this morning. What was up? [clarifying question]
>
> *Cindy:* I tried to get you to talk about that tax-related thing, and you just blew me off. Why do I keep trying?
>
> *Randy:* (*pausing*) So you were frustrated with me. You wanted me to get it done. [paraphrasing]
>
> *Cindy:* (*still irritated*) Yes, of course I did! And I've asked you a million times.
>
> *Randy:* (*Nods.*) Yes, I understand that gets frustrating. But partly it's because I'm having a tough time concentrating. Are you concerned that I won't get it done? [clarifying question]
>
> *Cindy:* (*Softens.*) Maybe I came down too hard on you, but the question is, when are we gonna do it? The 15th is coming up pretty quick.

Randy's reflective listening and validation of Cindy's point of view helped reduce her irritation and the antagonism that had built up between them. Ideally, this discussion would then merge into problem solving, another skill that will help you negotiate a more productive relationship with your spouse or parent (explained later in this section).

Skill No. 2: Positive Requests for Change

Another way to reduce tension and avoid the verbal attacks that can turn into full-scale war is to phrase your comments to family members as *positive requests for change*. This involves stating, *specifically and diplomatically,* what you'd like to see happen differently in your interactions with your relative. Criticisms tell people what they have done wrong—"I resent that you always bring up my illness when my friends are around"—and naturally generate defensiveness. Stating the same thought in a positive way—"It's very important to me that when we're with our friends, we talk about things we're all interested in other than my illness"—is almost certain to reduce your spouse or partner's defensiveness, even though it's not guaranteed to prevent it altogether. If you're not entirely sure of the difference between the two, note that positive requests usually ask someone to do something new and positive, whereas criticisms usually involve telling someone to stop doing something that is unpleasant to you.

After being hospitalized for a mixed episode of her bipolar disorder, Carol returned to her apartment, only to discover that her father, Roy, was constantly coming over unannounced and then criticizing her for how messy she kept her living room. This surveillance was a particularly sensitive issue for Carol, who felt strongly that her autonomy and independence were important to her recovery. For his part, Roy had become hypervigilant and worried that she would descend into another state of depression. He felt that his concerns were justified by the fact that she'd had three mood episodes in the past year.

During their initial family therapy sessions, Carol said things like "Just don't come over here anymore" or "Why don't you leave me alone?" to which her father responded, "I do it because I don't think you can take care of yourself." The therapist encouraged Carol to try transforming her criticisms into positive requests for change. At first she had trouble with this communication tool, saying things like "Dad, could you leave me alone more? That'd make my life much better." With coaching, she was able to word her request more diplomatically, and her father responded more positively as a result:

Carol: Dad, will you please call me before you're going to come over? That'd give me the chance to clean up first.

Therapist: Good, Carol. And tell him how that would make you feel.

Carol: I'd like it, and I'd probably feel grateful that you cared about me and what I need. It'd also be nice to see you.

Making a Positive Request

■ Look at your family member.

■ Say exactly what you would like him or her to do.

■ Tell your family member how it would make you feel.

■ Use phrases such as:

"I would like you to _____."

"I would really appreciate it if you would _____."

"It's very important to me that you help me with the _____."

Adapted by permission from Miklowitz (2010). Copyright © 2010 by The Guilford Press.

Therapist: That was excellent. Roy, what did you think about what Carol just said?

Roy: Much better, easier to hear. And I might even do it! (*Laughs.*) [From Miklowitz, 2010, p. 228]

Your family members are often doing their best to try to help you. They may benefit from knowing, in a constructive way, what they can do differently. Making positive requests may feel artificial at first, but it will help you make your needs known without alienating your relatives.

Skill No. 3: Problem Solving to Defuse Family Conflicts

Some of the arguments you have with your family members can be reduced to a specific problem that can be solved. As you know, mood episodes sometimes generate practical problems that need to be addressed by the whole family or both members of the couple. These can include financial problems, difficulties related to resuming your work or family roles (for example, child-rearing), problems related to your treatments or medications, or relationship and living situation conflicts. Often, unresolved problems fuel your relatives' expressions of criticism or resentment. The more you can help direct conversations with your family members toward identifying and solving specific problems, the less tension there will be during your recovery period.

The steps in the Problem-Solving Worksheet on pages 337–338 provide a structure for resolving your disagreements. (You may want to make extra copies; see the information at the end of the Contents to download and print the form.) Let's imagine, for example, that you got into an argument with your spouse or partner about the lack of intimacy in your relationship since your last episode of depression. You might find yourself getting increasingly irritated, especially if you were unclear about what your spouse wanted. First, define the problem (Step 1): Can the broad issue of intimacy be redefined as a more specific problem (for example, lack of time spent together away from the kids)? Try to get your spouse to slow down and help you define what the disagreement is about. Use your listening skills to help your spouse/partner define what is really bothering him or her.

Next, encourage your spouse to suggest as many solutions as possible to the problem you've defined (Step 2). Let's imagine you've defined it as lack of time spent together. Potential solutions could include cordoning off an hour or more of your time during the evening when the kids are not allowed to disturb you, arranging a weekly night out together, exercising together once or twice a week, or having one meal at home each week without the kids (or the parents) present. When generating solutions, be careful not to evaluate whether they are good or bad ideas just yet. It's important to get all of the ideas out on the table first.

Problem-Solving Worksheet

Step 1: Ask, "What is the problem?" Talk and listen, ask questions, and get everybody's opinion.

_____

_____

_____

_____

Step 2: List all possible solutions, even ones that don't seem feasible. Do not evaluate the pros or cons of any solution yet.

1. _____

2. _____

3. _____

4. _____

5. _____

Step 3: Discuss and list the advantages and disadvantages of each possible solution.

Advantages   _Disadvantages_

1. _____   _____

2. _____   _____

3. _____   _____

4. _____   _____

5. _____   _____

Step 4: Choose the best possible solution or solutions and list. Include combinations of possible solutions.

_____

_____

_____

_____

(continued)

Step 5: Plan how to carry out the chosen solutions, and set a date to implement them.

Date _____

List who will do what.

_____

_____

List what resources you'll need (for example, money, a babysitter, access to a car, reservations).

_____

_____

Step 6: Implement the chosen solution and praise each other's efforts.

Step 7: After you've implemented the solution, go back to Step 1 and decide whether the problem was solved. If not, try to redefine the problem and come up with solutions that will work better.

In Step 3, weigh the advantages and disadvantages of each proposed solution. For example, a weekly night out together has the advantage of being fun and pleasurable; its disadvantages might include its costs, or feeling too tired at the end of the day to enjoy it. Then try to choose one solution or a combination of solutions based on your mutual discussion of the pros and cons of each possibility (Step 4). For example, you may agree that going out once a week is too costly but that a meal at home together while the kids are at a babysitter's house achieves the same objective (bringing the two of you closer) at a lower cost.

In Step 5, think about the tasks involved in making the solution work. In this example, you'll need to choose a night to have dinner together, buy food to cook, and arrange a babysitter. You will find it easier to implement the solution—and the result will probably be more satisfying—if you divide up the tasks such that you do some of them and your spouse/partner does some of them.

In Step 6, try implementing your solution and see if the original problem has improved at all. Problem solving does not guarantee that you'll come up with a solution that works (or it may work once and not on other occasions). Nonetheless, give your spouse some encouragement and express gratitude, even if you don't feel the problem of intimacy is solved. For example, say, "I'm really glad you're working with me to solve this. It makes me feel good that you care." Your relatives need to know when they are doing things right, and it's important to tell them so as often as possible.

You may go through a problem-solving exercise only to discover that the original problem was not defined adequately in the first place. For example, the problem might be the lack of personal, intimate conversations between you and your spouse rather than simply not having enough time away from the kids. If so, try redefining the problem and going through the solution steps again (Step 7). You may be more successful the second time around.

Some families or couples find it useful to select a weekly time to sit down and solve problems that have cropped up during the week. Often they deal with problems such as household chores, managing finances, or planning social events. The structure of a regular meeting helps ensure that certain nagging disagreements, even if trivial, get discussed and, hopefully, resolved.

Communicating and Problem Solving with Relatives Who Are Overprotective

"Bipolar illness is so taxing emotionally to the family, and most families don't have the skills for knowing how to deal with it. We feel overwhelmed and our skills are exceeded, and we can't get answers from the mental health system. All the while we see our loved one in pain. Who wouldn't get overprotective under those circumstances?"

—A 34-year-old son who took care of his mother
during her manic and depressive episodes

Communication and problem solving can help you negotiate the difficulties that arise when your relatives start to *overmonitor* your behavior, such as taking your "emotional temperature" too often or worrying excessively about whether you've taken your medicines or gotten enough sleep. Your first task is to try to understand the underlying causes of their behavior. Overmonitoring is usually due to a relative's anxiety. If you've been ill recently, your relative is probably very concerned that you'll become ill again. He or she may fear that you will kill yourself, hurt someone, impulsively leave the family, spend a lot of money, or otherwise damage yourself or others. This anxiety can result in a desire to overcontrol things, which leads to overprotective behavior.

Use active listening as you gently encourage your relatives to recognize and verbalize their fears about your future if they haven't made these clear to you already. Reassure them that you'll work hard to manage your disorder on your own. For example, you might say, "I know you're afraid I'm going to become ill again and that things will be hard for our family [validating their feelings]. I am taking care of myself, though, and the best way you can help me is to let me do as much as I can on my own." They may be relieved to hear you say this. You may also be able to use your positive request skills to set more specific boundaries with them, as Carol did with her father.

Consider the role of problem solving when dealing with relatives who overmonitor your behavior. Can you develop agreements with them in which you do something to allay their anxiety, and they, in turn, agree not to watch you so closely? Bart, 18, was being constantly reminded by his mother, Greta, to take his medication and get his blood level checked. He got his revenge in a rather unproductive way: leaving lithium tablets around the house for her to find (for example, on the kitchen floor, behind the toilet, or under her pillow). Greta then became more annoyed and anxious and increased her monitoring of his behavior. Bart said that he was willing to take his medication and even have his blood level checked, but not if it meant that his mother "follows me around with pills in her hand." Understandably, he wanted to feel like taking medication was his own decision. Greta expressed doubt that he would take lithium without her vigilance. She complained, "How can I know if he's taking it if I don't ask?"

Through problem solving, Bart and his mother generated a list of possible scenarios: Bart taking full responsibility for his medication, Greta taking all the responsibility, Greta reminding him only once per day, Greta having more phone contact with his physician. Eventually they agreed that Greta would place Bart's four daily lithium tablets on a plate for him in the morning. He agreed to take them during the day, and she agreed not to mention his medication unless she found pills on the plate or lying around the house by the day's end. They also agreed that she could see his lithium level lab report whenever it became available. This agreement worked well for both of them.

What if it is your spouse who is behaving in an overprotective way? Some of my patients say that their spouses feel less anxious if they are allowed to co-attend the pharmacotherapy visits with the psychiatrist. There are some advantages to doing this: Your spouse will feel more secure if he or she has input into your care and has a connection with your physician (which can be helpful in emergencies). Your spouse may also remember certain of the physician's recommendations that have slipped your mind (and likewise, you may recall things that your spouse has forgotten). If you decide to go this route, you may want to establish some agreements ahead of time about what role you want your spouse to play in these medication visits. For example, you might say, "I want to invite you to my next medication session, but I need to do most of the talking about my state and what the medication is doing. You can chime in, but it's really me who has to describe my own experiences." Your spouse may feel less of a need to closely monitor your behavior if his or her opinions are heard and, when appropriate, incorporated into your treatment plan.

Troubleshooting Your Use of Communication and Problem-Solving Skills

Putting communication and problem-solving skills into practice after an acute episode presents some challenges. As I mentioned previously, even the healthiest of families can have trouble communicating clearly and efficiently. But when you are also dealing with dysregulations in your mood and thought processes, it can be even harder to step back and phrase your statements to your relatives in the ways that I've outlined, or take a step-by-step approach to problem solving. You will probably feel easily provoked and impatient. As a result you may quickly abandon the skills when in conflict with your spouse or relatives, which will then keep the negative cycles going.

There are several things you can do to address problems in implementing the skills. First, try to flag those instances when you are getting too upset to listen effectively or solve problems and then diplomatically exit the situation. Consider the scenario in which your relative is being critical and accusatory and the thought "this is so unfair" keeps going through your mind. *If you feel the heat rising and can tell that the conversation is going in a negative direction, ask for a "time-out."* For example, you might say, "I don't think I can discuss this right now. Let's talk later, when we're both calmed down." A time-out gives you breathing room so that you can think about what you do and don't want to say to your parent, spouse, or sibling. It also enables you to examine what is happening inside you that is making you so upset and in turn, what might be happening inside your relative (see the box on page 342).

You may want to resolve the disagreement with your relative later or perhaps just drop it, if it doesn't seem worth the cost of another argument. There may be a period after the time-out when things are awkward and icy in your household, but this probably would have occurred anyway if you had let the argument continue along its destructive path.

Here's another difficulty you might experience: You know the steps of a skill (for example, making a positive request) but then forget them as soon as an argument starts. It is hard to remember to draw on communication skills when you are angry and in the midst of a conflict with someone who is angry at you. When you recall the conversation later on, you may think of a number of things you could have said to help defuse the argument.

If this difficulty sounds familiar, practice using the skills first with people outside the family who don't provoke you and with whom you're generally comfortable. For example, make a positive request of a coworker ("I'd really appreciate it if you could cover for me next weekend so that I can take some time off") or try paraphrasing the statements of a friend who has described to you a problem he or she is having (for example, "Sounds like you're going through a rough time").

Now consider the scenario in which you are doing your best with the communication tools but there seems to be little impact on your relationship. You may feel annoyed that you are the only one who is trying to use communication skills or solve problems effectively, whereas others seem to keep doing whatever they've been doing. For

> **Effective solution:** You may find that when you practice a skill in nonthreatening circumstances, it becomes easier to remember to apply it when the stakes are higher.

Mentalization-Based Therapy

The process called *mentalization* is often described in forms of psychotherapy for people who have problems with emotion regulation (Bateman & Fonagy, 2010). According to Bateman and Fonagy, many problems with emotion regulation can be traced to *failures of mentalization*—when individuals misread the emotions or intentions of others. To function well in a relationship (in or outside of the family), you have to be able to identify significant feelings and impulses in yourself and how they may drive you in your interactions with another person. Then you need to step outside of yourself and think of what might be going on in the mind of the other person that makes him or her respond in a certain way. If there is enough trust in the relationship, you can check out the accuracy of your percep-tions with the person directly. Difficulties in mentalizing are sometimes at the core of one's problems in relationships with family members, friends, or one's spouse or partner.

> Latisha, age 18, was convinced that others in her school were gossiping about her, making up stories that impugned her reputation, and shunning her when she tried to be friendly. She described several such instances, usually when she was already feeling quite anxious and depressed about her social skills. She got the feedback from one of her friends that when she was in this anxious state she came across as confrontational (for example, asking "Were you guys just talking about me?") and that others would reflexively pull away. In therapy, she learned that her predictable sequence of feeling anxious, confronting others, and then trying to make sense of their withdrawal contributed to her depressed mood. Her mantra was to "become curious" about her peers' states of mind, even if it sometimes meant asking them personal questions. This helped her chip away at the assumption that they were always thinking about her and judging her harshly.

example, you may be quite diplomatic in asking your close relatives to change their behavior, yet the way they ask you to do the same continues to sound challenging and demeaning. Of course, if you were to ask your family members for their view of this problem, they might say that they try to be diplomatic but that you get defensive in return.

If you find yourself in this stalemate, consider the long-term benefits of "uni-lateral change." In other words, try to change your own behavior in relation to your partner or relatives first, with the expectation that, with time, they will change their behavior toward you. In other words, keep trying! Your repeated attempts at problem solving or diplomacy (for example, continuing to validate other people's emotions even when they refuse to do so for you) will eventually have an impact on their responses, especially if you are able to stick with the formats outlined on pages 333–336 (for active listening or making positive requests for change). Of course, this requires a high tolerance for frustration, but there is potentially a high payoff as well.

To increase the chances that your relatives will improve their way of communicating with you, be sure to praise them for even minor attempts on their part (for example, "Thanks for asking me if I was upset after our conversation—I'm glad you noticed that it bothered me," or simply, "Thanks for listening"). The chances are high that, over repeated discussions with your relatives, they will do or say something helpful or that shows an awareness of your viewpoint. Be ready to acknowledge their attempts to make things better, even if these attempts seem overshadowed by everything else they did that made you feel worse. Remember the cardinal rule of behavior modification: people increase the frequency of those behaviors that get rewarded by others.

You may feel that the communication or problem-solving strategies outlined here are artificial or superficial. If you are still hypomanic or energized, it may feel stifling to talk in this very measured, careful way. What happened to the exciting, spontaneous interchanges you used to have with your partner or your siblings? Remember that you are trying to improve life during a specific interval—your recovery period. This period requires that you be extra efficient in your communication and problem-solving styles, above and beyond what is required of others who do not have to cope with bipolar disorder. Think of incorporating these skills as if you were trying on a new pair of shoes. At first they won't fit or feel comfortable. If they're still uncomfortable after you've worn them for a while, you may decide you don't like them and take them off. But they have the potential to work well for you if you break them in. Practicing the skills repeatedly will eventually make them feel like second nature and will probably lead to changes in the way your family members respond to you. As you recover and your family relationships improve, you may be able to return to more spontaneous ways of communicating or making your needs known.

Reestablishing Physical Intimacy with Your Partner after an Episode

In the previous section, you saw an example of problem solving related to emotional intimacy in a couple's relationship. As for physical intimacy, you and your partner/spouse will probably need some time to get reacquainted with each other after an illness episode. If you both would like to reinitiate a physical relationship, consider getting the help of a couple counselor who specializes in sex therapy. Traditional sex therapists encourage couples to take part in *sensate focus* exercises that they do together at home (that is, *without* the therapist!).

After Mara's bipolar mixed episode, she and her husband, Kevin, abandoned their sex life. In a marital therapy session, Kevin explained, "Our primary goal as a couple is Mara's recovery." In their sessions, they both recognized that sex had become frightening to them and that the illness had become an excuse for not dealing directly with each other. Once they agreed that they wanted to reestablish a romantic life, their counselor encouraged them to take small steps, in between sessions, toward greater intimacy. They started by going out together on an evening date one week, giving each other back rubs the following week, hugging and kissing the next, taking a bath together the next, and gradually working back up to a sexual relationship. This relaxed, step-by-step approach was very important for Mara and Kevin in regaining the trust and intimacy they had shared prior to her episode.

You may feel that the guidance of a couple therapist is not necessary. But many couples do have significant anxiety concerning sex. If so, a therapist can teach you relaxation and desensitization techniques (like those above) to practice with your spouse between sessions.

The most important point to remember is that anxiety or discomfort about being close is a natural part of coping as a couple during the recovery period. People are afraid of getting hurt—your spouse may fear that your sudden interest in him or her is a sign of your mania or that you will be more attracted to other people. You may feel bad about your body or feel that your spouse is judging you. What once felt natural and automatic can take on a scripted quality. One person with bipolar disorder put it this way: "It's like the caterpillar who's asked to explain how he moves all his 1,000 legs at once and then can't do it anymore." Many couples can overcome this discomfort by moving slowly, not expecting too much from each other at first, and being willing to try again if their first attempts at sexual intimacy are not as satisfying as they had hoped.

Bipolar Disorder and the Work Setting

Louise, a 35-year-old woman with bipolar I disorder, had a manic episode that led to a 5-day hospitalization. Prior to the development of her episode, she had worked as a paralegal in a law firm. The trigger for her hospitalization appeared to have been a legal case. The firm had insisted that she work late at night for several weeks to help prepare the attorneys' arguments for the case.

Her illness episode kept her out of work for almost a month. When she had mostly recovered, she returned to her job. She decided not to tell her employers that she had been in the hospital and instead explained that she had had an unnamed physical illness, and did not elaborate further. But she became physically uncomfortable, easily fatigued, and irritable after her second week on the job, when her employers started to increase her workload again. They expected her to work late shifts one night and early-morning shifts the next. She found that she couldn't function mentally at work the morning after a night shift. Even worse, they assigned her a new task upon arriving at work in the morning: calling clients who were delinquent on their bills or who hadn't responded to letters. She summarized her experience this way:

> "It was a bad idea for me to do something like that first thing in the morning. It made it hard for me to even get up to go to this job. My body was slow, my mind was slow. It took me a long time to come out of my haze. If I got to work at 9, I had to be up by 6 just to get my mind rolling. I felt rushed, irritable, then depressed. My boss got controlling and started criticizing my work . . . I got stressed out and anxious, and then I would try to calm down and couldn't. I tried to make myself busy, but then I felt even more lethargic and couldn't get the job done."

Louise was on the verge of quitting her job when she decided to have an open conversation about her bipolar disorder with one of the partners in the law firm, a woman who, she felt, had been on her side. Louise apologized for her irritability and fatigue, and explained that she needed more consistent work hours, adding that the unpleasant tasks she had been assigned in the morning were better off assigned to the afternoon. The law partner was unwilling to compromise on the amount of work assigned to Louise or the quality she expected. But given that Louise was a valued employee, the partner did compromise on some other issues: limiting the number of late nights she would have to work, allowing her to do some of her work at home, and deferring the unpleasant tasks until later in the day. These adjustments made a big difference to Louise. She eventually decided to cut to a half-time work week, which was much better from the standpoint of her mood stability and health.

How Common Are Job Problems?

Job problems affect the majority of people with bipolar disorder, with unemployment as high as 65% and impairments in job performance as high as 80%, even though people with the disorder have higher average levels of education than the general public (O'Donnell et al., 2017a, 2017b). The two biggest reasons for vocational impairments will not be surprising: being depressed and having cognitive impairments (Gitlin & Miklowitz, 2017). We've seen in prior chapters that ongoing, subthreshold depressive symptoms are more often the rule than the exception in the course of bipolar disorder. The category of cognitive impairments includes problems in mental flexibility (that is, when examining a problem, the ability to generate several ideas and alternative responses at once), verbal memory, and recall (Bonnín et al., 2010).

Despite these somewhat depressing findings, there is an upside: if you have bipolar disorder, you can still be successful in your chosen career. A survey done by the Center for Psychiatric Rehabilitation at Boston University discovered that out of 500 professionals and managers previously diagnosed with a serious psychiatric illness (including nurses, newspaper reporters, corporate executives, lawyers, and professors), 73% were able to maintain full-time employment in their chosen occupations (Ellison, Russinova, Lyass, & Rogers, 2008). Of the respondents to the survey, 62% had worked in their position for more than 2 years, and 69% had increased their level of responsibility in their jobs. Most (84%) were taking some kind of psychiatric medication. Above all, respondents said that getting back to their jobs was important to their recovery.

As the story of Louise illustrates, people with bipolar disorder face significant challenges in the workplace. Some of these challenges arise from the stigma of bipolar disorder and the reactions of others. Stigma after disclosures of illness is closely associated with unemployment in bipolar disorder (O'Donnell et al., 2017a, 2017b). Stigma usually means that you experience rejection or judgment based on your illness, leading to feelings of alienation and social conditions that make doing your best difficult if not impossible. Not surprisingly, interpersonal conflicts with colleagues can directly affect your work functioning (Michalak, Yatham, Maxwell, Hale, & Lam, 2007; O'Donnell et al., 2017a, 2017b).

For many of my clients, the biggest challenge is finding a job that is satisfying and stimulating and supports their efforts at managing the disorder. The key is finding the right balance of stability in work hours, levels of stress and stimulation, social support from coworkers and supervisors, and satisfaction with the directions in which your job is taking you. I am optimistic that you can find this balance. In this section, I discuss some self-care strategies to help you get back into the working world after an episode.

New research: Creativity

It has long been known that people with bipolar disorder are more likely than people without bipolar disorder to be in creative occupations (for example, music or art), but are people in creative occupations more likely to be bipolar? In a "total population" study of over 1 million people in Sweden, people in creative professions (for example, writers, musicians) were more likely to have bipolar disorder than people in a matched control group (Kyaga et al., 2013). This connection with creativity, however, did not appear to be limited to bipolar disorder: the first-degree relatives of people with bipolar or major depressive disorder, schizophrenia, anorexia nervosa, and autism were more likely to be in creative professions than the first-degree relatives of healthy people, even though these relatives were not diagnosed with anything. Creativity seems to be a salient characteristic of people with vulnerabilities to a variety of psychiatric disorders.

"How Will Bipolar Disorder Affect My Job Performance?"

"I was hypomanic all last weekend, really pushing the envelope. Me and my buds were up partying and drinking until 3 in the morning both Friday and Saturday nights, and then I slept until 11 Sunday, even though I knew it was a bad idea because I had to get up at 6 for work on Monday. I forgot to take my medications on Sunday morning, and I didn't sleep that well Sunday night. By Monday I was tired, grouchy, withdrawn, snappy with my boss, and just really wasn't all that efficient. My boss reacted, mentioned that I seemed like I was in a bad mood, hinted that maybe in those circumstances I should just take the day off. He didn't know about my bipolar disorder. I could just feel the old 'authority figure' stuff coming up again, but I also recognized I was having a depression hangover of sorts. I took it easy after work Monday afternoon, did some low-stress stuff like talking on the phone and going for a run, had dinner, and went to bed at the usual time. I slept fine and was back in the swing of things by Tuesday. I apologized to my boss, and everything was OK after that, but I realized that, at some point, I might have to tell him about my problems."

—A 27-year-old man with bipolar II disorder

Getting a job is one challenge in bipolar disorder; keeping it and "moving up the ladder" is quite another. As is true for most people, your mood state will influence your day-to-day job performance. This man's cycle of sleep deprivation, alcohol use, and overstimulation followed by irritability, lethargy, and depression could have described almost anyone. The difference is that this cycle is magnified in bipolar disorder, and the intensity of your resulting mood can affect your work performance more than would be the case for the average person.

How are bipolar symptoms expressed in the work setting? Manic or hypomanic reactions can take the form of flying off the handle at things that normally wouldn't annoy you or being preoccupied by so many ideas that concentrating on one task for your job becomes difficult. You may start more projects than you can possibly complete, darting from task to task without accomplishing what you originally set out to do (multitasking). During hypomanic intervals, you may be prone to arguments with irritating coworkers or confrontations with your boss (a client said, "I usually just *think* my coworkers are idiots. When I'm manic, I also *tell* them so"). You may be inclined to talk excessively or interrupt your coworkers.

When you're in a depressed phase, your physical state is a lot like a severe case of the flu. At these times you will not be able to expect much from yourself, nor will others. Your thinking and physical responsiveness (for example, your typing speed) may be slower. You may be less likely to maintain eye contact or to hold up your side of conversations. You may also suffer from considerable anxiety, which can interfere with your concentration.

On the other side, some people report that their bipolar disorder enhances their job performance. Many persons with bipolar disorder work in high-level business or government positions and are known for their high work output. They report that when they have a major writing project to do, an oral presentation, or an important sales meeting, they use the "adrenaline rush" of hypomania to their advantage.

As you've learned in previous chapters, one of the most salient characteristics of bipolar disorder is its instability and unpredictability. Your work performance may suffer most from its lack of consistency. You may wonder how you can promise consistency and accountability when you don't know what your mood will be like on any given day. Your boss may complain that he or she can't be sure whether a project will be done on time, forgetting that, during your hypomanic or manic phases, or even your between-episode healthy periods, you may be more productive than others in the same firm. You may resent the implication that only your depressed side is being acknowledged. A good strategy is to keep track of your work output (for example, what tasks you completed and when; how many customers you worked with) so that if you need to, you can document your overall output during a more extended period (Michalak et al., 2007).

In my experience, people with bipolar disorder benefit from hypomania in the work setting only if they can harness it. Harnessing hypomania includes learning to recognize when you are moving or speaking too fast, setting limits on yourself when work starts to make you overly goal driven, trying to accomplish only one task at a time, accepting feedback from others about how you are coming across, and backing off when people seem to be reacting to your intensity. It may indeed be possible to translate your increased energy into work productivity, but also be aware of when you need to slow down and take a break.

Self-Disclosure in the Workplace: "Should I Tell People about My Illness?"

Can bipolar disorder be kept a secret? In my experience and that of many of my colleagues, people with bipolar disorder usually adopt one of five solutions regarding disclosure:

1. They tell everybody about it, including their boss and coworkers.
2. They disclose their illness to the human resources department so that accommodations can be arranged.
3. They tell one or more trusted coworkers who do not carry positions of authority over them.
4. They do not tell anybody, but do admit to bipolar disorder on their work-sponsored health insurance claims, leaving open the possibility that their employer could find out (although this is less risky since the advent of HIPAA).
5. They do not tell anyone at work, and they do not use their work-sponsored insurance to cover their psychiatric costs.

There is no single solution that is right for everybody (although in most cases I'd encourage you to avoid the first option). Let me go through the pros and cons of telling employers or coworkers about your disorder to help you decide which option seems best for you in your current or future work environment.

What Are the Disadvantages of Disclosing?
The Risk of Job Discrimination

If you are currently employed, the most obvious disadvantage of disclosing your disorder is that you may get fired or demoted or denied a promotion or a raise. Likewise, telling a prospective employer about your disorder introduces the possibility that he or she will decide against hiring you, without telling you why.

Some people with bipolar disorder, including some of my clients, have reported job discrimination. It is unclear how often this occurs. In a study by Nicholas Glozier (1998) of the Institute of Psychiatry in London, 80 British personnel directors were asked to evaluate two hypothetical job candidates who, based on a written profile, were described in an identical manner (for example, as having a good prior work record). One was described as having had a diagnosis of depression and the other as having diabetes. Personnel directors were less likely to hire the applicant with depression and more likely to believe that his or her performance in an executive job would be impaired compared to the applicant with diabetes. In other words, we have a long way to go in educating employers about depression and bipolar disorders, their similarity to other medical disorders, and how they will, and will not, affect job performance. It is not clear whether an unwillingness to hire a hypothetical candidate translates into discrimination once a real person with depression or bipolar disorder is hired.

If you are fired or are not hired because of your bipolar disorder, the law is on your side. In the United States, under the Americans with Disabilities Act (*www.eeoc.gov/eeoc/history/35th/1990s/ada.html*), it is unlawful to discriminate against a "qualified individual with a disability," meaning a person who, "with or without reasonable accommodation, can perform the essential functions of the employment position that such individual holds or desires" (42 U.S. Code § 12102). Bipolar disorder does qualify as a disability, which is defined as "a physical or mental impairment that substantially limits one or more of the major life activities of such individual." Discrimination refers to prejudicial behavior on the employer's part in job application procedures, hiring practices, promotion or discharge, pay, or training. You cannot legally be denied an equal job for equal pay, be segregated from others, or be classified such that your opportunities for advancement are limited (for example, demoted to working in the mail room) because of your psychiatric disorder.

If you are qualified for a job, "reasonable accommodations" can be required of the employer. For a person with bipolar disorder, certain job accommodations have been found to be useful (Tremblay, 2011; see the box on pages 356–357). For example, some people do better when they are allowed to complete some of their work at home or when they have "flex time." Of course, the employer has to know about your disorder to make such reasonable accommodations. Your employer cannot legally fire you or refuse to hire you because you need a reasonable accommodation, unless he or she can prove that such an accommodation would pose an undue hardship for the business (for example, place the firm deeply in debt, require moving to another facility). Be aware that accommodations can create a stigma of their own: your coworkers may feel jealous that you are being given special treatment and not convinced that you really have a disability.

Consider the experience of Janine, a 37-year-old woman who worked at an advertising firm.

> Janine was a valued employee of her firm because of her high productivity. She said that she had always been somewhat hypomanic by nature and that this hypomania had served her well in her high-demand workplace. Her first major bipolar episode was a depression with symptoms of paranoia that developed gradually and significantly interfered with her work productivity. She took a leave of absence but didn't know at the time that she had bipolar disorder. Following successful medical treatment with mood stabilizers and antipsychotic agents, she wrote a letter to her firm explaining what had happened. Upon learning of her disorder, her employer summarily dismissed her. She consulted an attorney and challenged this move on legal grounds. After several back-and-forth legal communications, she was invited back to work at the firm but was told she could do so only if she was interviewed for and offered a job in a different department. She was not happy with the other options offered to her, and ultimately decided that she did not want to work in a firm that held these attitudes toward her. She is now working in another firm that is more sympathetic to her needs.

Proving that job discrimination occurred can be difficult. If you think you are being discriminated against because of the disclosure of your disorder (whether it was you or someone else who made the disclosure), I would advise you to consult an employment attorney and the Equal Employment Opportunity Commission. They can help you determine if a legal action should be taken against your current or former employer.

Janine could have pursued legal action against her former employer but decided that doing so would be too stressful. Deciding whether or not to pursue a legal case is very much a personal and often a family decision. Consider its potential impact on your mood stability as well as the likely outcome of the case (for example, being reinstated in your old position, which you may no longer want or feel comfortable in). Be prepared for a long period of frustrations and high economic costs before your case is resolved. Nonetheless, after weighing all of the relevant factors you may well decide that pursuing your case is worth it.

"Can My Employer Ask Whether I Have Bipolar Disorder?"

The Americans with Disabilities Act makes it clear that employers are not to ask direct questions about your disability or require their own psychiatric examination for a job application or during the course of your employment, "unless such examination or inquiry is shown to be job-related and consistent with business necessity." They can require a medical examination after a job offer has been made if one is required of all new employees or as part of an employee health program (an example would be a physical exam required for all new personnel at a nursing home). However, they cannot use the results of this exam to change their mind about the offer.

Your employer would have to prove that inquiring about your mental health status is essential to knowing whether you can perform your job duties or whether you would endanger others. In most cases, having bipolar disorder does not mean that others are at risk, unless you have a documented history of violence or also have an alcohol or drug abuse problem. These associated problems could jeopardize the safety of others (for example, if you work at a child care facility, operate heavy machinery, or drive a vehicle).

If the business to which you're applying does require a medical exam, it has to collect this information in a form that can be treated as a confidential medical record, meaning that you would have to give a signed release of information before your records were sent to anyone. However, the doctor or nurse who examines you can inform a supervisor or manager of work accommodations required by your disorder, as revealed in the medical exam. Likewise, if your firm has safety or first-aid personnel, they may be informed that your bipolar disorder could require emergency treatment. These disclosures may or may not occur in your work setting and, in any case, cannot legally be used to discriminate against you.

What should you do if your current or potential employer asks about your psychiatric history, either directly or on a job application? You can say that you don't wish to answer the question (or leave the question blank) or point out that the question is inappropriate (Court & Nelson, 1996). If your employer presses you, you don't have to lie about having the disorder. Just say you'd rather not discuss this matter or that you want to get a consultation before you discuss it.

A potential employer can refuse to hire you upon learning of your disorder, but only if he or she can prove that the disorder will interfere with your job functions and that no reasonable accommodations can be made. In most cases, he or she will have a tough time proving these points just because you have bipolar disorder. Of course, you would need to initiate legal action against your prospective employer to make your case.

Disadvantages of Disclosure: Dealing with Stigma at Work

If your coworkers learn that you have a mood disorder, you may experience a feeling of stigma—the sense that your behavior is being viewed negatively in light of your illness. Usually this stigma will be most salient to you right after a major bout of mania or depression, in part because you will still be depressed or hypomanic and possibly more attuned to the reactions of others. But even people whose bipolar disorder has been stable can feel stigmatized at work. For example, imagine that your illness is "leaked" by a coworker to others in your office. Julie, age 55, became quite angry with a coworker one day, and the coworker left the office crying. Julie had earlier disclosed her illness to another woman in the office whom she considered to be a close friend. After the incident, this friend told others in the office about Julie's illness, as a way of explaining why Julie had responded so seemingly irrationally. After that, Julie felt that her coworkers viewed her with apprehension and avoided giving her tasks that required working closely with others.

Disclosing your illness to a coworker can lead to responses that may feel stigmatizing to you, even when you are telling the best intentioned of people. For example, their response may be "my mom had that" or "my grandmother was bipolar." They are probably trying to say that they understand what you're going through, but you may not like being compared to their ill relatives, especially if they have previously described these relatives as being abusive or emotionally draining.

The stigma you experience at work may feel similar to the stigma you experience in your family. For example, coworkers may interpret problems in your work as stemming from your illness, even when you can point to other employees who have the same problems (for example, being late with assignments, reacting irritably to a disorganized or harsh boss). You may also find that your coworkers become distant or overly cautious in their interactions with you. Coworkers may even react by doting on you or becoming overly solicitous (for example, frequently asking if you want to talk about your problems, repeatedly reminding you that "I'm there for you"). All of these responses can feel unhelpful, and eerily similar to the things that annoy you most about how your family members respond. To be fair, coworkers, like family members, are often struggling to figure out how to be helpful.

On a more hopeful note, mood disorders carry less of a stigma than they used to. Because of the bravery of many public figures who have talked openly about their experiences of bipolar disorder or unipolar depression (for example, Kay Jamison, Carrie Fisher, Patty Duke, Jane Pauley, Margot Kidder, Catherine Zeta-Jones, Demi Lovato, Mike Wallace, William Styron), and because of events such as National Depression Screening Day, the public has an increased awareness and a greater acceptance of mood disorders. As a result, you may get more understanding from others than you expected.

What Are the Advantages of Disclosing Your Disorder?

There are arguments in favor of being open about your disorder as well. First, disclosing can be destigmatizing and increase your own acceptance of the illness. You may feel that bipolar disorder is not so shameful if you tell a coworker who does not have a strong negative reaction. Upon learning of your disorder, a coworker may open up about their own problems with depression. Some of my clients have chosen one trusted person at work to tell about the disorder. Sharing this kind of personal information helps to increase mutual trust and can create an atmosphere of support within the work setting. But deciding to whom you disclose requires careful thought. In *An Unquiet Mind*, Kay Jamison (1995) describes the reactions of coworkers upon learning of her disorder, which varied from empathic acceptance to outright rejection and insensitivity.

When considering whether or not to disclose your disorder to a coworker or employer, first ask yourself several questions (Court & Nelson, 1996):

"Why do I want him or her to know?"

"How will it make my life at work easier—will it lead to specific work accommodations?"

"Will it be helpful for someone to know about my disorder if there is an emergency at work?"

"Will I feel closer to this coworker—is he or she a potential friend?"

"Will telling my boss about my disorder help me explain absences or lapses in my work productivity?"

"If there is no reason to expect that the illness will impair my work, why does she need to know?"

There are ways to tell people of your disorder without actually using the label *bipolar*. For example, your disorder can be described as "a chemical imbalance that affects my mood" or "a medical problem related to my energy levels that can affect my work and concentration." Simple explanations like these may be all that employers or coworkers require to understand why your work performance has shifted, or why you have been irritable, withdrawn, or absent lately.

Disclosing to your boss early on may set the stage for later changes in

> **Effective solution:** If you decide to disclose your disorder to your boss or someone else at work and it seems appropriate, use the Quick Fact Sheet (on pages 330–331) intended for family members to help you explain the illness. Also, the human resources department in some companies may be willing to support you with coaching on how to present your disorder and need for accommodations to your employer or by attending a disclosure meeting to document any legal issues.

the structure or demands of your job (see the box on pages 356–357). You may have more legal protection if you disclose your bipolar disorder when you are well. If your employer knows ahead of time, you can problem-solve together about what accommodations seem reasonable during your periods of illness and once you have begun to recover (as Louise did).

There may be instances when you feel you must disclose the disorder to your boss, such as when you've had multiple absences or a clear deterioration in your work productivity. Some people wait to see if their performance actually does slip and then disclose the disorder to the boss when asking for time off or other work adjustments. This can be a sensible plan, but timing is important: Your boss may feel annoyed by this disclosure if it occurs while you are trying to meet an important deadline. Also, when you are in an active period of illness, you may not be able to tell if your work performance has changed or if you need accommodations.

Self-Care Strategies for Coping Effectively in the Work Setting

Adjusting the Work Setting to Your Disorder

There is virtually no research literature on what kinds of jobs are best for people with bipolar disorder. We suspect that people with the disorder should avoid jobs that involve sudden bursts of social stimulation with little downtime in between (for example, being a waitress at a bar with a "happy hour"), frequent travel across time zones, or consistently stressful interactions with others (for example, working in a hospital emergency room or managing the complaint desk at the phone company). We also suspect that people with the disorder do better with consistent work hours and predictable workdays than in jobs requiring unpredictable and constantly shifting schedules (for example, working on weekdays one week and then weekends the next or working evening shifts followed immediately by morning ones). Jobs in restaurants, manufacturing, nursing, and retail sales often require variable shifts, whereas jobs in accounting, computer programming, banking, and schools are usually more consistent. But if the jobs in the former category appeal to you, you may not have to rule them out. Pursue them, but try to determine whether you can obtain some of the accommodations listed in the box on pages 356–357.

What Are Reasonable Accommodations?

These are innovations or modifications in your job requirements or work schedule that give you a better shot at successful employment. Reasonable accommodations are usually requested by you as the employee and are generally not offered up front by the employer. Remember that your employer cannot be expected to provide accommodations without knowing about your disorder and why these accommodations are required.

The box on pages 356–357 lists examples of accommodations that might be reasonable to request of an employer. These items are not meant to reflect adjustments that all people with bipolar disorder should expect. Rather, they are meant as examples of things you can ask for. Try to determine which of these are negotiable for you and which are not. It is highly unlikely that any employer would grant all or even a majority of them (and some may be against the nature or policies of the firm). Nonetheless, your employer might approve enough of these adjustments to help you function better at work. Note that some accommodations would also benefit employees who do not have bipolar disorder but are seeking ways to manage stress.

It is not always possible to know in advance which accommodations will work for you, but your employer will probably be most open to these requests once you have been offered the job and are in the negotiation phase. Some of the items (for example, changing from full-time to part-time work, negotiating leaves of absence, the style of employer/employee performance evaluations, asking that your office be moved) may need to be negotiated later, once you have worked at the job for a period of time and have identified problems with the existing structure.

> Ralph, 52, worked as the primary short-order cook in a fast-food restaurant, where he supervised two other cooks. He determined that he was prone to hyperactivity, irritability, and inefficiency on nights when the restaurant activity reached a certain volume. With the support of his employer, he learned to delegate the task of supervising food preparation to one of the other cooks at those times. He would then continue his shift in the role of the secondary cook and would take over again as primary cook the next day.

> Tina, age 59, worked as a photo editor for a firm that assigned employees to closely interconnected cubicles (or "pods," as they were called). One of her coworkers insisted on listening to his radio while working, which was not against company policy but was very disturbing to Tina. She became unable to concentrate. She tried to reason with the coworker, begging him to use headphones; he expressed mock sympathy and then went back to playing his radio. She began to have intrusive thoughts about killing him. She became more and more irritated and noticed that her thoughts had begun to race. She eventually consulted her boss about the problem without explaining that she had bipolar II disorder. Her boss felt that Tina was a good employee and decided to let her move to a smaller room where she would have less contact with others. This adjustment helped Tina restore her previous level of productivity.

> Beth, a 34-year-old woman with bipolar I disorder, discovered that her mood swings were at their worst at the onset of her menstrual period. She worked at a news office with variable shifts; she had been unable, for a variety of financial and personal reasons, to obtain regular hours. Despite the loss of pay, she

Reasonable Workplace Accommodations for Persons with Bipolar Disorder

Work Hours

- Working regular daily or nightly hours rather than variable night/day work shifts
- Being assigned work shifts that fit best with your circadian rhythms (for example, 10 A.M.–7 P.M. instead of 8 A.M.–5 P.M.; working 3-hour shifts for 5 days rather than 5-hour shifts for 3 days)
- Avoiding work early in the morning if you suffer from "medication hangovers"
- Reducing work hours or changing from full-time to part-time when having mood fluctuations
- Being excused from (or getting reductions in) overtime work
- Completing some of your tasks at home versus at work

Stress Management

- Being allowed to share responsibilities for projects with others
- Being placed in an office or cubicle that has a degree of distance from noise and stimulation
- Restructuring your work environment to avoid overstimulation (for example, working in well-lit, uncrowded rooms)
- Being excused from certain work assignments that historically have been triggers for your mood swings
- Obtaining support or counseling from an employee assistance program
- Leaving work for breaks or lunch to decompress, exercise, walk, meditate, or use relaxation techniques
- Taking a greater number of short breaks rather than two long breaks during an 8-hour work shift
- Being given autonomy in matters of goal setting

Absences from Work

- Being granted brief absences for medical appointments, with chances to make up the hours
- Being granted extended leaves of absence with a doctor's note
- Being allowed to leave work early when having difficult mood swings or anxiety/stress reactions

(continued)

Reasonable Workplace Accommodations for Persons with Bipolar Disorder *(continued)*

Communication with Your Employer about Performance Evaluations

■ Having regular and open communication with your employer about your job performance

■ Hearing what you're doing right as well as what you're doing wrong

■ Being judged by overall productivity and task completion or other, more individualized measures of productivity, instead of being judged only by the number of hours worked

■ Revisiting these accommodations from time to time to determine if they are enabling you to be productive and remain stable

---

decided each month to request two days off just prior to the expected onset of her menstrual period. She resumed work at her normal pace once the worst mood swings associated with her menstrual cycle were over.

Balancing Work Time against Downtime

One work-related difficulty I've heard expressed by a number of people with bipolar disorder is the feeling of being wired and driven at work and then feeling spent, exhausted, or depressed once home for the night. Their problems are compounded on the weekend if there is little to do and they feel like their body and brain have shut down. As a result, some people feel hypomanic when they're working and depressed when they're not.

This form of cycling is most likely to happen when you start a new job. Like most other new employees, you probably want to perform at your peak and begin pushing yourself hard. But a cycle can occur in which, at the beginning of a new job, you try to produce at your maximum level and are quickly rewarded with praise, compensation, or advancement by an appreciative boss. This reward may make you drive yourself even harder, leading to more rewards but also more hypomania or even mania. As I mentioned in Chapter 5, goal attainment events (events that involve reward or advancement and that increase your confidence and drive toward other goals) are particularly potent in precipitating manic or hypomanic episodes

Effective prevention: When you start a new job, keep a regular daily and nightly routine and set limits on the workload you initially accept. These adjustments can help keep the job from triggering hypomania during the workday and depression after work.

> **PERSONALIZED CARE TIP:**
> ## Adjusting levels of stimulation and structure in your off hours
>
> When you get home from work, allow yourself to relax but also introduce some structure (see Chapter 8) and a degree of low-key stimulation. Avoid scheduling lots of demanding social activities for weekday evenings. During weekends, avoid "sleep bingeing" (for example, sleeping 12 or more hours and getting up in the afternoon) to counteract your fatigue from getting up at 6 A.M. every morning during the week. Instead, keep your bedtimes and wake times during the weekend to within 1 hour of your times during the week. Plan a social activity or exercise for one or both weekend mornings to ensure that you'll be out of bed by a certain time. That way, your internal clock will stay regulated as you transition from the workweek to the weekend.

(Johnson et al., 2008). Unfortunately, these manic states are often followed by depressive or mixed episodes, along with negative thoughts and feelings about your capabilities ("I used to be able to accomplish so much"). In turn, your boss, who may not know about your disorder, may compare your performance when depressed to the way you performed when you first started the job (rather than to the performance of other workers in your firm). He or she may wonder what happened to you.

When you first start a job, try to take a more cautious, measured approach. Turn in a consistent work performance and get your footing in the new job, but don't try to be a superstar at the outset. Know when you are overstressing yourself. It's better to be a consistent employee than a "start–stop" employee, on whom others are unsure they can depend.

These recommendations may sound rigid, but they will help you function in the early stages of your new job. Once you have worked at a job for a while and have settled into a routine, you may be able to introduce more flexibility into your daily habits without sacrificing mood stability. This balance varies considerably from person to person, so take your time to find the solution that works best for you.

Employee Assistance Programs

One potential resource is your employer's human resources department and/or its employee assistance program, which are in part designed to help employees cope with health problems that affect their job performance. They may offer job assessments, counseling, recommendations for accommodations, or help in communicating with your immediate supervisor about your needs. Although people have variable experiences with these programs, they represent an important protective body between you and your employer and may have ideas that others won't think of.

Using Vocational Rehabilitation Support

If you have been having trouble finding a job that is suitable for you, or trouble keeping jobs, you may want to consider vocational counseling. Most states have a division of vocational rehabilitation devoted to helping people with disabilities. Generally, you will not have to pay for these services. To locate these services in your area, call the local mental health center or your city or town's chamber of commerce or look online using the search term "vocational rehabilitation" and the name of your state.

Vocational rehabilitation specialists can help you develop a plan for finding and performing successfully in a job. These plans are focused on what you want to achieve (for example, part-time versus full-time employment; people-oriented versus more solitary work settings). Rehabilitation can involve *vocational testing* (for example, questionnaires regarding your interests, environments you enjoy, or job skills); training in *job-seeking skills* (for example, writing a résumé, making initial telephone calls to an employer, and effective interviewing strategies); and *job development* (locating jobs in the community or sometimes even designing them to fit your aptitudes and skills).

Job coaching is often the most active component of vocational rehabilitation. A job coach goes with you to a new job site, helps you learn the required tasks, and encourages you to stay motivated. He or she can facilitate difficult communication between you and your boss. A job coach may help explain your disorder to your supervisor and clarify any special considerations you may require (for example, a work environment with as few distractions as possible).

Employers may listen and respond more readily to a job coach than to an employee.

Jamal, a 25-year-old man with bipolar I disorder, became stressed by his job at an auto parts store after being switched from one sales area to another. He didn't like his new supervisor, whom he found sarcastic and unsympathetic to the limitations imposed by his mood states. Just as he was about to quit, Jamal's job coach interceded and explained the disorder to this supervisor. They agreed on rules for their working relationship and strategies by which Jamal could temporarily leave the setting when he felt overwhelmed by it. He eventually left this job and found a new one, but he felt empowered by the fact that by the time he left, his supervisor's style of dealing with him had changed.

PERSONALIZED CARE TIP:
Volunteer work

In my experience, people with bipolar disorder who have volunteered at an agency, shelter, or mental health facility while on disability or medical leave from their previous job almost invariably say that it was an important component of their recovery. When you are questioning why you should still be alive and wondering why your days seem monotonous and meaningless, volunteering in a "socially conscious" position can do much to lift your mood. Work can enhance your life in many ways even if you are not being compensated—by helping you structure your schedule and build new friendships and giving you a greater sense of purpose. Also, you may pick up some job skills and experience in working with other staffers, or even a letter of recommendation, that will be useful when you return to paid work.

Annie, age 30, had a great love of animals, particularly dogs; her family had bred dogs when she was a child. She was less enthusiastic about her relationships with people, especially after her most recent mood crash, which had involved the breakup of a serious relationship and conflict with her parents. Once she felt up to it, she began volunteering at an animal shelter, at first for only 2 hours a week. The shelter director quickly recognized her passion and ability and suggested that she come aboard in a paid position. Although Annie preferred to volunteer until she felt better, the warm atmosphere of the shelter, combined with her enhanced feelings of self-worth, were essential components of her recovery.

Job coaches can also be helpful if you need a leave of absence from work. If you need to be hospitalized for a manic or depressive episode, you may not be in a condition to ask your employer for a leave. A job coach can write a letter or call your employer to advocate on your behalf.

Applying for Disability

If you have had a series of illness episodes or unremitting symptoms and have been unable to function at work, you may want to apply for disability payments. If you have previously paid for short-term or long-term private disability insurance through your employer, you may be eligible for payments with an accompanying doctor's order. You may also apply for disability payments through the Social Security Administration. Social Security payments are not large (for example, about $500 per month), but they can help support you during a period of work disability.

Usually, you apply for disability through a liaison at your local Social Security office. The application process can be long (about 6 months) and frustrating. The procedure usually requires that your doctor and psychotherapist provide medical records and answer questions about your ability to work. If you are in touch with a vocational rehabilitation counselor, he or she may be able to acquaint you with the application procedures or recommend someone who can. Because of the length of the process, you may be more stable by the time your payments arrive than you were when you first applied!

Receiving disability payments does not mean you have to abandon the idea of working in the future. You can be on disability for a period of time (for example, during a long-term depression that is not responding well to medications) and then reconsider the working world once you have recovered. *Being on disability should not have to be stigmatizing or shameful.* In fact, many people with bipolar disorder and other medical disorders conclude that they need this kind of support. In the Boston University survey of professionals and managers, one-third had received disability payments at some point in their past (Ellison et al., 2008).

• • • • • • • • • • • • • •

Despite the toll that bipolar disorder can take on your family and work life, I strongly believe that you can learn to cope effectively in both settings as well as in the broader community. As you've just seen, coping involves being comfortable with your own understanding of the disorder, educating others about it, knowing your limitations, setting appropriate expectations for yourself, and trying to adjust your environment to maximize the chances that you'll function at your best. Remember to rely on the help of others (friends, family, and coworkers) for support when it seems appropriate. Constance Hammen and her colleagues at UCLA (Hammen, Gitlin, & Altshuler, 2000) found that the people with bipolar disorder who did best within the work setting were those who had strong social and relationship support outside of work.

This book has emphasized self-management of the illness. But what should you (or your family members) do if you think one of your children has bipolar disorder, or is at risk for it? When do the same diagnostic criteria, prognosis, treatments, or illness management strategies apply, and when do they need to be different? This is the topic of the final chapter of this book.

CHAPTER 14

"Does My Child Have Bipolar Disorder?"

How Would You Know and What Should You Do?

Up to this point I've been talking about how to cope with your own bipolar disorder. But what if you think you're observing the early signs of bipolarity in one of your kids—what should you do with this information?

Bipolar disorder has long been known to run in families. You may be concerned about what this means for your children or for children you may have in the future. Some people with bipolar disorder wonder whether they should even have children. This is likely to be an especially salient issue if you've just been diagnosed (or your spouse or partner has) and are just starting a family. Nonetheless, many people who have had the illness for a long time have the same questions. If neither you nor your spouse has bipolar disorder but other first- or second-degree relatives of your child have it—siblings, aunts or uncles, grandparents—you may worry that one or more of your children has inherited these genes and will develop bipolar disorder later in life.

These concerns are understandable. A mood disorder is one of many things we worry will affect our children, and when bipolar disorder runs in your family these worries are intensified. The prospect of passing on the disorder to the next generation may generate feelings of anxiety or guilt, even though, as I've said in prior chapters, we have no control over the genes we pass on. In this chapter, I hope to answer some of the questions you have about the risk to your children of bipolar disorder and its associated symptoms and about what you can expect if your child is diagnosed.

Let's start with the question I hear most often: ***"If I have bipolar disorder, will my children develop it?"***

Researchers talk about risk for an illness in a number of ways, but usually they mean the lifetime percentage likelihood that you or someone related to you will develop a particular illness. It's hard to quantify risk for bipolar disorder because there are many different subtypes and comorbid disorders, as discussed throughout this book. Nonetheless, knowing the actual risks and what factors increase that risk will make you feel more in control of the outcome of your own or your child's mood disorder.

In the general population, between 1 and 2% of adults have bipolar disorder. An aggregation of clinical studies in the United States, Europe, and Asia, all of which used structured interviews and systematic diagnostic methods, found that across 17 studies with 31,443 kids (ages 7–21), 576 (1.8%) had some form of bipolar spectrum disorder (bipolar I, II, and unspecified or "not otherwise specified" bipolar disorder; see below) (Van Meter, Burke, Kowatch, Findling, & Youngstrom, 2016).

If you're a mother and have bipolar disorder, the chances that your child will develop it are about 10%. The risk goes up to about 25% if we include risk for mood disorders in general, including major depression without mania and unspecified bipolar disorder, as well as the traditional bipolar I and II conditions (Craddock & Sklar, 2013). Importantly, the children of bipolar parents are more likely to develop depressive disorders over time (30–40% in some studies) than full bipolar I or II disorder (Duffy et al., 2014; Hillegers et al., 2005). Some studies find that the risk to offspring is higher when the parent developed bipolar disorder earlier (under age 21) rather than later (Hafeman et al., 2016; Vieta et al., 2018).

These statistics reflect averages over a number of studies. You may find the relatively low percentages comforting, or they may raise additional questions: Is there anything I can do to further decrease my child's risk? If she has depression now, will she have mania later? How do I know what is a sign of bipolar disorder and what is related to a commonly comorbid disorder like ADHD—or just teen angst? If my child is diagnosed—or even if he has a lot of the features of bipolar disorder but doesn't currently qualify for a diagnosis—how will he function at school, at home, or with peers in the future?

In this chapter, you'll learn:

- How to recognize the symptoms of bipolar disorder in children and teens: how they're different from symptoms of other disorders or from ordinary child or teen moodiness

- How to spot the early warning signs of episodes of depression or mania and what to do with that information

- What kinds of outcomes we can expect when a child is diagnosed with bipolar disorder
- The nature of cognitive impairments in pediatric bipolar disorder and how they contribute to social or academic problems
- What treatments are most effective

As you'll soon see, I recommend starting with a full psychiatric evaluation of your child from a knowledgeable practitioner (see details on how to find one below). Some of your questions may be answered by this evaluation, although you may also be mystified by the terms your practitioner uses to describe your child (for example, disruptive mood dysregulation disorder [DMDD] or "bipolar unspecified"). You may wonder about the validity of these diagnoses or what they imply in terms of treatment and long-term care. Hopefully, the diagnostic terms will be less confusing after you've read this chapter, and the connection between these diagnoses and recommended treatments will be clearer.

Finally, I hope to help you balance your awareness of the signs and symptoms of bipolar disorder in your child with avoidance of "helicopter parenting." I've seen many loving parents become hypervigilant when they first learn that their child is showing low-level symptoms and start scrutinizing the child for even minor mood shifts. They may ask teachers, friends' parents, or athletic coaches to notify them of any explosive outbursts, tears, or irritability; or instances of talking fast, bragging, or doing too much. This approach is certainly understandable given the risks involved, but it has its downsides. It can lead you to exaggerate the significance of what you're seeing and creates unnecessary strain on the child. In this chapter my goal is to give you an understanding of what to look for and what to do about your observations *without* centering your family's life around the anticipation of an emerging illness.

Bipolar Disorder in Children: A Brief History

When you're worried that a child in your family might already have bipolar disorder or get it someday, it's helpful to know how our understanding of bipolar disorder in children has evolved. It's only been in the last few decades that children and teens have been recognized as even having depression. Before then, psychologists and psychiatrists believed that before adolescence kids' emotional and cognitive development had not matured to the point that they could experience disabling sad moods. We now know this isn't true; children can be diagnosed with bipolar disorder and depression as young as age 5 (Luby & Navsaria, 2010). One large-scale community study found that 28% of people with adult bipolar disorder had developed it before age 13 and another 38% between ages 13 and 18 (Perlis et al., 2004).

Studies in the United States

In the early 1980s, two investigators at UCLA, Michael Strober and Gaye Carlson (Carlson, 1990; Strober & Carlson, 1982), looked at 60 teenagers (ages 13–16) who had been diagnosed with major depression. At that point, depression was recognized in children, but bipolar disorder was not. They found a distinctive set of factors that predicted the onset of bipolar disorder in the 20% of kids who developed it over the next 3–4 years. These included (1) the presence of bipolar disorder in each of three previous generations; (2) several features of the child's illness, including episodes of depression that appeared suddenly, severe lethargy, or psychotic symptoms (delusions or hallucinations); and (3) hypomanic or manic reactions to antidepressants. Their study was the first to suggest that the early signs of bipolar disorder could be observed during the teen years, before the onset of the full illness.

Barbara Geller, a child psychiatrist at Washington University in St. Louis, did much to clarify the boundaries of childhood bipolar disorder in preadolescent and adolescent children (mean age 11) who came to treatment for a manic episode. She found that, like its adult counterpart, bipolar I disorder in kids waxed and waned between recurrences and recoveries, and kids were affected in their academic and social functioning (Geller et al., 2000). However, only 44% of the children Geller studied had a manic recurrence at an 8-year follow-up, when they were between the ages of 18 and 21. These findings suggest that, either because of treatment, environmental protective factors (for example, a warm family), or the natural developmental course of the illness, kids' outcomes can be more positive than expected (Geller et al., 2008).

During the last three decades, childhood diagnoses of bipolar disorders have exploded, particularly in the United States. With this sudden interest came haphazard and sloppy diagnoses. Many kids were now called bipolar when other diagnoses (for example, major depression, generalized anxiety disorder, or ADHD) were probably correct. In the United States, during the interval between 1994/1995 and 2002/2003, the number of outpatient medical visits in which bipolar disorder was diagnosed increased 40-fold in patients under age 20, whereas the increase was less than twofold among adults age 20 or older (Moreno et al., 2007).

What was happening? It is likely that, during the intervals surveyed, physicians believed that pediatric-onset bipolar disorder was reflected in near-constant states of irritability interspersed with angry or explosive outbursts. Some doctors interpreted the symptoms of ADHD as being early presentations of mania. Rather than diagnosing kids with chronic aggression or irritability with oppositional defiant disorder (ODD) or conduct disorder—as might have been done in previous eras—psychiatrists were now using the bipolar disorder label and prescribing the same medications as for bipolar adults. As a result, many children and adolescents in the United States did not get appropriate treatment, although we do not know how frequently this occurred.

These views have changed substantially in recent years. Nowadays, practice guidelines say that kids should not receive a bipolar diagnosis unless they clearly cycle in and out of manic/hypomanic and depressive episodes characterized by multiple symptoms that change together (Goodwin et al., 2016). Chronic irritability is no longer thought to be a defining feature of bipolar disorder.

The Reaction in Europe

European psychiatrists came down hard on the childhood bipolar movement in the United States, claiming that American clinicians were misdiagnosing children. Some European investigators suggested that American psychiatrists were using too many stimulants or antidepressants and causing mania to occur in kids who were just depressed or had ADHD (Reichart & Nolen, 2004). Some believed that U.S. pharmaceutical companies were pushing the diagnosis to sell more drugs. Some even thought that pediatric bipolar disorder was unique to the United States. In an international symposium in 2003, when I described the features of bipolar children we were seeing in our studies, a child psychiatrist from Ireland asked me, "I've never seen one of these kids in my 30 years of practice. Is this something you guys cooked up across the pond?"

These clashes in perspective may have other roots. For example, the way illnesses are identified and treated differs greatly between the United States and Europe. In the United Kingdom, for example, mental health practitioners don't always give a diagnosis but may list the child's problem areas in order of significance. Having a mood disorder may not be high on a problem list that includes physical abuse, school truancy, and parental alcoholism, and so the existence of bipolar disorder in a child might not be a focus of attention.

There are also population differences between the United States and Europe. American psychiatrist Robert Post and his colleagues in the Stanley Research Consortium found that a family history of bipolar illness was more common among adults with bipolar disorder in the United States than in Europe, as was having childhood experiences of abuse or co-occurring medical illnesses (for example, thyroid disease) (Post et al., 2017). They also pointed out that medical illnesses in general were more common among children in the United States than in Europe, a difference that is influenced by many factors, including exercise and diet.

My own view of this controversy is that, at least in the 1990s and early 2000s, practitioners in the United States probably overdiagnosed bipolar disorder in kids, whereas those in Europe underdiagnosed it. There are pros and cons to both positions: by overdiagnosing the disorder, we in the United States may have given kids unnecessary medications, notably SGAs, that led to significant weight gain and metabolic problems. The European tendency to underdiagnose bipolar disorder may have meant that school failure, disrupted peer relationships, and suicide attempts went unexplained or were attributed to some other diagnosis like ADHD. Treatments that might be effective for these children—both medical and psychological—were passed up (Youngstrom, Findling, Youngstrom, & Calabrese, 2005).

Nowadays, practitioners in the United States are more wary of diagnosing children with bipolar disorder (or routinely accepting the bipolar diagnosis in a child referred for treatment). However, there are still diagnostic and treatment biases. For example, practitioners may still apply the label because the disorder has clearer treatment guidelines than many others: you can treat a child with bipolar disorder with a mood stabilizer or an SGA and, if he or she does not fully respond, follow up with antidepressants, other mood stabilizers or antipsychotics, or psychotherapy (Schneck, Chang, Singh, Delbello, & Miklowitz, 2017). The pharmacological treatment algorithms for children with ODD or conduct disorder are less obvious.

Moving Forward to Help Children and Teens

While controversies over the diagnosis continue to roil clinicians and researchers on both sides of the Atlantic, the field is moving past questions about whether childhood bipolar disorder exists to address the clinical needs of children or teens who clearly have it or are at high risk of developing it (B. I. Goldstein et al., 2017). You can be more confident now than 10–20 years ago that a standard psychiatric evaluation with an experienced practitioner will lead to an accurate diagnosis. *Therefore, as a first step, seek an evaluation from a clinician who is familiar with childhood bipolar disorder and has a firm grasp of normal child development, so that age-appropriate behaviors don't get attributed to the illness.*

A good evaluation may help determine whether other DSM-5 disorders better capture the symptomatic picture (DMDD, for one) or whether your child meets criteria for a comorbid disorder (for example, ADHD, ODD, or generalized anxiety disorder) as well as bipolar disorder. Generally, this evaluation should be done by a psychiatrist, psychologist, psychiatric nurse, or social worker; it is not usually the province of a family physician.

"What Should We Be Looking For?"

Francine, a 42-year-old mother, described her 10-year-old son Trevor as moody, brooding, ruminative, impulsive, sad, and at times preoccupied with violence and death. She felt strongly that his moodiness affected his school performance and ability to maintain friendships, a view that was consistent with what she had heard from his teachers and school counselor. She feared that Trevor would never have close friendships or stable relationships and would not be able to finish school. She sought help from the school district to help him get learning accommodations; her advocacy led to an individualized education program (IEP) for him.

Dan, 37, was concerned that his daughter Justine, 14, might be thrown out of school. At the beginning of the school year she had had a 2-week medical absence due to a depressive episode. With only 1 week left to go in the fall semester, she was routinely skipping classes (citing her hatred for various teachers as the reason), becoming more verbally combative at home and at school, and staying up later and later at night. Given her family history of mania, Dan became worried that she was developing bipolar disorder but was more immediately concerned that she would be expelled from school. He explained to the school administration that she had never fully stabilized after her last depressive episode and requested that she be given a degree of latitude on her attendance record.

How Severe Are Your Child's Mood Swings?

In deciding whether to pursue a psychiatric evaluation, it's best to have a brief "case summary" in mind that you can use to explain whether your child's symptoms are severe enough to warrant a diagnosis, treatment, or both. Consider whether your child has the telltale signs of mood and energy instability that often predate a bipolar diagnosis. Both of the cases just presented showed these signs, although neither had the diagnosis yet.

As a first step, try completing the Parent's General Behavior Inventory—10 item Mania (PGBI-10M) scale on pages 369–370. The PGBI-10M is a screening instrument, not a diagnostic instrument. It won't tell you whether your child has bipolar I, II, or unspecified disorder. Instead, it provides a dimension along which the severity of mood swings can be quantified (recall the discussion of dimensions vs. diagnostic categories in Chapter 3). Indeed, many of the diagnostic disagreements between practitioners come down to where one puts the cut point between having an illness and not having it. Scores of 15 or above on the PGBI-10M indicate a high risk of bipolar diagnosis (that is, a high chance that a child has it now or will develop it in the future).

Notice that the scale items emphasize that symptoms are a change from your child's usual self, last a few days or more, and reflect moods that vary from one extreme to the other. Both Trevor and Justine experienced significant changes in their mood states that were noticeable not only to parents but to school personnel as well; both would have scored above 15. In contrast, kids who are irritable by temperament, or those who show manic-like behaviors for only a few hours a day, would not score high on the PGBI-10M. The practitioner you consult may or may not know this scale, but take the completed form along to the first meeting—it may save time and help you zero in on the symptoms you want to explain.

Here are some questions about behaviors that occur in the general population. Think about how often they occur for your child. Using the following scale, select the number that best describes how often your child experienced these behaviors **over the past year:**

0	1	2	3
Never— or hardly ever	Sometimes	Often	Very often— almost constantly

Keep the following points in mind:

Frequency: you may have noticed a behavior as far back as childhood or early teens, or you may have noticed it more recently. In either case, estimate how frequently the behavior has occurred **over the past year.**

For example: if you noticed a behavior when your child was 5, and you have noticed it over the past year, mark your answer **"often"** or **"very often—almost constantly."** However, if your child has experienced a behavior during only one isolated period in his/her life, but not outside that period, mark your answer **"never—hardly ever"** or **"sometimes."**

Duration: many questions require that a behavior occur for an approximate duration of time (for example, "several days or more"). The duration given is a **minimum** duration. If your child usually experiences a behavior for shorter durations, mark the question **"never—hardly ever"** or **"sometimes."**

Changeability: what matters is not whether your child can get rid of certain behaviors if he/she has them, but whether these behaviors have occurred at all. So even if your child can get rid of these behaviors, you should mark your answer according to how frequently he/she experiences them.

Your job, then, is to rate how frequently your child has experienced a behavior, over the past year, for the duration described in the question. Please read each question carefully, and record your answer next to each question **by placing an "X" in the appropriate box.**

0   1   2   3

☐   ☐   ☐   ☐   1. Has your child experienced periods of several days or more when, although he/she was feeling unusually happy and intensely energetic (clearly more than your child's usual self), he/she was also physically restless, unable to sit still, and had to keep moving or jumping from one activity to another?

☐   ☐   ☐   ☐   2. Have there been periods of several days or more when your child's friends or other family members told you that your child seemed unusually happy or high—clearly different from his/her usual self or from a typical good mood?

(continued)

0	1	2	3	
☐	☐	☐	☐	3. Has your child's mood or energy shifted rapidly back and forth from happy to sad or high to low?
☐	☐	☐	☐	4. Has your child had periods of extreme happiness and intense energy lasting several days or more when he/she also felt much more anxious or tense (jittery, nervous, uptight) than usual (*other than related to the menstrual cycle*)?
☐	☐	☐	☐	5. Have there been times on several days or more when, although your child was feeling unusually happy and intensely energetic (clearly more than his/her usual self), he/she also had to struggle very hard to control inner feelings of rage or an urge to smash or destroy things?
☐	☐	☐	☐	6. Has your child had periods of extreme happiness and intense energy (clearly more than his/her usual self) when, for several days or more, it took him/her over an hour to get to sleep at night?
☐	☐	☐	☐	7. Have you found that your child's feelings or energy are generally up or down, but rarely in the middle?
☐	☐	☐	☐	8. Has your child had periods lasting several days or more when he/she felt depressed or irritable, and then other periods of several days or more when he/she felt extremely high, elated, and overflowing with energy?
☐	☐	☐	☐	9. Have there been periods when, although your child was feeling unusually happy and intensely energetic, almost everything got on his/her nerves and made him/her irritable or angry (other than mood swings related to the menstrual cycle)?
☐	☐	☐	☐	10. Has your child had times when his/her thoughts and ideas came so fast that he/she couldn't get them all out, or they came so quickly that others complained they couldn't keep up with your child's ideas?

_____ Total Score

Interpretation Guide:

Total Score: Add up the items so that you get a score between 0 and 30. Scores are used to indicate risk for bipolar disorder rather than whether a child has bipolar disorder or not. Scores of 0 are considered Minimal Risk; 1–4, Mild Risk; 5–14, Neutral Risk; 15–17, High Risk; 18+, Very High Risk.

> ### PERSONALIZED CARE TIP:
> ## "Should we be concerned about 'subthreshold' symptoms?"
>
> Your child may have some manic or depressive symptoms and not others. He may have multiple symptoms of mania, but they may not be severe enough or last long enough to interfere with his ability to function at school. His mood may bounce back and forth between elation, irritability, and sadness without staying at one pole long enough to meet the full diagnostic criteria. If your child has several of these low-level symptoms, he may have subthreshold or unspecified bipolar disorder (also see Chapter 3). If bipolar disorder also runs in your family, it's best to get an evaluation for your child to see if treatment is warranted now. The early treatment may or may not involve mood stabilizers or SGAs. There are family psychoeducation and skill-training programs (see Chapter 6) that may be relevant to you (Fristad & MacPherson, 2014; Miklowitz et al., 2013).

The Nature of Bipolar Diagnoses in Children

The General Behavior Inventory gives you an idea of the main symptom features taken into account when diagnosing children with bipolar disorder. First, the clinician needs to establish whether the child's manic, hypomanic, or depressive symptoms cluster together in *episodes* that are of a certain minimal *duration* and whether the symptoms within these episodes are impairing, intense, and frequent (Fristad & Goldberg Arnold, 2003). Your child's doctor should not issue a diagnosis of mania unless your child has had elevated or intensely irritable mood and increased activity (for example, moving faster, or with "grander" movements) every day for at least 1 week or less if a hospitalization was necessary, plus at least three of the following: grandiose thinking, decreased need for sleep, rapid or pressured speech and/or "flight of ideas," racing thoughts, distractibility (attention easily drawn to irrelevant stimuli), excessive goal-driven activity, and impulsive or reckless behavior (American Psychiatric Association, 2013). Second, the changes in your child's mood or behavior have to be severe enough for episodes to be clearly distinguishable from his or her usual self. Third, the symptoms must be noticeable to other people and present across settings (not just at home) and, in the case of full bipolar I mania, result in a deterioration in functioning across settings (such as an inability to keep up with schoolwork or personal hygiene). Impairment is not required for diagnosing hypomania in bipolar II disorder.

If your daughter is depressed, she'll probably have trouble finishing homework or may sleep through classes. If your son is manic or hypomanic, he will talk fast, jump from topic to topic (usually interrupting others in the process), tell wild and heroic stories, or get in trouble in public places, all of which may alienate his peers. These are the diagnostic signs that, either singularly or collectively, point to the need for a professional evaluation.

The Role of Comorbid Disorders

There are many nuances to diagnosing bipolar disorder in children and adolescents. You can only supply information from your own observations, but these observations will be given maximal weight by the practitioner—you know your child better than anyone else does.

One area where your input will be particularly helpful is in diagnosing comorbid disorders. Perhaps you know from your child's prior school performance that he or she has significant attentional or learning difficulties, but it may be unclear whether these problems worsen alongside the mood disorder episodes, in which case the attentional problems are considered part of a comorbid condition like ADHD. Your child may have a speech or language disorder that is largely independent of his or her mood disorder. A significant number of kids describe anxiety problems that may worsen with depressive or manic episodes, but they may also persist between episodes, warranting a separate diagnosis.

Information about comorbid disorders is also critical to whether we apply the label of bipolar disorder or not. Consider a 10-year-old boy who is described as distractible, nervous, and agitated. To diagnose bipolar I or II disorder, his mania/hypomania symptoms must be above and beyond what would be expected for ADHD or an anxiety disorder alone. To include distractibility or agitation as manic symptoms, we'd need to know whether it reflects a significant departure from his usual self (has he always been distractible or just recently?) and whether it worsens along with other symptoms of mania (for example, decreased need for sleep) that are worsening at the same time. If this 10-year-old has never had a manic episode before, it may not be possible to know whether distractibility and agitation reflect a mood disorder or other disorders (like ADHD) that sometimes "travel" with bipolar disorder.

More complexity is added when one considers the child's age and developmental stage. For example, many girls develop depression after the onset of puberty, but they may develop anxiety or attentional problems at a much younger age. Hypersexuality, a key symptom of mania or hypomania, may not be fully observable until adolescence, but it may be present in milder forms in childhood (for example, speech that references sexual acts, drawing pornographic pictures).

Symptoms in Children versus Adults: Are They Different?

Diagnoses are additionally challenging because mood symptoms may not have the same frequency, severity, or duration in children as in adults. An example is a mixed episode or a rapid cycling presentation: in a child we may see significant mood shifts over only a day or two, rather than over the 1- or 2-week-long episodes common in adults. Nonetheless, you should be able to observe mood episodes in your child even though they may be very short. Mixed or rapid cycling presentations are not the same as irritability or temper outbursts, which are very common in young people and often signal other problems, including ADHD or anxiety disorders. On the whole, pediatric-onset bipolar disorder is characterized by the same mood symptoms and episodes seen in adulthood, even though the symptoms may be more childlike in appearance and may not last as long.

Moods and associated symptoms have to be understood in relation to age group—it may be normal for an 8-year-old to have an imaginary playmate, but a similarly aged child who says she has "500 brothers who live on the moon" may be grandiose and even delusional. In an adult, elevated mood may appear as unusual jocularity, speaking and laughing loudly, excessive optimism and bragging, or physical intrusiveness. For a child, elevated mood may come across as silliness, sloppy and erratic movements, uncontrollable laughing, or sudden outbursts of tears.

Are there any differences in the course patterns of children and adults? One study that looked across time found that (1) kids with bipolar spectrum disorders had more time with subthreshold mood symptoms than adults; (2) kids have longer intervals with mixed symptoms (that is, manic or hypomanic symptoms simultaneous with depression); and (3) children and adolescents have more "polarity switches" than adults, meaning, for example, switches from depressed to manic and back to depressed again (Birmaher et al., 2006). It's important to keep these features in mind if you're thinking about how your child's behaviors compare with yours or those of other adult family members with bipolar illness. For example, the fact that your child's mood episodes are very short but also change polarity quickly may be more typical of his or her age group.

Core Symptom Features of the Early Stages of Bipolar Disorder

There is a recognizable set of core symptoms during the early stages of bipolar disorder, regardless of whether the onset is in childhood or adolescence. If your child or teen has developed one of these core symptoms—especially if he or she has developed more than one symptom in tandem—this is a good time to seek a professional evaluation. Some of these core symptomatic features have been discussed in relation to adults in Chapters 2 and 3, so I am going to emphasize those symptom patterns that are most common in children or teens.

If symptoms are caught early, there may be opportunities to try behavioral interventions such as sleep–wake cycle regulation (Chapter 8), behavioral activation (Chapter 10), or family psychoeducation (Chapter 13). In a study of children with a first-degree relative with bipolar disorder, we found that children who had prodromal symptoms of depression or hypomania had better outcomes over 1 year if they and their parents received 12 sessions of family education and communication skills training as compared to a briefer educational treatment (Miklowitz et al., 2013).

Early Warning Signs of a First Episode

Earlier in this book I talked about being alert to "prodromal" (early warning) signs of new episodes of mania or depression so you can minimize their negative effects on your life. Are there specific prodromal signs and symptoms that appear before the first full episode that you could watch for in your child or teenager? A meta-analysis by Anna Van Meter and colleagues (2017) found that the average length of symptoms before the full onset of the illness was 27.1 months. That's a long time in the life of a child and presents challenges to parents who are trying to figure out whether they have reason to be concerned. In the meta-analysis, the most common early warning signs of a first manic episode were having too much energy, followed by pressured speech, being talkative, elated mood, or being overly productive or goal directed. These symptoms were present in muted form in at least 50% of kids who went on to a full manic episode. For example, a kid in the prodromal phase might be getting only 5 hours of sleep a night without feeling tired the next day; during a full manic episode, he might not sleep at all for nights on end. For an initial episode of depression, the most common early warning signs are a diminished ability to think or concentrate, indecisiveness, academic or work difficulties, insomnia, and depressed mood (Van Meter, Burke, Youngstrom, Faedda, & Correll, 2016).

The Dutch Bipolar Offspring Study, in which a cohort of adolescents and young adults (ages 12–21) with bipolar parents was followed over 12 years, found that 88% had a depressive episode as their initial episode of bipolar disorder (Mesman, Nolen, Reichart, Wals, & Hillegers, 2013). A unique study of offspring of bipolar parents within the Amish population of Pennsylvania found that anxiety, hyperalertness, physical complaints during preschool, and more fluctuations in mood, crying, sleep disturbance, and fearfulness during the school years were associated with developing bipolar I disorder 16 years later (Egeland et al., 2012).

Other research has shown that mood instability in childhood or early adolescence—the constant swinging back and forth of moods, from depressed to irritable, to elevated, to anxious or depressed—is often a forerunner of having full manic or depressive episodes later on (Hafeman et al., 2016). In other words, the most common early warning signs of mania or depression are muted symptoms of mania or depression! Nonetheless, learning to recognize milder forms of these symptoms in your child may help you spot the early stages of an episode on its way up; an earlier intervention, in turn, may lead to a shorter and milder episode.

Learning to recognize and track your child's symptoms has one negative side effect: it can lead to your child complaining that you're watching her too closely. Your spouse may be saying, "Leave her alone; she's just a kid." You may begin to feel very alone in attempting to keep your child well. If this pattern describes you, see the following box.

PERSONALIZED CARE TIP:
Avoiding hypervigilance

How do you learn as much as you can about bipolar disorder and watch for changes in your child's moods or sleep–wake patterns without becoming a hypervigilant or overly controlling parent? This is a balance that many parents I've worked with have struggled to find. The following strategies have worked for many parents, with adjustment depending on the child's age, level of illness, and presence of other family supports:

1. Make sure that your interactions with your child do not become all about moods or other symptoms. Spend plenty of time talking about the child's interests, friends/playdates, sports, upcoming school events—without veering off into the buzzwords that may have become a threat to your child: unstable moods, depression, mania, rapid cycles, meltdowns, or mixed episodes.

2. Explain to your spouse or partner the difficult position you find yourself in, between trying to monitor your child's moods and observe changes in your own moods and stress levels, while also being an everyday parent. Be direct about how you want your partner to help.

3. Think about whether your hypervigilance has roots in your own childhood. Possibly, you want to provide your child with the parent that you never had when you were little—one who put her kids' needs first. Keep in mind that most kids do best with "scaffolding." Scaffolding means offering the child structured support when she is first learning a task (for example, how to manage her moods), and then gradually removing this support as the child learns to do the task on her own.

4. Use support groups, such as the Depression and Bipolar Support Alliance (*www.dbsalliance.org*) and its subsidiary, the Balanced Mind Parent Network (*http://community.dbsalliance.org/welcome.htm*), or the International Bipolar Foundation help site (*www.ibpf.org*), for suggestions and support regarding the difficult role of parenting a child with bipolar disorder.

5. Make sure you are taking time for yourself, which can take various forms, including time with your spouse, time with friends, or personal activities (for example, going to the gym). The key is to emphasize parts of your life that don't necessarily involve kids. Most of us who have kids know the importance of personal time in maintaining balance.

Subthreshold Bipolar Disorder: Early Warning Sign or Primary Diagnosis?

If your child has *unspecified bipolar disorder* or *cyclothymic disorder,* he or she will have brief but recurrent periods of subthreshold mania (or even full mania) that last 1–2 days each, with increased activity, irritable or elevated mood, decreased sleep, rapid speech, and signs of poor judgment. These periods cause impairment at school, with friends, or with family. Kids with subthreshold conditions often have histories of depression and associated symptoms that may include anxiety, aggressiveness, or self-injurious behavior. It's important to know about these diagnoses, because the practitioner you consult may use them and because they can indicate a heightened risk of developing bipolar I or II disorder in the next 4–7 years (Axelson, Birmaher, Strober, et al., 2011; Hafeman et al., 2016; Kochman et al., 2005). Not surprisingly, the risk for bipolar I or II is greatest among those youth with more severe (but subthreshold) hypomanic symptoms.

A diagnosis of unspecified bipolar disorder or cyclothymic disorder—like bipolar I or II disorder—presumes that your child's changes in mood and behavior are not typical of her when she is feeling well. The changes also have to be more extreme than what is developmentally typical. For example, pretending to be friends with people in outer space is probably age appropriate for an 8-year-old. Climbing up on the roof in the middle of the night to wave hello is probably not.

Many children with unspecified bipolar disorder or cyclothymic disorder never actually develop the full bipolar syndrome. The rates of conversion differ if the child has a bipolar parent or full sibling—in which case his or her chances of developing bipolar I or II disorder hover around 58.5% in 5 years—but they are lower (35.5%) if there is no bipolar relative (Axelson, Birmaher, Strober, et al., 2011). In other words, your child's symptoms may stay at a subthreshold level without ever progressing to bipolar I or II.

Common Attributes of Childhood Bipolar Disorder

As discussed earlier, the early warning signs of bipolar disorder in children are often just muted forms of core manic or depressive symptoms. What are the most common attributes of childhood bipolar disorder that help to define the syndrome? And what attributes are also features of other disorders, like ADHD?

Irritability: Bipolar Symptom or Distress Signal?

Although it is often a symptom of manic and hypomanic episodes in children, irritability is also a symptom of other psychiatric disorders, including generalized anxiety disorder, autism spectrum disorders, ADHD, ODD, and major depression. It may be best thought of as a distress signal—a way for the child to communicate that he or she is anxious, depressed, confused, frustrated, or stressed from being unable to fulfill adult expectations. As noted earlier in the chapter, irritability is one of the key causes of the diagnostic confusion about childhood bipolar disorder: **Manic episodes should not be confused with episodes of explosive anger.** Anger outbursts are often precipitated by certain situations or stressors (such as sudden changes of plans) and may reflect an inability to regulate emotions (see the discussion of disruptive mood dysregulation disorder below). Be very skeptical if a mental health professional tells you your child is bipolar because he or she has rage attacks.

Currently, we think that irritability in a child is associated with mania only when it represents a clear departure from the child's usual state and is *episodic*, meaning that it waxes and wanes in conjunction with other symptoms that define manic or depressive episodes. When irritability is chronic, we think it is likely to be a precursor of major depressive disorder or anxiety disorders in adulthood (Leibenluft, Cohen, Gorrindo, Brook, & Pine, 2006).

Ultra-rapid and Ultradian Cycling

Although these terms are often used interchangeably, *ultra-rapid cycling* refers to having episodes monthly, whereas ultradian cycles are multiple mood switches within a single episode. Some kids have *ultradian cycles* that go from full depressive moods to manic/elevated moods within 24 or 48 hours. They may have extreme

---

PERSONALIZED CARE TIP:
Dealing with your child's mood instability

If your child is regularly showing wide mood changes throughout the day and evening, here is a "litmus test" for whether you need to take him in for an additional (or a first) psychiatric visit: Do his mood swings disrupt family functioning, so that it becomes harder to make dinner, get the kid (or his siblings) ready for school, or get homework done? If not, does it disrupt school functioning, such as being unable to sit through classes or getting in fights at school?

If your child is already taking mood stabilizers, he will probably need to have these medications adjusted because they are not providing the control that you and he should be able to expect. If his mood shifts are predictable, occurring only at certain events or times, you may want to choose your responses accordingly. That might mean, for example, ignoring outbursts of irritability that occur when he first wakes up or helping him find more structured activities in the evening if that is when he is most likely to become bored or depressed. If he becomes anxious and irritable over an upcoming exam, some low-key downtime and encouraging words may be all that's necessary.

changes in energy or activity levels that parallel these mood changes, or their speech may swing from pessimistic to grandiose. In other words, we might say that the child had a monthlong mixed episode, but during that period he or she cycled back and forth on a daily basis between depressed and hypomanic moods. These patterns appear to be more common in children than adults (Birmaher et al., 2006).

Sleep Disturbance and Decreased Need for Sleep

Like adults, children with bipolar disorder have significant problems falling or staying asleep, especially during a depressive episode. They may complain that they can't sleep, wake up feeling unrested, and have to drag themselves through the school day. They may nap as soon as they get home. Absences from school due to not feeling well become increasingly common.

During mania, children or teens may get along with very little sleep. They may be up late at night text-messaging friends or in online chat rooms, playing video games, watching livestream shows, or talking on the phone to friends who are also up all night. They may not go to sleep at all. The next day they may say that they don't feel tired despite getting only a few hours of sleep. This is what we call *decreased need for sleep*—it is different from insomnia or other sleep problems that might leave the child feeling tired the next day.

> **Effective treatment:** Sleep disturbance
>
> If your child is in a depressed or manic state, it will be very hard for you to legislate sleep and wake times—your child's circadian rhythms may be on their own trajectory. Sleep disturbances are one of the main reasons that some parents decide it's time for their child to try antipsychotic medications (for example, quetiapine or Seroquel), which can help the child fall and stay asleep. There are also cognitive-behavioral programs that can be useful for managing sleep (for example, Ehrnstrom & Brosse, 2016; or *www. sleepio.com*). Although focused on adults, these programs have exercises your child can try (for example, keeping the room darkened and free of electronic devices).

Depression and Suicidal Thoughts and Behaviors

Depression in youth is similar to depression in adults, but it may be of quicker onset and offset. Your child may wake up severely depressed one day and then snap out of it equally rapidly. In kids with severe bipolar I disorder, depression can be associated with delusional thinking, often centered on morbid themes such as "my body is rotting" or "I'm being punished." Teens with bipolar depression are at an especially high risk for attempting suicide.

It's important to know about sex differences in who reports depression, either as part of bipolar disorder or as part of a unipolar depressive illness. Depression is equally common in boys and girls during the period up to puberty. After puberty, depression becomes three times more common in girls than boys (Hankin & Abramson, 2001). Boys may not admit to depression at all and instead describe feeling bored or empty. They may express their unhappiness through aggression, withdrawal, or substance abuse. Girls are more likely to ruminate over problems related to peers, romantic relationships, and body image. But suicidal ideation and behaviors are not limited to teenagers. In a study of younger bipolar patients (ages 7–13), nearly 50% had active suicidal ideation or behaviors (West et al., 2014).

The reality is that suicidal thoughts are very common in teens and do not usually portend a suicide attempt (Hawton, Sutton, Haw, Sinclair, & Harriss, 2005). Nonetheless, in the interests of long-term prevention, every threat needs to be taken seriously. If your child is saying things like "I don't know why I'm here" or "My life is worthless" but says nothing about hurting herself, you should nonetheless contact her psychiatrist and therapist. If your child does not have any providers, the appearance of suicidal thoughts is a good reason to initiate contact with one.

If the thoughts become more specific, such as when teens express a concrete plan for hurting or killing themselves using resources that they already have (overdosing on sleeping medications, for example), consider initiating a psychiatric hospitalization to keep the teen safe over a short interval. Hospitalizations are frightening to teens and parents, but they often provide a short-term solution to a high-risk situation. Make sure to limit the teen's access to pills, knives, or guns. Review Chapter 11 for other strategies to use when your son or daughter becomes suicidal. Most of the coping methods applicable to adults—such as the "Reasons for Living" and "Improving the Moment" strategies—are also valuable for children and teens.

> Kaitlyn, age 17, had bipolar I disorder that was diagnosed when she was 13. She had been thinking about suicide almost daily before she started family-focused treatment with her family members. She denied that she wanted to kill herself but had made two prior attempts, both involving overdosing on pain relievers. Surprisingly, her parents did not know that these attempts had occurred until they took her to a clinic for an evaluation. Her mother downplayed the significance of her suicidal thinking, saying, "All teenage girls think that way." During their first family session, Kaitlyn's 15-year-old brother rolled his eyes and refused to take the issue seriously. He and his mother seemed to agree that Kaitlyn was a "drama queen." Her father, who had experienced his own father's suicide, was much more inclined to take the threats seriously.
>
> During a series of family therapy sessions, Kaitlyn clarified that her two prior attempts had been related to loss or separation experiences. In one case she had broken up with her boyfriend, and in the other her parents had undergone a brief separation.
>
> The treatment "contract" involved several agreements between Kaitlyn, her parents, and the therapist. First, Kaitlyn agreed to contact her father at work (or approach him at home) if her suicidal thoughts started again, and especially if she felt they were getting out of control. They agreed to have a

discussion about what was upsetting her, and he agreed to help her find temporary ways to distract herself from her thoughts. Previously, she had found that when at home, dancing to hip-hop music in her room and "screaming into my pillow" temporarily defused the thoughts.

Kaitlyn expressed the wish that her parents would avoid being so critical of her and blaming her for her "bad feelings." The clinician worked with Kaitlyn and her family on ways to communicate and express support for each other, especially when Kaitlyn expressed self-injurious thoughts. Her parents had their own wishes, such as wanting her to call her therapist when she felt suicidal for help understanding where her thoughts were coming from. In a medication management session, her psychiatrist recommended she try a higher lithium dosage. She was not thrilled by this idea but agreed to try it for 3 months. Between the support of her family and the extra protection afforded by medications, Kaitlyn became more stable. By the end of family treatment she remained mildly depressed but had not made any more suicide attempts.

This illustration is not meant to suggest that all teens showing signs of bipolar disorder are thinking about suicide, but it is a feature to be aware of since it can remain hidden. If one parent has the child's trust (even if only temporarily), that parent may be in the best position to help the teen manage self-harming impulses, which can be very hard for the teen to ignore.

Self-Injury

Separately from suicide attempts, self-injurious behavior (for example, self-cutting) is an increasingly common behavior in teens and appears to be more common in bipolar disorder than in major depression (Weintraub, Van de Loo, Gitlin, & Miklowitz, 2017). Sometimes self-cutting reflects self-destructive impulses, or

Effective treatment: There are treatment programs that focus on preventing self-injury in teens who are prone to it. The most promising appears to be dialectical behavior therapy (DBT; Linehan & Wilks, 2015), which has a strong evidence base across a number of psychiatric disorders, including bipolar disorder (T. R. Goldstein et al., 2015). DBT involves both individual and group (or family) treatment and uses a skill-training format to teach coping strategies related to managing one's emotions, such as acceptance, mindfulness, distress tolerance, and interpersonal effectiveness. Another treatment, mentalization-based therapy, focuses on clarifying the teen's feelings about herself and encouraging her to become curious about others' emotions and motivations and how they differ from her own. This treatment, usually given individually or in an individual and family format, has been found to be effective in treating adolescent self-harm (Rossouw & Fonagy, 2012).

it may be associated with other high-risk behaviors (for example, driving while intoxicated, doing dangerous moves on a skateboard, staying out late to meet up with people met on the Internet). Some promising treatment programs for self-injury in teens are described in the box on the facing page.

Cognitive Problems

Usually, cognitive problems are assessed with neuropsychology tests, such as repeating back a list of words or copying a figure drawing. These studies do not always find the same thing when comparing bipolar and healthy children. Nonetheless, the majority of studies indicate that, when compared with healthy volunteers of the same age, children with bipolar disorder have problems with memory for words or stories, attention, working memory, executive functioning (skills such as planning, ordering, and decision making), visual perception, and visual memory (Pavuluri, West, Hill, Jindal, & Sweeney, 2009; Walshaw, Alloy, & Sabb, 2010). Some studies find problems with reading and verbal fluency as well (Joseph, Frazier, Youngstrom, & Soares, 2008).

Neuroimaging studies find that kids with bipolar disorders have less activation of the prefrontal areas of the brain (involved in executive functioning, memory, goal-directedness, and emotional control). Prefrontal cortical deficits may show up as problems remembering what a story was about, understanding the steps in accomplishing a task, staying on task, or regulating emotional reactions. Kids with bipolar disorders often have correspondingly more activation of the lower-brain "limbic" areas, such as the amygdala, which plays a key role in emotion regulation. The idea here is that abnormal development of the amygdala may lead to problems processing emotions in the circuit connecting the amygdala and the prefrontal cortex, also known as the "affective control" circuit (Townsend & Altshuler, 2012). In children without bipolar disorder, the prefrontal cortex has better control over inputs from the amygdala, leading to more restraint in expressing emotions. Pharmacological treatments, and even some psychosocial treatments, may operate by improving the ability of the prefrontal areas to modulate the amygdala and other limbic areas (Chang, Saxena, & Howe, 2006).

These research findings can be quite disheartening to parents, who wonder if their child has been consigned to a life of mediocre cognitive functioning. However, there is quite a bit of variability in the academic and social functioning of kids who have bipolar disorder. Some children show significant improvements in cognition when they take mood-stabilizing or antipsychotic medications. Furthermore, skill deficits are not always stable over time: impairments seen at one age may not necessarily be seen later.

The important thing to remember is that the child's academic difficulties are rarely due to inadequate motivation. In the absence of clear mood symptoms, it is easy to believe that your child should be able to put in more effort. Consider the likely possibility that he is actually trying very hard, but cognitive limitations asso-

> **PERSONALIZED CARE TIP:**
> ## "Do my child's cognitive problems indicate bipolar disorder?"
>
> If you observe that your child is having problems with verbal memory, maintaining attention, or visual processing, these may not be caused by the same underlying vulnerabilities that cause bipolar disorder. In fact, they may be due to another disorder entirely, or one that is comorbid with bipolar disorder, like ADHD. A full battery of neuropsychological tests from a qualified psychologist—usually accompanied by a report in lay language—will answer many of your questions about the origins of your child's cognitive impairments and what to expect over time. The battery will not tell you if your child has bipolar disorder, but it can clarify areas that will be hardest for him in school, and help identify accommodations that could be made in an individualized educatinal plan (IEP). You can ask for an MRI, but it may not be worth the time and money. MRI brain scans are not designed as diagnostic instruments. More generally, be skeptical of any provider who claims that neurological or neuropsychological tests of any sort can determine whether your child has a "bipolar brain."

ciated with his mood disorder or a comorbid disorder affect his performance even when his mood symptoms are not obvious.

There are treatments that emphasize cognitive retraining and remediation, and some of these have been shown to be effective, at least for adults with bipolar disorder (for example, see Torrent et al., 2013; Deckersbach et al., 2010). For kids, it may be most useful to work with the school first to determine what kinds of accommodations can be made in an individualized educational plan. School psychologists may also refer you to local practitioners who work with kids with attentional or memory problems. The Juvenile Bipolar Disorder Research Foundation has an excellent set of articles for families who are trying to ensure their child's success in the school system, including what accommodations will be helpful (*www.jbrf.org/page-for-families/educational-issues-facing-children-with-bipolar-disorder*).

"What Should We Do If We're Worried?"

With the overview of childhood bipolar disorder you now have, you're in a better position to judge whether you have anything to be concerned about. If you think you do, the first step is to have your child evaluated by a practitioner who has a good working knowledge of bipolar disorder in kids, even if this is not his or her specialty.

"What Should We Expect from a Comprehensive Evaluation?"

In the UCLA Child and Adolescent Mood Disorders clinic (*www.semel.ucla.edu/champ*), we start with structured diagnostic interviews of the child and, separately, at least one parent who can report on the child's symptoms and history. In three or four meetings of 1–2 hours each, our child psychiatrists and psychologists evaluate the child's symptoms of mood disorders, psychosis, ADHD, eating disorders, anxiety disorders, autism spectrum disorders, oppositional or conduct disorders, and substance abuse or dependence. We take a thorough developmental history (When did your child start talking, walking? When did you first notice problems?), social history (for example, your child's strengths vs. difficulties in making friends and keeping them), and family history (whether any psychiatric disorders run in the family). We take note of any adverse childhood experiences—such as physical or sexual abuse, trauma, severe physical illness, or loss of a parent or a sibling—that may be causing anxiety or posttraumatic stress symptoms. During a feedback session for the family at the end, we offer our diagnostic impressions, review any conclusions from a medical evaluation and any other testing results, and present our formulation as to how environmental stressors—present and past—may be affecting the child. We also review the medical and psychosocial treatment options that are available locally.

Of course, what I'm describing here is the "Cadillac model" of diagnostic evaluation. There may be few practitioners in your area who specialize in childhood mood disorders, or those that are available may be under the gun to see as many kids as possible in a short time. You may want to explore going to one of the many specialty mood disorder centers around the country, usually located in major cities (see the Resources section on National and International Organizations).

Diagnostic ambiguity and disagreement is a cause of considerable anxiety for parents, who, understandably, want answers. But it is important to wait until the practitioner offers a diagnosis with a reasonable degree of certainty before proceeding with treatment. The diagnostic evaluation should not only arrive at a presumptive diagnosis; the provider should offer guidance about treatment directions. He or she may weigh in on whether your child will benefit mostly from medications or whether therapies that are available in your locale would help. The clinician may recommend that you start with medications (accompanied by medication management sessions with a psychiatrist), family support sessions, individual therapy for the child, or even "watchful waiting," which means keeping an eye on your child's symptoms and consulting the provider if they get worse. As you'll learn later in the chapter, there are no treatment recommendations that work for every child with or at risk for bipolar disorder. If you aren't comfortable with the recommendations, seek a second opinion.

"What Kind of Practitioner Should We Consult?"

Where you live, your finances, your health insurance policy, and the availability of local practitioners are more likely to determine who your child sees than any decisions you make about who is the most appropriate provider. Here are some questions to keep in mind as you and your child seek an evaluation. Although you may not be able to ask the practitioner these questions before the first appointment, you will probably have a good idea of the answers by the end of that appointment.

1. *How does the provider approach the evaluation?* Ideally, the practitioner evaluates the time course of mood symptoms over your child's lifetime, such as when they began, whether symptoms have ever gone away for an extensive period (for example, 6 months), and when (or how frequently) symptoms have returned (recurrences). Bipolar disorder is a cyclic illness, and the only way to establish that feature is to understand the onset, course, and duration of prior episodes and whether there have been periods of healthy functioning in between.

2. *How does the provider explain why bipolar disorder (vs. another disorder) is the right diagnosis for your child?* Can the clinician explain, at a level that you (and ideally, your child) can understand, how the diagnosis of bipolar disorder differs from other associated disorders? Or does the provider say something like "I don't use the DSM-5 system" or "I don't find diagnoses helpful"? If he or she emphasizes dimensions instead of categories (for example, "I think your son is on the autistic spectrum" or "she has a moderate level of depression but it's not severe"), that's fine, but the practitioner should be able to clarify what dimensions are most relevant to your child, how he or she determines where to place your child on these dimensions, and how these dimensions inform treatment. You may ask whether the provider thinks your child's behaviors are due to a mood disorder, reactions to environmental events (for example, a recent move, an illness in the family), or even normal development. If you have an alternative explanation for your child's behavior, offer it.

3. *Does the provider have a good working knowledge of normal youth development?* He or she should be able to answer questions like "How do we know if he's showing mood symptoms as opposed to just normal teenage behavior?" Or "Can these highs and lows be explained by reaching puberty?" Or "How do we know whether these are really delusions or just fanciful beliefs that kids can have?"

4. *Does the provider inquire as to any family history of psychiatric disorders?* Some practitioners ask only one question: Does bipolar disorder run in your family? In most cases that won't really clarify your child's family history. We know that the presence of mania in a first- or second-degree relative puts the child at a substantially increased risk for bipolar disorder (Axelson, Birmaher, Strober, et al., 2011). So, your provider should be inquiring about both sides of the family, aunts/uncles, and two generations removed from your child (for example, grandparents). He should also be asking about depression, alcoholism, schizophrenia, criminal behavior, psychiatric hospitalizations, and other disorders in the family as well as bipolar disorder.

PERSONALIZED CARE TIPS:
Finding the right provider

■ Look for a practitioner who takes his or her time to evaluate your child's symptoms and functioning. You should not feel like you're being rushed through the interview. A clinician who diagnoses your child and makes medication recommendations in 45 minutes is probably someone to avoid.

■ On the flip side, don't expect that you will walk out of the first psychiatry appointment with a prescription and treatment plan. It is unusual for physicians to make determinations that quickly. The only scenario in which this might happen is if your child is already being successfully treated with a certain drug and you are wanting to keep the regimen but need to switch practitioners.

■ Is the practitioner a child or an adult psychiatrist? Adult psychiatrists may be quite competent in diagnosing children, but they sometimes miss the important role of developmental milestones (for example, language delays) in interpreting a child's history.

■ Make sure the practitioner has worked with children with mood disorders. Some psychologists and psychiatrists have never seen a bipolar child before, but they will not advertise this. Ask, "Do you feel comfortable diagnosing kids with bipolar disorder? Is it an area of specialty for you, or is there someone else you'd recommend?" In my experience, this background is far more important than whether the practitioner has an MD, a PhD, or a social work or nursing degree.

■ Is the provider willing to write a report on his or her findings that you can share with other practitioners or school authorities? These reports may cost extra and take time, but if they are well done, they will prevent a lot of problems later on.

■ What if you have doubts about the practitioner's conclusions? You should express those doubts and ask for answers. It's often a good idea to get a second opinion, even though going through another psychiatric evaluation may feel burdensome to you and your child. Second practitioners often see things that the first did not, and together they may offer different but possibly complementary treatment options.

"How Do I Know If My Child Has Bipolar Disorder and Not Something Else—or Bipolar Disorder *and* Something Else?"

Hopefully, your practitioner will help you determine whether your child has bipolar disorder or another disorder, such as ADHD or anxiety. As you know from other chapters, there are other psychiatric disorders that are often mistaken for bipolar disorder or can co-occur with it. Comorbidity is the rule rather than the exception in childhood bipolar disorder—most kids who have it also have at least one other illness. This makes diagnosing children and teens even more challenging.

> Julie, age 12, was initially diagnosed with social anxiety disorder because she feared being around peers who might judge her. A group of girls at school had ganged up on her and written slurs on her Facebook page. Shortly after this event she had fallen into a deep depression. Her first doctor recommended that she attend social skill training groups. However, her mother was never convinced of the social anxiety diagnosis because Julie had previously had friends and was even occasionally the "life of the party." When it became clear that Julie was socially anxious only when she was depressed, her anxiety diagnosis was dropped and treatment began to focus on alleviating her depressive symptoms. When she recovered from her depressive episode, she felt much more able to connect with others, although a residual feeling of mistrust of her peers continued to bother her. Her final diagnosis was major depressive disorder.

Comorbid disorders are important to flag during the initial evaluation of your child because they can worsen the course of bipolar disorder and may indicate the need for more intensive (or a different kind of) treatment. Kids with bipolar disorder have high rates of comorbidity with ADHD (about 60%; Lan et al., 2015) and anxiety disorders (30–40%; Sala et al., 2010; Yen et al., 2016). A child who has bipolar disorder that is comorbid with ADHD or anxiety disorder will have inattention, distractibility, or physical states of anxiety in between manic or depressive episodes. If these symptoms occur only when the child is manic or depressed (for example, in Julie's case), they may just be manifestations of mood disorder.

ADHD

The section in Chapter 3 on misdiagnosis and comorbid disorders (see page 58) describes many of the ways we distinguish adult bipolar disorder from other disorders, most of which also apply to children and teens. The table on page 387 summarizes some of the key differences between bipolar disorder and ADHD.

As you can see from the table, several symptoms occur in both disorders: irritability, rapid speech, distractibility, and increased energy. Other symptoms—such as grandiosity and elated mood—are key features of bipolar disorder and occur

Symptoms That Distinguish Childhood Bipolar Disorder from ADHD

Symptom	Bipolar disorder	ADHD
Elated mood and grandiosity	Common during mania	Rare
Decreased need for sleep	Common during mania	Rare
Flight of ideas	Common during mania	Rare
Ultradian cycling	Common	Rare
Hypersexuality	Fairly common during mania	Rare
Psychosis	Common during episodes	Rare
Irritability	Common during episodes	Ongoing problem
Rapid speech	Common during mania	Ongoing problem
Distractibility	Common during mania	Ongoing problem
Increased energy and activity	Common during mania	Ongoing problem

Sources: Geller et al. (1998); Kim and Miklowitz (2002).

only rarely in ADHD. Kids with ADHD usually are distractible, but kids with bipolar disorder may experience distractibility only when manic or hypomanic. To make sense of these differences, the clinician has to consider the course of the illness over time: bipolar disorder is *episodic,* whereas ADHD is believed to be a fairly constant state of disrupted cognitive functioning (unless the child is benefiting from treatment with psychostimulants or other agents).

Disruptive Mood Dysregulation Disorder

You may have already heard of DMDD, especially if your child is male and has temper outbursts. This disorder was introduced in DSM-5 to provide a "diagnostic home" to children who were explosively angry and chronically irritable but did not otherwise fit the bipolar disorder criteria. This diagnosis has several core features in children and teens: (1) severe and recurrent temper outbursts that are clearly disproportionate to the situation, with verbal rages and/or physical aggressiveness (for example, breaking a window when denied a snack); (2) the temper outbursts are inconsistent with developmental level (the child is too old to have this kind of tantrum); (3) the outbursts occur, on average, three or more times per week; and (4) in between these outbursts, the child is irritable, angry, sad, or anxious virtually every day for most of the day (American Psychiatric Association, 2013).

You can see how this disorder could be confused with bipolar disorder. In fact, the overall intent of this diagnosis is to reduce the frequency with which mental health professionals diagnose bipolar disorder, and presumably reduce the number of kids who are erroneously given second-generation antipsychotic medications. There are some problems with the diagnosis of DMDD, however. First, a significant proportion of kids who have DMDD also have ODD or conduct disorder (Axelson, Birmaher, Findling, et al., 2011). So, a child with a complex symptomatic picture may end up with the diagnosis of DMDD and ODD or conduct disorder instead of bipolar disorder, which doesn't add a great deal of clarity.

A bigger problem is that the expected course and treatment of DMDD are unclear. Some long-term data suggest that it is not stable over time (Axelson et al., 2012). Furthermore, when a child is explosive and angry, often the best medication options are second-generation antipsychotics or antidepressants, the same drugs that are used in bipolar disorder. In the short time since DMDD became an official diagnosis (2013) there has been a reduction in childhood bipolar diagnoses but no significant changes in medication recommendations (Faheem, Petti, & Mellos, 2017). If your child is diagnosed with DMDD, you may want to ask the practitioner what implications this diagnosis has for treatment: How will it differ from the treatment of a child with bipolar disorder?

Keep in mind that irritability can be of a manic variety (for example, "I want to do great things, and my parents are getting in my way"), but it can also be a sign of depression (for example, "I just want to be left alone; I don't want to talk to anyone"). By itself, without other mood or behavior changes, irritability is not very diagnostically useful.

Drug and Alcohol Use Disorders

Although not a symptom of the bipolar syndrome, substance use disorders are very common in teenagers with bipolar disorder. Some teens take drugs like methamphetamine, Ecstasy, cocaine, or crack or are abusing prescription stimulants like Adderall or narcotic pain medicines like oxycodone (OxyContin, Percocet), hydrocodone (Vicodin), or fentanyl. They may report that they enjoy the high periods of mania and hypomania and seek drugs as a way of bringing them on.

More common in our clinic are kids who smoke marijuana every day or several times a week. They may approach their doctors asking for a medical marijuana license because they think it will help their bipolar disorder, or because of anxiety, pain, headaches, or a host of other reasons. Their argument is often that marijuana stabilizes their moods better than mood stabilizers like lithium and lamotrigine do. They may try to rope you into getting marijuana for them or making their case to the doctor, especially if they know you smoke it yourself.

My opinion on this is going to sound old-fashioned: ***Do not go along with it. There is no evidence that marijuana is a good treatment for bipolar disorder in kids or adults.*** In fact, bipolar people who are in and out of hospitals are often smoking marijuana regularly and using other drugs (Strakowski et al., 2000). Marijuana appears to interfere with the biological effects of mood stabilizers or second-generation antipsychotics, so it doesn't make sense to be taking those medications and smoking marijuana heavily at the same time. Be skeptical of claims that medical marijuana is the treatment of choice for psychiatric disorders—the evidence is just not there, and, as is true of pharmaceuticals in general, there are business interests underlying its widespread use.

Comorbid Physical Problems

Comorbid physical disorders are also common in early-onset bipolar disorder. Your child may be obese or have risk factors for cardiovascular disease, such as high blood pressure or glucose values. Kids with bipolar disorder are also at risk for accelerated atherosclerosis (narrowing of the arteries from fatty deposits) (B. I. Goldstein et al., 2015) due to poor diet and high cholesterol. We don't know for sure whether these problems emerge as part of bipolar disorder (for example, a depressed and sedentary lifestyle associated with overeating) or reflect a reaction to its treatments (for example, weight gain on antipsychotics). There may also be genes that affect both mood and physical health.

What can you do as a parent? As is true for any child, it is essential to encourage healthy eating habits at home, such as not using eating as a way of modulating anxiety, avoiding the urge to satisfy carbohydrate cravings, and avoiding snacking between meals. Needless to say, with teens this is easier said than done. Additionally, having depression can make the drive toward carbohydrates even stronger. I recommend Linda Craighead's self-help guide, the *Appetite Awareness Workbook* (Craighead, 2006), as a place to start in helping your child learn strategies to control overeating.

"So, Aren't All Teenagers Bipolar?"

After having their child undergo a full psychiatric evaluation, and after reviewing the myriad diagnostic uncertainties that often accompany it, some parents of adolescents feel like they have circled back to one of the key questions they had originally: How do we know this isn't just teenage angst, or the ups and downs of adolescent hormones? What's being a bipolar teenager and what's being a normal teenager? It's a question I've had myself when treating some families of kids with mood instability or early warning signs of bipolar disorder.

I've heard this question so many times that I put together a list that explains some of the key behavioral differences between "healthy teens" and bipolar teens; see the table on page 390. Notice that bipolar disorder and teenage behavior are on a continuum: many mood symptoms can be found in isolation in ordinary teens, but without the other symptoms or functional impairments associated with full manic or depressive episodes.

When you find yourself wondering about this question, try consulting the table to see whether the behavior you have just witnessed is consistent with

What's Bipolar versus Being a "Normal" Teenager?

Healthy Teen	Bipolar Teen
Increases in risk taking, mood instability, and family conflict	Same three factors but much more impairing; risk taking can get them arrested, and family conflicts can become violent
Excitement is usually appropriate to context (e.g., being "hyper" at Christmas)	Excitement is often inappropriate to context and alienates others
Occasional sexual experimentation	Has had several instances of unsafe or impulsive sex, has had many partners
Has "bad days" with a single mood symptom, but functioning is stable	Has clusters of mood symptoms that co-occur, last for several days, and impair functioning
Occasionally has sleep irregularities	Has persistent difficulty with insomnia when depressed, has no regular sleep schedule, or sleeps too little or not at all when mood is elevated
Argumentative, opinionated, and rebellious but can be reined in	When in episode, can be overtly hostile or physically assaultive to parents, teachers, or other authority figures

other signs of bipolar disorder or seems more like teenage mood variability. It may be both, in that bipolar disorder will exaggerate some of the features that we usually associate with adolescence—unstable moods, risk taking, and family conflicts.

"What Can We Expect over Time?"

As mentioned earlier, a psychiatric evaluation can produce a number of results, from a definitive diagnosis of bipolar disorder to a diagnosis of another disorder, a tentative diagnosis, a wait-and-see plan, or a conclusion that you have nothing to worry about. If the clinician agrees that there is cause for concern about bipolar disorder in your child, you will undoubtedly have questions about what the future holds. What happens to children or teens with bipolar disorder over time?

> Zadie, now age 20, had been a rebellious, angry, and impulsive teenager. According to her parents, her problems began shortly after she reached puberty at age 12. Her menstrual periods were associated with wide mood swings and intense anger; on one occasion she struck her younger brother. An endocrinologist was consulted, but nothing abnormal was found that would explain her moodiness. Her outbursts began to invade the time between her menstrual periods as well.

At age 15, she became involved with a girl she met at a community house. As the relationship became more intimate, she became increasingly hostile toward her parents. She began to disappear overnight, crawling out through her bedroom window to meet her partner and their other friends. She smoked marijuana nightly but denied drinking alcohol—"it made me sick." After Zadie was away from home all night for several nights without answering her phone, Zadie's parents called the police. The police eventually found her walking down a highway; she tried to run away and was wrestled into the back of a police car. At the county jail, she ran back and forth in her cell, hit her head against the wall, threw water from the toilet at people nearby, screamed at the top of her lungs, and sang songs so loudly that other inmates told her to shut up. She said she had not ingested anything other than marijuana.

Her manic episode lasted 2 weeks and required a hospitalization. During the inpatient stay and its aftermath, her psychiatrist treated her with risperidone, valproate, and alprazolam (Xanax) for sleep. A few weeks after discharge, she swung into depression, and her parents took her out of school for the semester. Zadie's beliefs about herself and her future became increasingly negative: "I've blown it already, so why even try? College is out!" were common thoughts. She broke up with her girlfriend, which contributed to her depression. Wellbutrin was added, along with individual therapy, with some modest success.

Zadie had one more major depressive episode shortly after she turned 16. However, that year things began to turn around. She decided she did want to go to college and began spending time after school with a theater group. Her mood began to lift. She stuck with her medications even though they had annoying side effects and made her gain weight. When she turned 17, she began studying for the SATs. She graduated high school on time and was admitted to a state university. During the summer before college she had two short (1- to 2-day) intervals of "hyper" behavior but nothing that required emergency treatment. At a follow-up interview conducted when she was 20, she reported having no additional mood episodes or symptoms since age 16. Her parents verified her report.

Do Bipolar Kids Become Bipolar Adults?

We usually describe bipolar disorder as a lifelong illness, so giving a child a bipolar diagnosis can cause understandable distress for both parents and child. Parents ask, "What will he be facing in the future? If he's bipolar now, or may develop bipolar disorder soon, what will it be like when he's an adult? Won't it get worse?"

A recently published study of children of bipolar parents gives partial answers to these questions. In an 8-year follow-up of children with and without bipolar parents, Danella Hafeman and colleagues at the University of Pittsburgh (2016) found that children with certain characteristics (mood instability, depression and anxiety, and a bipolar parent whose illness began before age 18) had a 50% chance of developing bipolar disorder, compared to only 2% of kids who did not have any of these attributes. This research, although pointing to factors that clearly predispose kids to bipolar disorder, also point to the heterogeneity in the outcomes of kids who are genetically at risk.

What about kids who already have bipolar disorder—do they continue to have manic episodes as they age? Barbara Geller (mentioned earlier) and her colleagues followed a group of 115 children who had full manic or mixed episodes in childhood or early adolescence (average age 11) over the next 8 years (Geller et al., 2008). Of these kids, most (73%) had a relapse of mania during the 8-year followup. At 8 years, 54 of the participants were now adults between the ages of 18 and 21; of these 54, only 44% had recurrences of mania after age 18. Thirty percent had depression and 35% had substance use disorders after age 18. It appears that the course pattern shown by Zadie, who had her most extreme episodes in midadolescence and then "mellowed" with age, is not atypical: children with bipolar I disorder do not always go on to a lifetime of regular recurrences (Axelson, Birmaher, Strober, et al., 2011; Birmaher et al., 2014) (see the box on page 393).

The good news, then, is that not all bipolar children grow up to be bipolar adults. Nor is it a given that your child will get worse with time or have ongoing impairments. Unfortunately, we do not have enough long-term data to say with certainty which kids will go on to have more mood episodes or how often the bipolar syndrome is a time-limited adolescent phenomenon. However, the great heterogeneity in outcomes in nearly every study suggests that there are risk or protective factors (see Chapter 3) that affect some kids more than others. The goal of personalized medicine is to find out what treatments fit best with which risk or protection profiles to maximize the chances of your child having the best possible outcome.

Long-Term Functioning in School and Work

Stella, age 19, had subthreshold mixed symptoms characterized by impulsive behavior, trouble sleeping, suicidal thoughts, and near-constant fatigue. After multiple interviews, she got a job as a hostess at a local restaurant. However, in the first week of the job she experienced a worsening of her depressive symptoms. She called in sick three times and in one case missed a shift without calling. At the beginning of the next week she was notified of her dismissal.

Children and teens who grow up with bipolar spectrum disorders struggle with social and academic functioning, although again, there is considerable variability from child to child. Sometimes the impairments are due to their comorbid disorders, like ADHD; in other cases, their intervals of wellness are not long enough to allow them to catch up in school. Some children suffer with depressive symptoms that affect their ability to study, stay focused, or keep up with the requirements of a job. They may not be able to tell you that they have ongoing

New research: Do kids with bipolar disorder ever become free of symptoms?

The Course and Outcome of Bipolar Youth (COBY) study has examined what happens to bipolar kids over time using a dimensional measure of illness course—the number of weeks they spend well. After all, an illness can be tolerable if the worst symptoms are only present for a few weeks of the year. The study, conducted in three university settings, followed 367 children and adolescents with bipolar spectrum disorders (bipolar I, II, or unspecified) over 4 years (Birmaher et al., 2014). Birmaher and colleagues found that the kids could be classified according to their 4-year course patterns, as follows: (1) a group labeled "predominantly euthymic" (24% of the sample) was free of symptoms for an average of 84.4% of the weeks of follow-up; (2) a group called "moderately euthymic" (34.6%) was well for 47.3% of the weeks of follow-up; (3) a group that was "ill with an improving course" (19.1% of sample) was well for 42.8% of the weeks; and (4) a group of "predominantly ill" youth (22.3%) was free of symptoms for only 11.5% of the weeks.

What does this all mean? Once again, child outcomes are very heterogeneous: in the COBY study, about one in four children who were diagnosed with a bipolar spectrum disorder went on to be symptom-free for most of the next 4 years. The kids who went on to be predominantly euthymic had a later age at onset of mania (12 years) compared to kids who went on to have different courses of illness (9–11 years). Kids with more euthymic courses of illness also had (1) less severe depressive symptoms at study entry, (2) less of a family history of psychiatric disorders, and (3) a lower incidence of childhood sexual abuse. Some of these factors may be amenable to change. For example, if we can catch depression early enough, we can work toward helping children remain symptom free by making adjustments to their medications or combining medicines with evidence-based forms of psychotherapy (discussed later in this chapter). We can encourage people in the family who have psychiatric disorders to obtain treatment so that they can be more effective caregivers.

depressive symptoms (for example, rumination, lack of concentration) that interfere with their performance.

There is a particularly important thing to keep in mind when your child is navigating social relationships, academics, or the job world: she did not ask to have bipolar disorder and may be doing her best to regulate her moods. Her problems in functioning may be well beyond her personal control. If she is unwilling to take medications, you may believe that she isn't taking the illness seriously and could do more to enhance her functioning. While this may be true, most teens or young adults do experiment with going off their medications from time to time. They may need to prove to themselves that medications are necessary and not just a feature of their childhood.

If your child is struggling with these issues—which are as much about her sense of self as about her medications—try to be patient with the decision-making process. Express your concerns, notify her doctors, and, if she thinks it would be useful, remind her to take medications. Otherwise, avoid getting into power struggles with her about treatment.

The Effects of Childhood Bipolar Disorder on the Family

If I've convinced you of one thing, it's that parenting a child with bipolar disorder requires a very difficult balance. Parents often report high levels of distress and physical health problems (Perez Algorta et al., 2017). If you have bipolar disorder yourself, you may experience more symptoms when your child is symptomatic (like the bumper sticker that reads, "Mental illness is inherited—you get it from your kids"). And, as I said earlier, it's equally true that children whose parents have mood disorders are more stable when their parents are more stable (Weissman et al., 2015). We don't know which direction the causal arrow goes—from parent to child or child to parent—but in all likelihood it's bidirectional.

You may also be concerned about your other children, who may not have developed any symptoms yet. The risk of bipolar disorder in a sibling of a child with bipolar disorder averages 10–15%, similar to the rate of parent-to-child transmission (Craddock & Sklar, 2013). Siblings, however, may develop mental health disorders other than bipolar disorder—they may have acute stress reactions, depression, or anxiety that can be tied directly to what is happening with their brother or sister.

It's important to educate your other children about their sibling's bipolar disorder. If your children are old enough, you may be able to use the Quick Fact Sheet in Chapter 13, which is designed to help family members understand bipolar disorder. If your children are younger, you will have to explain it in language they can understand. You may have to explain it to them several times and in different ways, but eventually they will absorb it. In my experience, children understand a lot more about mental health than we give them credit for.

The key point is to communicate that the "well sibling" is not responsible for how her brother is acting (unless you suspect that she is purposely taunting him). Tell the sibling that you understand how hard it is when her brother has a "meltdown" or rages at her in a way that is out of proportion to the slight. "Your brother has problems with his moods. He gets really mad or really sad sometimes and he may take it out on you—but it's not his fault and it's not yours either" are good concepts to emphasize.

If one of your children asks why his brother has to take pills, you may want to explain this in a general and nontechnical way: "He takes pills for making his moods better, and they help but they don't always help right away." Of course, your bipolar child may feel stigmatized by these conversations, so avoid getting into his personal details with siblings. Instead, give them enough information to enable them to try to empathize with their sibling's emotional pain.

Finally, if one of your non-bipolar children states that she is feeling neglected, or if her behavior is a transparent attempt to draw your attention, comment in a supportive way: "I know that sometimes we act like we aren't listening when you tell us what's going on with you, or you may think it's unfair that we worry about Brad so much. I can understand why you feel that way, but Brad is having an especially rough time right now. We love you very much, and you can always tell me (us) about things that are important to you, good or bad."

"How Can We Help as a Family?"

In my experience, parents are very conscientious about getting access to needed treatments and school services for their child, as long as these services are available in their locale. What they can underestimate is the importance of helping the child understand his own disorder: what's happening to him and how to accept it. Let's consider how to discuss the diagnosis with your child, some good ways to track her mood states over time, and how to handle her oppositional behavior or outbursts within the family.

Discussing the Diagnosis with Your Child

Understandably, kids often have strong feelings about psychiatric diagnoses, depending on their level of comprehension. If your child has just received a bipolar diagnosis for the first time, try to get her to discuss it with you. Avoid expressing alarm or making strong statements about what it will mean for her future. Try to present your understanding in an innocuous way that doesn't make her feel different or disabled: "It means you have some problems with your moods going up and down, like when you can't sleep, or feel sad, or start feeling mad at everyone, or have too much energy. Lots of kids have mood swings—you may not know whether other kids have them unless they tell you." Emphasize that having bipolar disorder doesn't mean your child is doing anything wrong.

Whether to discuss medications with your child right away is a judgment call. If your child is a teenager, the doctor will probably have told him directly about the mood stabilizers or SGAs she is recommending. If so, you can ask "What did you think (or feel) when the doctor told you that?" If your child is younger, the doctor may or may not spend time explaining the medications. With teens, avoid saying that medications are an absolute necessity, even if you think they are. Instead, say "Taking medicines is something we should discuss. I know you have some strong feelings about it." If needed, frame taking medications as an experiment: "Let's try it for 3 months and see if it makes a difference. What would you think about that?"

Tracking Symptom States with a Mood Chart

In Chapter 8, we discussed the importance of keeping a daily mood and sleep chart to augment medication visits. The best way to do this is for both you and your child to keep a weekly chart of changes in her moods and sleep–wake cycles. If your child is willing, ask her to keep her own mood chart and then compare yours with hers at the end of each week. Tracking moods may help you and your child's doctor know when an emergency intervention—including a hospitalization or an increased dosage of a medication—is necessary to stave off a full episode. Having a regular mood chart may even help you distinguish between a new illness episode and mood swings that fall within her normal range.

On page 397 you'll find a chart that we have used successfully in our clinic. It was designed by a 13-year-old girl! You can copy and fill in the chart as you see fit (the form is also available online; see the end of the Contents for information). On page 398 you will find an example of how one child filled hers out. If your child is willing to do the mood-tracking task, ask her to help you choose words that describe her different mood states, preferably words that distinguish highs from lows. For example, the 13-year-old described her mood on any given day as follows: super-hyper (fully manic in both mood and energy); energized (hypomanic, elevated, or irritable in mood but not out of control); balanced (even keel, "my usual mood"); down (depressed, pessimistic, have little energy and don't enjoy things); and angry (which, she felt, was her most impaired state). Note that she also filled in when she woke up and went to bed, as well as phrases to describe her different moods (for example, "I want to live in a bubble").

Make sure to use mood descriptors that you and she will agree on. Words like *chaotic* or *amped* may be better than *hyper,* and *chill* may be better than *balanced,* but make sure she is thinking of the same state that you are when she uses that term. If you see many changes in the course of a single day, ask her to make separate ratings for the morning and evening. A rating may simply be an X at the relevant point on the shaded lines.

Medications for Childhood Bipolar Disorder: Why, When, and Which Ones?

Allison, a 17-year-old with bipolar I disorder, was treated with several different medication "cocktails" during her teen years. Her regimen had at various points included lithium, Depakote, Seroquel, Wellbutrin, and Adderall. She complained frequently about her side effects. She had a therapist that she felt was helpful, but as high school graduation approached she was still depressed and anxious. She had had several hypomanic episodes between lengthy stretches of depression, with no consistent return to normal moods in between.

How I Feel

Put an X on the line next to the term that describes how you felt that day. You can use an X and a Y if you want to make a separate rating for morning and night. Feel free to use different mood terms than the ones provided.

	Monday	Tuesday	Wednesday	Thursday	Friday	Saturday	Sunday
Super-Hyper							
or: _____							
Energized							
or: _____							
Balanced							
or: _____							
Down							
or: _____							
Angry							
or: _____							
I woke up at:							
I went to bed at:							

397

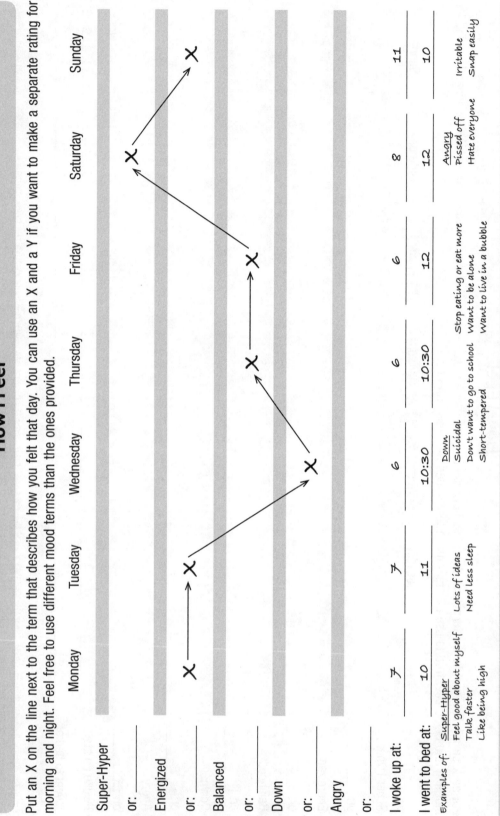

How I Feel

Put an X on the line next to the term that describes how you felt that day. You can use an X and a Y if you want to make a separate rating for morning and night. Feel free to use different mood terms than the ones provided.

	Monday	Tuesday	Wednesday	Thursday	Friday	Saturday	Sunday
Super-Hyper							
or: ___							
Energized		X				X	
or: ___							
Balanced	X				X		
or: ___				X			
Down							
or: ___			X				
Angry							
or: ___							
I woke up at:	7	7	6	6	6	8	11
I went to bed at:	10	11	10:30	10:30	12	12	10

Examples of:

Super-Hyper
Feel good about myself
Talk faster
Like being high

Lots of ideas
Need less sleep

Down
Suicidal
Don't want to go to school
Short-tempered

Stop eating or eat more
Want to be alone
Want to live in a bubble

Angry
Pissed off
Hate everyone

Irritable
Snap easily

In the summer before she began college, she saw a different psychiatrist who specialized in bipolar disorder. She was reluctant to see this new doctor, concerned that he would just add more drugs to her regimen. In fact, he recommended that, before leaving for college, she "wean herself off" all of her medications except lithium. He allowed her to keep a prescription for alprazolam (Xanax) for when she felt unusually anxious or couldn't sleep.

By the end of the summer, Allison felt better than she had ever felt, with no signs of hypomania or depression. Her parents worried that she might be cycling upward, but in fact her first semester of college went very well on lithium alone. She had some return of depressive symptoms when she went home for the holidays that were unpleasant but not crippling. Her doctor recommended more exercise in the morning (she selected a yoga class) and trying a "light box." She was able to get through her first year of college without any additional medications.

Let's say your child has undergone a full psychiatric evaluation, and the physician has made recommendations involving mood stabilizers, SGAs, or antidepressants. Should you follow these recommendations? Deciding whether or not to encourage your child to take psychiatric medications is very difficult. None of us want to see our kids experimenting with medications, especially when these medications have serious side effects and offer no guarantee of working. We hear stories of kids being on mountains of medications by the time they're 12. Why would anyone want to consign their child to a lifetime of polypharmacy? On the other hand, you may see how much your child is suffering and how much fuller her life could be if her moods were stable.

I have explained in prior chapters why most of us believe that medications are the first-line treatment for bipolar disorder. We know that psychotherapies and complementary or alternative treatments do not adequately treat bipolar disorder when given alone. Be skeptical of practitioners who tell you that "being bipolar isn't what I focus on . . . I care more about developing a relationship with the child and exploring his history" or "the majority of kids I see don't need medicines." This kind of stance may be music to your ears, but this doctor either doesn't see bipolar children regularly or sees only children who are more mildly or moderately ill, for whom medications are more a quality-of-life issue than a health necessity. If your child has true bipolar I or bipolar II disorder, there is a high likelihood that he will need to take medications before he'll be able to benefit from psychotherapy.

What if your child has a subthreshold condition like unspecified bipolar disorder? Decisions about taking medicine often depend on how much impairment is present. If she is missing school, complaining of lack of sleep, and appears irritable, withdrawn, disinterested, and unhappy, medications are probably necessary. If your child is activated and full of plans, takes on too much, and often gets a poor night's sleep, consider whether these symptoms are getting worse with time. Is she getting along at school, at home, and with peers, or are there increasing examples of problems in one or more of these contexts? Is she able to concentrate on school-work as soon as she gets to school? Can she complete homework assignments at night? Are family relationships on solid ground, or are her moods beginning to upset everyone else?

Acute Mania or Mixed Disorder: Which Medications?

The FDA has approved the following medications for the treatment of mania or mixed episodes in 10- to 17-year-olds: risperidone (Risperdal), aripiprazole (Abilify), quetiapine (Seroquel), olanzapine (Zyprexa), ziprasidone (Geodon), and (for 13- to 17-year-olds) asenapine (Saphris). Lithium has an FDA indication for both the treatment of acute mania and the prevention of recurrences in children age 12 or above (B. I. Goldstein et al., 2017). Note the absence on this list of val-proate (Depakote): the evidence for valproate in treating acute mania in children is weak at best.

As you have probably noticed, the medications recommended for childhood bipolar disorder are the same as those for adult bipolar disorder, with some impor-tant caveats. First, treatment decision making can be a tougher balancing act with kids than with adults. When do you start heavy-duty medications like antipsy-chotics? Young people are more susceptible than adults to metabolic side effects such as weight gain. Nonetheless, SGAs appear to be more effective than mood stabilizers like lithium for mania in children (Liu et al., 2011; Correll, Sheridan, & DelBello, 2010; see the box below).

Treatment of Acute Depression

As is true of adults, depression is harder to treat than mania in children. Cur-rently, the only medication that has an FDA indication for bipolar depression in 10- to 17-year-olds is the olanzapine/fluoxetine (Zyprexa and Prozac) combination,

Effective treatment: The Treatment of Early Age Mania (TEAM) study

In an 8-week treatment trial for 290 children between the ages of 6 and 15, all of whom were in acute manic or mixed episodes, Barbara Geller and her associates (2012) explored whether children's responses to mood stabilizers were comparable to their responses to SGAs. The study was unique in that most of the participants were school-age children. Over 8 weeks, the proportion of kids with a significant alleviation of symptoms was highest for risperidone (68%), an SGA, followed by lithium (35%) and valproate (24%). However, weight gain, body mass index, and prolactin levels were all higher for risperidone than for mood stabilizers. Results of the TEAM study suggest that there can be a trade-off between effectiveness and metabolic side effects when treating children with mania.

usually marketed under the name Symbyax. Few doctors prescribe it, preferring to prescribe the two individual medications rather than a combination pill whose dosage is harder to adjust. There is a smattering of studies supporting lithium and lamotrigine for kids with bipolar depression, but no randomized trials showing clear effects of any one agent versus placebo. Nonetheless, these are often the go-to medications used for depression in bipolar kids.

Although not FDA-approved yet, there is at least one large-scale trial indicating that lurasidone (Latuda) is more effective than placebo for bipolar depression in children (average age 14) over a 6-week period. That study indicated that Latuda was also effective in alleviating anxiety and improving functioning, without causing a significant amount of weight gain. Its most common side effects (compared to placebo) were nausea and sleeping too much (DelBello et al., 2017).

Most practitioners avoid using antidepressants for children with bipolar disorder, recognizing the risks of antidepressant-induced mania (see Chapter 6). It's not clear whether the risk is comparable in children and adults with bipolar disorders (Bhowmik et al., 2014). Nonetheless, practice guidelines recommend that, if your child with bipolar disorder is going to take an antidepressant for depression or anxiety, she should also take an antipsychotic or a mood stabilizer (Schneck et al., 2017). This combination may not eliminate the risk of mania, but it will lower it.

At the beginning of depression treatment, your child's doctor should obtain blood samples to determine whether she has a low level of thyroid hormone or whether certain metabolic levels (for example, fasting blood lipids) argue against the use of SGAs. Low levels of thyroid hormone are correlated with depression in adults, and lithium can suppress the thyroid gland.

Maintenance Care

As explained earlier, the medications used to stabilize the acute episode may not be the same as those used to prevent future episodes of depression or mania (maintenance treatment). Your child may be on multiple medications at high doses during the 9–12 months it may take to recover from a manic or mixed episode (Geller et al., 2008; Miklowitz et al., 2014), but her physician may be able to simplify the regimen before then. Many physicians recommend that children stay on SGAs in combination with mood stabilizers long enough to make sure the mania has cleared, after which they recommend discontinuing the antipsychotic during maintenance care.

Many children with bipolar disorder are maintained on medications for ADHD as well as mood stabilizers. The consensus is that kids who have both bipolar disorder and ADHD can be treated with mixed amphetamine salts (for example, Ritalin, Adderall) once they are in a stable mood state. Stimulants should be combined with mood stabilizers and/or SGAs rather than given alone (Scheffer, Kowatch, Carmody, & Rush, 2005). The guidelines for continuing a child on an antidepressant during maintenance care follow a similar set of rules.

New research: Omega-3 supplementation for kids with subthreshold bipolar disorder

Do kids with subthreshold bipolar disorder necessarily need the heavy-duty medications used with adults who have the full disorder? Mary Fristad and her group at Ohio State University College of Medicine conducted two randomized trials of omega-3 fish oil with children who had either major depression, unspecified bipolar disorder, or cyclothymia (Fristad et al., 2016; Vesco, Young, Arnold, & Fristad, 2018). They randomly assigned school-age kids (ages 7–14) to omega-3 with or without twice-weekly sessions of family-based psychoeducational therapy over 12 weeks or to placebo with or without psychoeducational therapy sessions. No other psychotropic drugs were allowed during the trial except for stimulants or sleep aids. Kids who got omega-3 (whether or not they also got therapy) showed greater improvement than those taking placebo in depression symptoms and parent-rated executive functioning scores (for example, emotional or behavioral self-regulation) over 12 weeks. These findings suggest that, at least for subthreshold conditions that have not progressed into full bipolar disorder, omega-3 may be a reasonable place to start.

PERSONALIZED CARE TIP:
Adjusting dosages

Medication dosages often need to be adjusted upward or downward, depending on the balance between benefits and side effects. When your child is getting more symptomatic, or is suffering from untoward side effects and you cannot reach the physician, you may be tempted to adjust medications yourself (for example, if she seems sedated, giving her an extra 5-mg tablet of Adderall). While it is understandable to want to do this, I would advise against it. There can be negative interactions among drugs that occur at higher but not lower dosages. In addition, it can be very difficult to know what medication is causing what side effect, or even whether the side effect is really due to the medications or to the disorder itself (for example, stimulants can cause irritability, but so can ADHD). It's better to leave an emergency message with the doctor, even if it's with an answering service. Explain what you need to know and why you think it's important to get an answer now instead of waiting for your child's next in-person session. If you feel your child is at risk for suicide or is becoming psychotic, take her to the nearest emergency room and inform her physician that you have done so.

"What Should I Know about Psychosocial Treatment?"

Psychosocial interventions clearly have a place in the treatment of childhood bipolar disorder. Some parents do not want their child touching any psychiatric medication and look to psychosocial interventions for stabilization. There are pros and cons to this position. As I discussed earlier, the decision of whether or not to try medicines should be based on the child's current level of impairment in school or at home: if she is truant from school, threatening or attempting suicide, self-cutting, provoking major family arguments, acting out sexually, or getting in fights, she will probably need to be stabilized with medications before she will benefit from psychotherapy.

The most well-established psychosocial treatments for pediatric bipolar spectrum disorders involve family psychoeducation and skill building. Several research groups, including my own at UCLA (and my earlier one at the University of Colorado Boulder), have shown that family interventions—provided together with medications—are associated with better outcomes of bipolar disorder than brief supportive treatments (for example, two to three educational sessions) with medications (Miklowitz & Chung, 2016). The ingredients of our treatment, family-focused therapy (FFT), include (1) acquainting the family and child with the signs and symptoms of bipolar disorder and helping them learn to recognize the child's early warning signs, (2) helping parents develop the skills needed to navigate the mental health system and intervene when the child's condition is worsening, and (3) showing parents and their child how to communicate and solve problems more effectively as a family.

What can you expect to gain from FFT or other forms of family psychoeducation? First, knowledge about the disorder is associated with obtaining higher-quality mental health services, and obtaining these services usually enhances the child's progress. Additionally, when parents and their children develop more open and flexible communication and problem-solving styles in family therapy, and when parents learn to label the positive as well as the negative attributes of the child's behavior, children have more favorable symptom trajectories than in comparison treatments (Fristad & MacPherson, 2014; MacPherson, Weinstein, Henry, & West, 2016; West et al., 2014; O'Brien, Miklowitz, & Cannon, 2014).

There is some initial evidence that family treatment can help stabilize children who are in the prodromal stages of illness. We studied 40 preadolescents and adolescents with major depression or unspecified bipolar disorder, all of whom had a first-degree relative with bipolar disorder. We considered this a "high-risk" sample. We randomly assigned half of the kids to 12 sessions of family-focused treatment over 4 months with their parents and siblings; the other half received a couple of sessions of diagnostic feedback and treatment planning. All children had the option of taking (or continuing to take) mood stabilizers or SGAs or stimulants, as managed by their own or a study psychiatrist; 60% opted to do so. Over 1 year, the kids in FFT showed more rapid recovery from their depressive symptoms and more improvement in hypomanic symptoms (Miklowitz et al., 2013). We do not know yet whether treatments like FFT, when added to medications, can prevent or at least delay the onset of bipolar disorder in adulthood, but that is a question we should be able to answer in the next few years (Miklowitz et al., 2017).

Conclusions and Directions

The recognition that children and teens can become bipolar is an advance in our field, and it may become easier to diagnose and treat bipolar spectrum disorders now that clinicians have access to more systematic ways of collecting diagnostic information and evaluating progress (for example, using structured interviews or online assessments of mood states). However, our better recognition of the illness has not enabled us to fit specific treatments to individual children and family situations. Whereas we know that the medications best for mania are often different from those best for depression, we also know that combinations of medications, psychosocial interventions, and parent advocacy (such as working with school systems) are crucial for children with the disorder. In the future, youth with bipolar disorder may receive combinations of medications and psychological treatments that are tailored to each stage of the illness, as well as to individual attributes of the child such as age, whether there is a family history of bipolar disorder, and patterns of comorbidities (Malhi, Morris, Hamilton, Outhred, & Mannie, 2017).

One of the biggest struggles for families has been the low availability of pharmacological and psychosocial treatments given by experts. Where do you go to get these treatments, or at least some approximation of them? The increasing availability of evidence-based care in many mental health centers, plus programs delivered online (for example, the Sleepio digital program for insomnia, at *www.sleepio. com*), is slowly changing the mental health landscape for the better. The Resources section that follows should get you started on locating providers, as well as online resources that should be helpful to you, your child, and your family.

• • • • • • • • • • • • • •

Bipolar disorder poses many challenges that are hard for anyone except those suffering from it to understand. Now that you are at the end of this book, I hope you have become convinced that the strategies recommended here—learning as much as you can about the disorder, getting consistent medical treatment, taking full advantage of psychotherapy, relying on your social supports, and using self-management tools—can help you cope with the disorder on a day-to-day basis. As articulately expressed by one of my patients who has been stable for some time, "I have learned to manage my disorder rather than being managed by it."

Resources for People with Bipolar Disorder

National and International Organizations

The following are comprehensive organizations that offer not just a wealth of online services and information but also in many cases community outreach services and phone/mail contacts.

Balanced Mind Parent Network (800-826-3632; *www.dbsalliance.org/site/PageServer?pagename=bmpn_landing*) is a parent-led program of the Depression and Bipolar Support Alliance (see listing on the next page). It provides information and support to family members, health care professionals, and the public concerning the nature, causes, and treatment of early-onset mood disorders and their comorbid conditions. The organization has a help line and various online support communities for parents. Particularly useful is information on how to locate a mental health provider in your area who sees children with mood disorders. The website also offers examples of mood charts, articles on how to prepare for initial doctor visits, and information on research studies.

Bipolar UK (11 Belgrave Road, London, SW1V 1RB, UK; 0333 323 3880; *www.bipolaruk.org.uk*) is a user-led charitable organization that offers self-help groups, publications, and other practical information for those living with bipolar disorder. There is a useful link for employment services and an "eCommunity" with online message boards.

Brain and Behavior Research Foundation (646-681-4888 or 800-829-8289; *www.bbrfoundation.org*) is the largest donor-supported, nongovernment organization in the United States dedicated to raising and distributing funds for research into the nature, causes, treatments, and prevention of severe mental illnesses, including bipolar disorder, schizophrenia, depression, and severe anxiety disorders. Its website includes up-to-date information about the diagnosis and treatment of severe psychiatric disorders.

Canadian Mental Health Association (CMHA) (416-646-5557; *https://cmha.ca/find-your-cmha*; email: *info@cmha.ca*) helps people with mental health conditions and addiction through self-help groups, peer support, written materials, workshops, and classes.

Depression and Bipolar Support Alliance (800-826-3632; *www.dbsalliance.org/FindSupport*), an organization I have always admired, is devoted to educating consumers and their family members about mood disorders (notably bipolar disorder), decreasing the public stigma of these illnesses, fostering self-help, advocating for research funding, and improving access to care. DBSA has chapters in many cities that offer free peer-led support groups. There are also online support groups. DBSA features a technology app called the Wellness Tracker, which won a "best app" award from HealthLine. If you would like to start a chapter of DBSA in your hometown, go to *www.DBSAlliance.org/StartChapter*.

International Bipolar Foundation (858-598-5967; *www.ibpf.org*) is an organization devoted to supporting people with bipolar disorder and their families, and educating the public to reduce stigma. There is a special emphasis on children and adolescents with the disorder and how to find care. One can communicate with other people who are coping with the same individual or family issues. There are over 40 bloggers who regularly write for this site, on relationships, medications, therapy, and effective coping strategies. Muffy Walker's award-winning *My Support Newsletter*, available on the site, has comprehensive coverage of recent studies, new treatments, upcoming events and lectures, and books.

International Society for Bipolar Disorders (*www.isbd.org* or email Jill Olds at *jillo@isbd. org*) aims to promote awareness of bipolar conditions in society at large, educate mental health professionals, foster research on bipolar disorder, and promote international collaborations. Its journal, *Bipolar Disorders: An International Journal of Psychiatry and Neurosciences*, is becoming a primary outlet for new research on the diagnosis, etiology, and treatment of bipolar conditions. It sponsors the International Conference on Bipolar Disorder, an outlet for the latest research findings. ISBD publishes a newsletter and has several online chat rooms, including an "ask the experts" exchange.

Juvenile Bipolar Research Foundation (914-468-1297; *www.jbrf.org*) actively promotes and supports scientific research focused on the cause of and treatments for bipolar disorder in children. JBRF investigators are confident that they have identified a brain-based, heritable condition, Fear of Harm (FOH), and have identified a treatment for the children who fit this specific profile. The JBRF website provides information on educational forums for parents and teachers; how to subscribe to professional email listservs for family members, physicians, and therapists; and new research studies and findings pertinent to childhood-onset bipolar disorder. Of particular help to parents is a section on educational concerns, including how to prepare an individualized education program for the child. There is also a quick, easy, and inexpensive screening tool to assist parents and medical professionals in evaluating children for bipolar disorder.

Mental Health America (800-969-6642; *www.mentalhealthamerica.net*) is the oldest and largest nonprofit organization in the United States that addresses all aspects of mental health and illness. Research information, legislative updates, and practitioner referrals are available on its website.

National Alliance on Mental Illness (800-950-NAMI [6264]; *www.nami.org*) is a grassroots self-help support and advocacy organization for people with severe mental illnesses (including bipolar disorder, recurrent depression, and schizophrenia) and their family members and friends. NAMI offers parent support groups and a structured educational program taught by parents of people with severe psychiatric disorders called "NAMI Family-to-Family."

National Institute of Mental Health (866-615-6464; *www.nimh.nih.gov/health/publications/index.shtml*) provides publications with up-to-date information on the symptoms, course, causes, and treatment of bipolar disorder. Topics include child and adolescent bipolar illness, suicide, medical treatments and their side effects, co-occurring illnesses, psychosocial treatments, sources of help for individuals and families, and clinical research studies.

National Network of Depression Centers (734-332-3914; *www.nndc.org*) is a collection of comprehensive care centers for depression and bipolar disorder across the United States, coordinated by the University of Michigan. It consists of a network of universities committed to implementing consistent, state-of-the-art treatment protocols and research. Referrals to specialty centers around the United States are available.

Organization for Bipolar Affective Disorders Society (403-263-7408; *www.obad.ca/about_us*) hosts a variety of support groups to help Canadians affected directly or indirectly by bipolar disorder, depression, or anxiety. Groups are in Calgary, Edmonton, and Alberta.

Websites

The following are Internet-only resources. They offer a variety of information and often have interactive features such as chat rooms and forums, but have no physical presence in the community and no phone contact (email contact is available where noted).

Bipolar Child (*www.bipolarchild.com*), developed by Demitri and Janis Papolos, is an online resource designed to accompany the book by the same name. It offers up-to-date research findings pertaining to children with bipolar disorder, a newsletter on new treatment approaches, samples of individualized educational programs, information on upcoming conferences, and tips on how to start a support group (see also *www.jbrf.org*).

Bipolar Significant Others (*www.bpso.org*) is a website and an email exchange group in which members—relatives or friends of persons with bipolar disorder—share information about the illness, provide support to one another, and solve problems about issues related to the impact of the illness on families and intimate relationships. The website contains much helpful information on treatment, book reviews, and links. Instructions for joining the listserv can be found at *www.bpso.org/subscrib.php*.

Bring Change to Mind (*https://bringchange2mind.org*) is devoted to combating stigma and discrimination and raising awareness related to mental illness. The organization was started by the actress Glenn Close, who has a sister with bipolar disorder (there is a video interview of Close and her sister). Among the various resource tools is an interactive talk tool with illustrations on how to talk to people about mental illness.

Harbor of Refuge Organization (*www.harbor-of-refuge.org*) provides peer-to-peer support for individuals diagnosed with bipolar disorder who are undergoing treatment. There is a discussion forum/chat room. Information is provided on self-care and illness management strategies. There is a frequently asked questions section that is a useful starting point for learning about the disorder.

Internet Mental Health (*www.mentalhealth.com*) provides a direct linkage between specific topics related to bipolar disorder and relevant published research abstracts. It is a particularly good site for new research on medications. Downloadable self-rated mood questionnaires and mood charts are available.

McMan's Depression and Bipolar Web (*www.mcmanweb.com*) is a comprehensive website with substantial links to current research, essays on first-person experiences, and an opinion page. The webmaster, John McManamy, is an award-winning mental health journalist and author.

Medline Plus (*www.nlm.nih.gov/medlineplus*) offers links to National Institute of Mental Health publications and clinical trials. It includes overviews of current bipolar research and information regarding children, teenagers, and seniors with the disorder. A link to the Medline search engine for the most recent research articles on bipolar disorder is provided.

Pendulum Resources (*www.pendulum.org*) offers information about the DSM diagnostic criteria for bipolar disorder, current medical treatments, books favored by mental health consumers and family members, articles on how to cope with depression or bipolar disorder in yourself or a loved one, writings and poetry by people with bipolar disorder, links to other relevant sites, and updates on research studies. One section compiles abstracts of research studies relevant to specific topics related to bipolar disorder.

Psycom.net (*www.psycom.net/depression.central.bipolar.html*) is an informational website that offers answers to frequently asked questions about bipolar disorder; discusses treatment guidelines; gives up-to-date information on topics such as novel medication approaches, differential diagnosis, adjunctive therapy, and suicide; first-person accounts; and a self-screening tool.

Books on Bipolar Disorder or Depression

Informational Volumes

Frank, E. (2007). *Treating bipolar disorder: A clinician's guide to interpersonal and social rhythm therapy.* New York: Guilford Press.

Goodwin, F. K., & Jamison, K. R. (2007). *Manic–depressive illness* (2nd ed.). New York: Oxford University Press.

Jamison, K. R. (1993). *Touched with fire: Manic–depressive illness and the artistic temperament.* New York: Macmillan.

Jamison, K. R. (2000). *Night falls fast: Understanding suicide.* New York: Vintage Books.

Jamison, K. R. (2004). *Exuberance: The passion for life.* New York: Knopf.

Miklowitz, D. J. (2010). *Bipolar disorder: A family-focused treatment approach* (2nd ed.). New York: Guilford Press.

Miklowitz, D. J., & Gitlin, M. J. (2014). *Clinician's guide to bipolar disorder.* New York: Guilford Press.

Papolos, D. F., & Papolos, J. (2007). *The bipolar child: The definitive and reassuring guide to childhood's most misunderstood disorder* (3rd ed.). New York: Broadway Books.

Whybrow, P. C. (2015). *A mood apart: Depression, mania, and other afflictions of the self.* New York: Basic Books.

Wilens, T. E., & Hammerness, P. G. (2016). *Straight talk about psychiatric medications for kids* (4th ed.). New York: Guilford Press.

Self-Help Guides

Amador, X., & Johanson, A. L. (2011). *I am not sick, I don't need help!* (10th anniversary ed.). Peconic, NY: Vida Press.

Basco, M. R. (2015). *The bipolar workbook: Tools for controlling your mood swings* (2nd ed.). New York: Guilford Press.

Bauer, M., Ludman, E., Greenwald, D. E., & Kilbourne, A. M. (2009). *Overcoming bipolar disorder: A comprehensive workbook for managing your symptoms and achieving your life goals.* Oakland, CA: New Harbinger.

Birmaher, B. (2004). *New hope for children and teens with bipolar disorder.* New York: Three Rivers Press.

Brondolo, E., & Amador, X. (2007). *Break the bipolar cycle: A day-by-day guide to living with bipolar disorder.* New York: McGraw-Hill.

Cohen, B. M., & Lowe, C. (2010). *Living with someone who's living with bipolar disorder: A practical guide for family, friends, and coworkers.* San Francisco: Jossey-Bass.

Copeland, M. E., & McCay, M. (2002). *The depression workbook: A guide for living with depression and manic depression* (2nd ed.). Oakland, CA: New Harbinger.

Ehrnstrom, C., & Brosse, A. L. (2016). *End the insomnia struggle: A step-by-step guide to help you get to sleep and stay asleep.* Oakland, CA: New Harbinger.

Fast, J. A., & Preston, J. D. (2004). *Loving someone with bipolar disorder: Understanding and helping your partner.* Oakland, CA: New Harbinger.

Fristad, M. A., & Goldberg Arnold, J. S. (2003). *Raising a moody child: How to cope with depression and bipolar disorder.* New York: Guilford Press.

Greenberger, D., & Padesky, C. A. (2015). *Mind over mood: Change how you feel by changing the way you think* (2nd ed.). New York: Guilford Press.

Miklowitz, D. J., & George, E. L. (2007). *The bipolar teen: What you can do to help your teen and your family.* New York: Guilford Press.

Phelps, J. (2006). *Why am I still depressed?: Recognizing and managing the ups and downs of bipolar II and soft bipolar disorder.* New York: McGraw-Hill.

Roberts, S. M., Sylvia, L. G., & Reilly-Harrington, N. (2014). *The bipolar II workbook.* Oakland, CA: New Harbinger.

Smith, H. T. (2010). *Welcome to the jungle: Everything you ever wanted to know about bipolar disorder but were too freaked out to ask.* Newburyport, MA: Conari Press.

Williams, M., Teasdale, J., Segal, Z., & Kabat-Zinn, J. (2007). *The mindful way through depression: Freeing yourself from chronic unhappiness.* New York: Guilford Press.

First-Person Accounts

Behrman, A. (2002). *Electroboy: A memoir of mania.* New York: Random House.

Cheney, T. (2009). *Manic.* New York: HarperCollins.

Fisher, C. (2016) *The princess diarist.* New York: Blue Rider Press.

Greenberg, M. (2008). *Hurry down sunshine: A father's story of love and madness.* New York: Vintage Press.

Hamilton, S. F. (2016). *Fast girl: A life spent running from madness.* New York: Dey Street Books.

Hines, K., & Reidenberg, D. J. (2013). *Cracked, not broken: Surviving and thriving after a suicide attempt.* Lanham, MD: Rowman & Littlefield.

Hinshaw, S. P. (2017). *Another kind of madness: A journey through the stigma and hope of mental illness.* New York: St. Martin's Press.

Hornbacher, M. (2008). *Madness: A bipolar life.* New York: Houghton Mifflin.

Jamison, K. R. (1995). *An unquiet mind.* New York: Knopf.

Jamison, K. R. (2017). *Robert Lowell, setting the river on fire: A study of genius, mania, and character.* New York: Knopf.

Pauley, J. (2005). *Skywriting: A life out of the blue.* New York: Ballantine Books.

Simon, L. (2002). *Detour: My bipolar road trip in 4-D.* New York: Washington Square Press.

Solomon, A. (2001). *The noonday demon: An atlas of depression.* New York: Touchstone.

Steele, D. (2000). *His bright light: The story of Nick Traina.* Des Plaines, IL: Dell.

Styron, W. (1992). *Darkness visible: A memoir of madness.* New York: Vintage Books.

Weiland, M. F., & Warren, L. (2009). *Fall to pieces: A memoir of drugs, rock 'n' roll, and mental illness.* New York: William Morrow.

References

Abbasi, J. (2017). Ketamine minus the trip: New hope for treatment-resistant depression. *Journal of the American Medical Association, 318*(320), 1964–1966.

Akiskal, H. S., Kilzieh, N., Maser, J. D., Clayton, P. J., Schettler, P. J., Shea, M. T., . . . Keller, M. B. (2006). The distinct temperament profiles of bipolar I, bipolar II and unipolar patients. *Journal of Affective Disorders, 92*(1), 19–33.

Ali, J., & Khemka, M. (2008). Hyperprolactinemia: Monitoring children on long-term risperidone. *Current Psychiatry, 7*(11), 64–72.

Allain, N., Leven, C., Falissard, B., Allain, J. S., Batail, J. M., Polard, E., . . . Naudet, F. (2017). Manic switches induced by antidepressants: An umbrella review comparing randomized controlled trials and observational studies. *Acta Psychiatrica Scandinavaca, 135*(2), 106–116.

Altman, E., Rea, M., Mintz, J., Miklowitz, D. J., Goldstein, M. J., & Hwang, S. (1992). Prodromal symptoms and signs of bipolar relapse: A report based on prospectively collected data. *Psychiatry Research, 41*, 1–8.

Altshuler, L. L., Cohen, L. S., Vitonis, A. F., Faraone, S. V., Harlow, B. L., Suri, R., . . . Stowe, Z. N. (2008). The Pregnancy Depression Scale (PDS): A screening tool for depression in pregnancy. *Archives of Womens' Mental Health, 11*(4), 277–285.

Altshuler, L. L., Sugar, C. A., McElroy, S. L., Calimlim, B., Gitlin, M., Keck, P. J., . . . Suppes, T. (2017). Switch rates during acute treatment for bipolar II depression with lithium, sertraline, or the two combined: A randomized double-blind comparison. *American Journal of Psychiatry, 174*(3), 266–276.

Altshuler, L. L., Suppes, T., Black, D., Nolen, W. A., Keck, P. E. J., Frye, M. A., . . . Post, R. (2003). Impact of antidepressant discontinuation after acute bipolar depression remission on rates of depressive relapse at 1-year follow-up. *American Journal of Psychiatry, 160*, 1252–1262.

American Psychiatric Association. (2000). *Diagnostic and statistical manual of mental disorders* (4th ed., text rev.). Washington, DC: Author.

American Psychiatric Association. (2013). *Diagnostic and statistical manual of mental disorders* (5th ed.). Arlington, VA: Author.

Amsterdam, J. D., Wang, G., & Shults, J. (2010). Venlafaxine monotherapy in bipolar type II depressed patients unresponsive to prior lithium monotherapy. *Acta Psychiatrica Scandinavaca, 121*(3), 201–208.

Andreasen, N. C. (2008). The relationship between creativity and mood disorders. *Dialogues in Clinical Neuroscience, 10*(2), 251–255.

Axelson, D. A., Birmaher, B., Findling, R. L., Fristad, M. A., Kowatch, R. A., Youngstrom, E. A., . . . Diler, R. S. (2011). Concerns regarding the inclusion of temper dysregulation disorder with dysphoria in the *Diagnostic and Statistical Manual of Mental Disorders*, Fifth Edition. *Journal of Clinical Psychiatry, 72*(9), 1257–1262.

Axelson, D. A., Birmaher, B., Strober, M. A., Goldstein, B. I., Ha, W., Gill, M. K., . . . Keller, M. B. (2011). Course of subthreshold bipolar disorder in youth: Diagnostic progression from bipolar disorder not otherwise specified. *Journal of the American Academy of Child and Adolescent Psychiatry, 50*(10), 1001–1016.

Axelson, D. A., Findling, R. L., Fristad, M. A., Kowatch, R. A., Youngstrom, E. A., Horwitz, S. M., . . . Birmaher, B. (2012). Examining the proposed disruptive mood dysregulation disorder diagnosis in children in the Longitudinal Assessment of Manic Symptoms Study. *Journal of Clinical Psychiatry, 73*(10), 1342–1350.

BALANCE investigators and collaborators, Geddes, J. R., Goodwin, G. M., Rendell, J., Azorin, J. M., Cipriani, A., . . . Juszczak, E. (2010). Lithium plus valproate combination therapy versus monotherapy for relapse prevention in bipolar I disorder (BALANCE): A randomised open-label trial. *Lancet, 375*(9712), 385–395.

Baldessarini, R. J., Tondo, L., Ghiani, C., & Lepri, B. (2010). Illness risk following rapid versus gradual discontinuation of antidepressants. *American Journal of Psychiatry, 167*(8), 934–941.

Baldessarini, R. J., Tondo, L., & Hennen, J. (1999). Treatment delays in bipolar disorders. *American Journal of Psychiatry, 156*(5), 811–812.

Barnett, J. H., & Smoller, J. W. (2009). The genetics of bipolar disorder. *Neuroscience, 164*(1), 331–343.

Barthelmess, E. K., & Naz, R. K. (2014). Polycystic ovary syndrome: Current status and future perspective. *Frontiers in Bioscience (Elite Ed.), 6*, 104–119.

Bateman, A., & Fonagy, P. (2010). Mentalization based treatment for borderline personality disorder. *World Psychiatry, 9*, 11–15.

Bauer, M. S., & McBride, L. (1996). *Structured group psychotherapy for bipolar disorder: The life goals program*. New York: Springer.

Beck, A. T., Rush, A. J., Shaw, B. F., & Emery, G. (1987). *Cognitive therapy of depression*. New York: Guilford Press.

Benazzi, F., Berk, M., Frye, M. A., Wang, W., Barraco, A., & Tohen, M. (2009). Olanzapine/fluoxetine combination for the treatment of mixed depression in bipolar I disorder: A post hoc analysis. *Clinical Psychiatry, 70*(10), 1424–1431.

Berk, M. S., Henriques, G. R., Warman, D. M., Brown, G. K., & Beck, A. T. (2004). A cognitive therapy intervention for suicide attempters: An overview of the treatment and case examples. *Cognitive and Behavioral Practice, 11*, 265–277.

Berrettini, W. (2003). Evidence for shared susceptibility in bipolar disorder and schizophrenia. *American Journal of Medical Genetics, Part C, 123C*, 59–64.

Bhowmik, D., Aparasu, R. R., Rajan, S. S., Sherer, J. T., Ochoa-Perez, M., & Chen, H. (2014). Risk of manic switch associated with antidepressant therapy in pediatric bipolar depression. *Journal of Child and Adolescent Psychopharmacology, 24*, 551–561.

Bilderbeck, A. C., Atkinson, L., McMahon, H., Voysey, M., Simon, J., Price, J., . . . Goodwin, G. M. (2016). Psychoeducation and online mood tracking for patients with bipolar disorder: A randomised controlled trial of Facilitated Integrated Mood Management versus Manualised Integrated Mood Management. *Journal of Affective Disorders, 205*, 245–251.

Birmaher, B., Axelson, D., Goldstein, B., Strober, M., Gill, M. K., Hunt, J., . . . Keller, M.

(2009). Four-year longitudinal course of children and adolescents with bipolar spectrum disorders: The Course and Outcome of Bipolar Youth (COBY) study. *American Journal of Psychiatry, 166*(7), 795–804.

Birmaher, B., Axelson, D., Strober, M., Gill, M. K., Valeri, S., Chiappetta, L., . . . Keller, M. (2006). Clinical course of children and adolescents with bipolar spectrum disorders. *Archives of General Psychiatry, 63*(2), 175–183.

Birmaher, B., Gill, M. K., Axelson, D. A., Goldstein, B. I., Goldstein, T. R., Yu, H., . . . Keller, M. B. (2014). Longitudinal trajectories and associated baseline predictors in youths with bipolar spectrum disorders. *American Journal of Psychiatry, 171*(9), 990–999.

Bonnín, C. D. M., Martínez-Arán, A., Torrent, C., Pacchiarotti, I., Rosa, A. R., Franco, C., . . . Vieta, E. (2010). Clinical and neurocognitive predictors of functional outcome in bipolar euthymic patients: A long-term, follow-up study. *Journal of Affective Disorders, 121*(1–2), 156–160.

Boufidou, F., Nikkolaou, C., Alevizios, B., Liappas, I. A., & Christodoulou, G. N. (2004). Cytokine production in bipolar affective disorder patients under lithium treatment. *Journal of Affective Disorders, 82*, 309–313.

Brohan, E., Gauci, D., Sartorius, N., Thornicroft, G., & GAMIAN-Europe Study Group. (2011). Self-stigma, empowerment and perceived discrimination among people with bipolar disorder or depression in 13 European countries: The GAMIAN-Europe study. *Journal of Affective Disorders, 129*(1–3), 56–63.

Bryant, F. B., & Veroff, J. (2007). *Savoring: A new model of positive experience.* Mahwah, NJ: Erlbaum.

Buoli, M., Serati, M., & Altamura, A. C. (2017). Biological aspects and candidate biomarkers for rapid-cycling in bipolar disorder: A systematic review. *Psychiatry Research, 258*, 565–575.

Cade, J. F. J. (1949). Lithium salts in the treatment of psychotic excitement. *Medical Journal of Australia, 36*, 349–352.

Carlson, G. A. (1990). Child and adolescent mania: Diagnostic considerations. *Journal of Child Psychology and Psychiatry, 31*, 331–342.

Carlson, G. A., & Goodwin, F. K. (1973). The stages of mania: A longitudinal analysis of the manic episode. *Archives of General Psychiatry, 28*, 221–228.

Carrà, G., Bartoli, F., Crocamo, C., Brady, K. T., & Clerici, M. (2014). Attempted suicide in people with co-occurring bipolar and substance use disorders: Systematic review and meta-analysis. *Journal of Affective Disorders, 167*, 125–135.

Carreno, T., & Goodnick, P. J. (1998). Creativity and mood disorder. In P. J. Goodnick (Ed.), *Mania: Clinical and research perspectives* (pp. 11–36). Washington, DC: American Psychiatric Press.

Chang, K., Saxena, K., & Howe, M. (2006). An open-label study of lamotrigine adjunct or monotherapy for the treatment of adolescents with bipolar depression. *Journal of the American Academy of Child and Adolescent Psychiatry, 45*, 298–304.

Chung, T. K., Lau, T. K., Yip, A. S., Chiu, H. F., & Lee, D. T. (2001). Antepartum depressive symptomatology is associated with adverse obstetric and neonatal outcomes. *Psychosomatic Medicine, 63*(5), 830–834.

Cipriani, A., Barbui, C., Salanti, G., Rendell, J., Brown, R., Stockton, S., . . . Geddes, J. R. (2011). Comparative efficacy and acceptability of antimanic drugs in acute mania: A multiple-treatments meta-analysis. *Lancet, 378*(9799), 1306–1315.

Cipriani, A., Hawton, K., Stockton, S., & Geddes, J. R. (2013, June 27). Lithium in the prevention of suicide in mood disorders: Updated systematic review and meta-analysis. *British Medical Journal, 346*, f3646.

Cohen, L. S. (2007). Treatment of bipolar disorder during pregnancy. *Journal of Clinical Psychiatry, 68*(Suppl. 9), 4–9.

Colom, F., Vieta, E., Martinez-Aran, A., Reinares, M., Benabarre, A., & Gasto, C. (2000). Clinical factors associated with treatment noncompliance in euthymic bipolar patients. *Journal of Clinical Psychiatry, 61*, 549–555.

Colom, F., Vieta, E., Martinez-Aran, A., Reinares, M., Goikolea, J. M., & Martínez-Arán, A. (2009). A randomized trial on the efficacy of group psychoeducation in the prophylaxis of bipolar disorder: A five year follow-up. *British Journal of Psychiatry, 194*(3), 260–265.

Colom, F., Vieta, E., Tacchi, M. J., Sanchez-Moreno, J., & Scott, J. (2005). Identifying and improving non-adherence in bipolar disorders. *Bipolar Disorders, 7*(5), 24–31.

Correll, C. U., Hauser, M., Penzner, J. B., Auther, A. M., Kafantaris, V., Saito, E., . . . Cornblatt, B. A. (2014). Type and duration of subsyndromal symptoms in youth with bipolar I disorder prior to their first manic episode. *Bipolar Disorders, 16*(5), 478–492.

Correll, C. U., Sheridan, E. M., & DelBello, M. P. (2010). Antipsychotic and mood stabilizer efficacy and tolerability in pediatric and adult patients with bipolar I mania: A comparative analysis of acute, randomized, placebo-controlled trials. *Bipolar Disorders, 12*(2), 116–141.

Correll, C. U., Sikich, L., Reeves, G., & Riddle, M. (2013). Metformin for antipsychotic-related weight gain and metabolic abnormalities: When, for whom, and for how long? *American Journal of Psychiatry, 170*(9), 947–952.

Coryell, W. (2009). Maintenance treatment in bipolar disorder: A reassessment of lithium as the first choice. *Bipolar Disorders, 11*(Suppl. 2), 77–83.

Coryell, W., Scheftner, W., Keller, M., Endicott, J., Maser, J., & Klerman, G. L. (1993). The enduring psychosocial consequences of mania and depression. *American Journal of Psychiatry, 150*, 720–727.

Court, B. L., & Nelson, G. E. (1996). *Bipolar puzzle solution: A mental health client's perspective.* Philadelphia: Taylor & Francis.

Craddock, N., & Sklar, P. (2013). Genetics of bipolar disorder. *Lancet, 381*(9878), 1654–1662.

Craighead, L. W. (2006). *The appetite awareness workbook: How to listen to your body and overcome bingeing, overeating, and obsession with food.* Oakland, CA: New Harbinger.

Dalai Lama. (1999). *Ethics for the new millennium.* New York: Riverhead Books.

Dalai Lama, & Cutler, H. C. (1998). *The art of happiness: A handbook for living.* New York: Riverhead Books.

Dalwood, J., Dhillon, R., Tibrewal, P., Gupta, N., & Bastiampillai, T. (2015). St John's wort: Is it safe in bipolar disorder? *Australian and New Zealand Journal of Psychiatry, 49*(12), 1226.

Davis, M., Eshelman, E. R., & McKay, M. (2008). *The relaxation and stress reduction workbook* (6th ed.). Oakland, CA: New Harbinger.

de Assis da Silva, R., Mograbi, D. C., Camelo, E. V. M., Peixoto, U., Santana, C. M. T., Landeira-Fernandez, J., . . . Cheniaux, E. (2017). The influence of current mood state, number of previous affective episodes and predominant polarity on insight in bipolar disorder. *International Journal of Psychiatry in Clinical Practice, 21*(4), 266–270.

Deckersbach, T., Nierenberg, A. A., Kessler, R., Lund, H. G., Ametrano, R. M., Sachs, G., . . . Dougherty, D. (2010). Cognitive rehabilitation for bipolar disorder: An open trial for employed patients with residual depressive symptoms. *CNS Neuroscience and Therapeutics, 16*(5), 298–307.

Deckersbach, T., Peters, A., Sylvia, L., Urdahl, A., Vieira da Silva Magalhaes, P., Otto, M. W., . . . Nierenberg, A. (2014). Do comorbid anxiety disorders moderate the effects of psychotherapy for bipolar disorder?: Results from STEP-BD. *American Journal of Psychiatry, 171*(2), 178–186.

DelBello, M. P., Goldman, R., Phillips, D., Deng, L., Cucchiaro, J., & Loebel, A. (2017). Efficacy and safety of lurasidone in children and adolescents with bipolar I depression: A double-blind, placebo-controlled study. *Journal of the American Academy of Child and Adolescent Psychiatry, 56*(12), 1015–1025.

Diav-Citrin, O., Shechtman, S., Tahover, E., Finkel-Pekarsky, V., Arnon, J., Kennedy, D., . . .

Ornoy, A. (2014). Pregnancy outcome following in utero exposure to lithium: A prospective, comparative, observational study. *American Journal of Psychiatry, 171*(7), 785–794.

Dimidjian, S., Goodman, S. H., Felder, J. N., Gallop, R., Brown, A. P., & Beck, A. T. (2016). Staying well during pregnancy and the postpartum: A pilot randomized trial of mindfulness-based cognitive therapy for the prevention of depressive relapse/recurrence. *Journal of Consulting and Clinical Psychology, 84*(2), 134–145.

Dmitrzak-Weglarz, M., Rybakowski, J. K., Suwalska, A., Skibinska, M., Leszczynska-Rodziewicz, A., Szczepankiewicz, A., & Hauser, J. (2008). Association studies of the BDNF and the NTRK2 gene polymorphisms with prophylactic lithium response in bipolar patients. *Pharmacogenomics, 9*(11), 1595–1603.

Duffy, A., Horrocks, J., Doucette, S., Keown-Stoneman, C., McCloskey, S., & Grof, P. (2014). The developmental trajectory of bipolar disorder. *British Journal of Psychiatry, 204*(2), 122–128.

Duncan, W. C., Jr., Ballard, E. D., & Zarate, C. A. (2017). Ketamine-induced glutamatergic mechanisms of sleep and wakefulness: Insights for developing novel treatments for disturbed sleep and mood. *Handbook of Experimental Pharmacology.* [Epub ahead of print]

Egeland, J. A., Endicott, J., Hostetter, A. M., Allen, C. R., Pauls, D. L., & Shaw, J. A. (2012). A 16-year prospective study of prodromal features prior to BPI onset in well Amish children. *Journal of Affective Disorders, 142*(1–3), 186–192.

Ehlers, C. L., Kupfer, D. J., Frank, E., & Monk, T. H. (1993). Biological rhythms and depression: The role of zeitgebers and zeitstorers. *Depression, 1*, 285–293.

Ehrnstrom, C., & Brosse, A. L. (2016). *End the insomnia struggle: A step-by-step guide to help you get to sleep and stay asleep.* Oakland, CA: New Harbinger.

Einarson, A., & Boskovic, R. (2009). Use and safety of antipsychotic drugs during pregnancy. *Journal of Psychiatric Practice, 15*(3), 183–192.

Eisenberger, N. I. (2015). Social pain and the brain: Controversies, questions, and where to go from here. *Annual Review of Psychology, 66*, 601–629.

El-Mallakh, R. S., Vöhringer, P. A., Ostacher, M. M., Baldassano, C. F., Holtzman, N. S., Whitham, E. A., . . . Ghaemi, S. N. (2015). Antidepressants worsen rapid-cycling course in bipolar depression: A STEP-BD randomized clinical trial. *Journal of Affective Disorders, 184*, 318–321.

Ellison, M. L., Russinova, Z., Lyass, A., & Rogers, E. S. (2008). Professionals and managers with severe mental illnesses: Findings from a national survey. *Journal of Nervous and Mental Disease, 196*(3), 179–189.

Faheem, S., Petti, V., & Mellos, G. (2017). Disruptive mood dysregulation disorder and its effect on bipolar disorder. *Annals of Clinical Psychiatry, 29*(2), 84–91.

Fawcett, J., Golden, B., & Rosenfeld, N. (2000). *New hope for people with bipolar disorder.* Roseville, CA: Prima Health.

Fears, S. C., Service, S. K., Kremeyer, B., Araya, C., Araya, X., Bejarano, J., . . . Bearden, C. E. (2014). Multisystem component phenotypes of bipolar disorder for genetic investigations of extended pedigrees. *JAMA Psychiatry, 71*(4), 375–387.

Forman, D. R., O'Hara, M. W., Stuart, S., Gorman, L. L., Larsen, K. E., & Coy, K. C. (2007). Effective treatment for postpartum depression is not sufficient to improve the developing mother–child relationship. *Development and Psychopathology, 19*(2), 585–602.

Fortinguerra, F., Clavenna, A., & Bonati, M. (2009). Psychotropic drug use during breastfeeding: A review of the evidence. *Pediatrics, 124*(4), e547–e556.

Frank, E. (2007). *Treating bipolar disorder: A clinician's guide to interpersonal and social rhythm therapy.* New York: Guilford Press.

Frank, E., Kupfer, D. J., Thase, M. E., Mallinger, A. G., Swartz, H. A., Fagiolini, A. M., . . . Monk, T. (2005). Two-year outcomes for interpersonal and social rhythm therapy in individuals with bipolar I disorder. *Archives of General Psychiatry, 62*(9), 996–1004.

Fraser, L. M., O'Carroll, R. E., & Ebmeier, K. P. (2008). The effect of electroconvulsive therapy on autobiographical memory: A systematic review. *Journal of ECT, 24*(1), 10–17.

Freeman, M. P., Smith, K. W., Freeman, S. A., McElroy, S. L., Kmetz, G. E., Wright, R., & Keck, P. E. J. (2002). The impact of reproductive events on the course of bipolar disorder in women. *Journal of Clinical Psychiatry, 63*(4), 284–287.

Fristad, M. A., & Goldberg Arnold, J. S. (2003). *Raising a moody child*. New York: Guilford Press.

Fristad, M. A., & MacPherson, H. A. (2014). Evidence-based psychosocial treatments for child and adolescent bipolar spectrum disorders. *Journal of Child and Adolescent Psychology, 43*(3), 339–355.

Fristad, M. A., Vesco, A. T., Young, A. S., Healy, K. Z., Nader, E. S., Gardner, W., . . . Arnold, L. E. (2016). Pilot randomized controlled trial of omega-3 and individual-family psycho-educational psychotherapy for children and adolescents with depression. *Journal of Child and Adolescent Psychology, 7*, 1–14.

Geddes, J. R., Calabrese, J. R., & Goodwin, G. M. (2009). Lamotrigine for treatment of bipolar depression: Independent meta-analysis and meta-regression of individual patient data from five randomised trials. *British Journal of Psychiatry, 194*(1), 4–9.

Geddes, J. R., & Miklowitz, D. J. (2013). Treatment of bipolar disorder. *Lancet, 381*(9878), 1672–1682.

Geller, B., Bolhofner, K., Craney, J. L., Williams, M., DelBello, M. P., & Gunderson, K. (2000). Psychosocial functioning in a prepubertal and early adolescent bipolar disorder phenotype. *Journal of the American Academy of Child and Adolescent Psychiatry, 39*, 1543–1548.

Geller, B., Luby, J. L., Joshi, P., Wagner, K. D., Emslie, G., Walkup, J. T., . . . Lavori, P. (2012). A randomized controlled trial of risperidone, lithium, or divalproex sodium for initial treatment of bipolar I disorder, manic or mixed phase, in children and adolescents. *Archives of General Psychiatry, 69*(5), 515–528.

Geller, B., Tillman, R., Bolhofner, K., & Zimerman, B. (2008). Child bipolar I disorder: Prospective continuity with adult bipolar I disorder; characteristics of second and third episodes; predictors of 8-year outcome. *Archives of General Psychiatry, 65*(10), 1125–1133.

Geller, B., Williams, M., Zimerman, B., Frazier, J., Beringer, I., & Warner, K. L. (1998). Prepubertal and early adolescent bipolarity differentiated from ADHD by manic symptoms, grandiose delusions, ultra-rapid or ultradian cycling. *Journal of Affective Disorders, 51*, 81–91.

Ghaemi, N., Sachs, G. S., & Goodwin, F. K. (2000). What is to be done?: Controversies in the diagnosis and treatment of manic-depressive illness. *World Journal of Biological Psychiatry, 1*(2), 65–74.

Ghasemi, A., Seifi, M., Baybordi, F., Danaei, N., & Samadi, R. (2018). Association between serotonin 2A receptor genetic variations, stressful life events and suicide. *Gene, 658*, 191–197.

Gignac, A., McGirr, A., Lam, R. W., & Yatham, L. N. (2015). Recovery and recurrence following a first episode of mania: A systematic review and meta-analysis of prospectively characterized cohorts. *Journal of Clinical Psychiatry, 76*(9), 1241–1248.

Gilman, S. E., Ni, M. Y., Dunn, E. C., Breslau, J., McLaughlin, K. A., Smoller, J. W., & Perlis, R. H. (2015). Contributions of the social environment to first-onset and recurrent mania. *Molecular Psychiatry, 20*(3), 329–336.

Gitlin, M. J., & Miklowitz, D. J. (2017). The difficult lives of individuals with bipolar disorder: A review of functional outcomes and their implications for treatment. *Journal of Affective Disorders, 209*, 147–154.

Glovinsky, P., & Spielman, A. (2006). *The insomnia answer: A personalized program for identifying and overcoming the three types of insomnia*. New York: TarcherPerigee.

Glozier, N. (1998). Workplace effects of the stigmatization of depression. *Journal of Occupational and Environmental Medicine, 40*, 793–800.

Goghari, V. M., & Harrow, M. (2016). Twenty year multi-follow-up of different types of hallucinations in schizophrenia, schizoaffective disorder, bipolar disorder, and depression. *Schizophrenia Research, 176*(2–3), 371–377.

Goldberg, J. F., Burdick, K. E., & Endick, C. J. (2004). Preliminary randomized, double-blind, placebo-controlled trial of pramipexole added to mood stabilizers for treatment-resistant bipolar depression. *American Journal of Psychiatry, 161*(3), 564–566.

Goldstein, B. I., Birmaher, B., Carlson, G., DelBello, M. P., Findling, R. L., Fristad, M. A., . . . Youngstrom, E. A. (2017). The International Society for Bipolar Disorders Task Force Report on Pediatric Bipolar Disorder: Knowledge to date and directions for future research. *Bipolar Disorders, 19*(7), 524–543.

Goldstein, B. I., Carnethon, M. R., Matthews, K. A., McIntyre, R. S., Miller, G. E., Raghuveer, G., . . . McCrindle, B. W. (2015). Major depressive disorder and bipolar disorder predispose youth to accelerated atherosclerosis and early cardiovascular disease: A scientific statement from the American Heart Association. *Circulation, 132*(10), 965–986.

Goldstein, B. I., Goldstein, T. R., Collinger-Larson, K. A., Axelson, D. A., Bukstein, O. G., Birmaher, B., & Miklowitz, D. J. (2014). Treatment development and feasibility study of family-focused treatment for adolescents with bipolar disorder and comorbid substance use disorders. *Journal of Psychiatric Practice, 20*(3), 237–248.

Goldstein, T. R., Fersch-Podrat, R. K., Rivera, M., Axelson, D. A., Merranko, J., Yu, H., . . . Birmaher, B. (2015). Dialectical behavior therapy (DBT) for adolescents with bipolar disorder: Results from a pilot randomized trial. *Journal of Child and Adolescent Psychopharmacology, 25*(2), 140–149.

Goodwin, F. K., Fireman, B., Simon, G. E., Hunkeler, E. M., Lee, J., & Revicki, D. (2003). Suicide risk in bipolar disorder during treatment with lithium and divalproex. *Journal of the American Medical Association, 290*, 1467–1473.

Goodwin, G. M., Bowden, C. L., Calabrese, J. R., Grunze, H., Kasper, S., White, R., . . . Leadbetter, R. (2004). A pooled analysis of 2 placebo-controlled 18-month trials of lamotrigine and lithium maintenance in bipolar I disorder. *Journal of Clinical Psychiatry, 65*(3), 432–441.

Goodwin, G. M., Haddad, P. M., Ferrier, I. N., Aronson, J. K., Barnes, T., Cipriani, A., . . . Young, A. H. (2016). Evidence-based guidelines for treating bipolar disorder: Revised third edition recommendations from the British Association for Psychopharmacology. *Journal of Psychopharmacology, 30*(6), 495–553.

Gordon-Smith, K., Forty, L., Chan, C., Knott, S., Jones, I., Craddock, N., & Jones, L. A. (2015). Rapid cycling as a feature of bipolar disorder and comorbid migraine. *Journal of Affective Disorders, 175*, 320–324.

Greenberger, D., & Padesky, C. A. (2015). *Mind over mood* (2nd ed.). New York: Guilford Press.

Grof, P. (2010). Sixty years of lithium responders. *Neuropsychobiology, 62*, 27–35.

Grof, P., Duffy, A., Alda, M., & Hajek, T. (2009). Lithium response across generations. *Acta Psychiatrica Scandinavaca, 120*(5), 378–385.

Grossman, D. C., Mueller, B. A., Riedy, C., Dowd, M. D., Villaveces, A., Prodzinski, J., . . . Harruff, R. (2005). Gun storage practices and risk of youth suicide and unintentional firearm injuries. *Journal of the American Medical Association, 293*, 707–714.

Grover, S., & Avasthi, A. (2015). Mood stabilizers in pregnancy and lactation. *Indian Journal of Psychiatry, 57*(Suppl. 2), S308–S323.

Grunze, H. (2014). Stimulants for treating bipolar disorder: Pro and con. *Harvard Review of Psychiatry, 22*(6), 358–362.

Hafeman, D. M., Merranko, J., Axelson, D., Goldstein, B. I., Goldstein, T., Monk, K., . . . Birmaher, B. (2016). Toward the definition of a bipolar prodrome: Dimensional predictors of bipolar spectrum disorders in at-risk youths. *American Journal of Psychiatry, 173*(7), 695–704.

Hamilton, S. F. (2016). *Fast girl: A life spent running from madness.* New York: Dey Street.

Hammen, C., Gitlin, M., & Altshuler, L. (2000). Predictors of work adjustment in bipolar I patients: A naturalistic longitudinal follow-up. *Journal of Consulting and Clinical Psychology, 68,* 220–225.

Hankin, B. L., & Abramson, L. Y. (2001). Development of gender differences in depression: An elaborated cognitive vulnerability–transactional stress theory. *Psychological Bulletin, 127*(6), 773–796.

Harlow, B. L., Wise, L. A., Otto, M. W., Soares, C. N., & Cohen, L. S. (2003). Depression and its influence on reproductive endocrine and menstrual cycle markers associated with peri-menopause: The Harvard Study of Moods and Cycles. *Archives of General Psychiatry, 60*(1), 29–36.

Harmanci, H., Çam, Ç. F., & Etikan, İ. (2016). Comorbidity of adult attention deficit and hyperactivity disorder in bipolar and unipolar patients. *Noro Psikiyatr Ars, 53*(3), 257–262.

Harrison, P. J., Geddes, J. R., & Tunbridge, E. M. (2018). The emerging neurobiology of bipolar disorder. *Trends in Neuroscience, 41*(1), 18–30.

Harrow, M., Grossman, L. S., Herbener, E. S., & Davies, E. W. (2000). Ten-year outcome: Patients with schizoaffective disorders, schizophrenia, affective disorders and mood-incongruent psychotic symptoms. *British Journal of Psychiatry, 177,* 421–426.

Harvey, A. G. (2011). Sleep and circadian functioning: Critical mechanisms in the mood disorders? *Annual Review of Clinical Psychology, 7,* 297–319.

Haskey, C., & Galbally, M. (2017). Mood stabilizers in pregnancy and child developmental outcomes: A systematic review. *Australia and New Zealand Journal of Psychiatry, 51*(11), 1087–1097.

Haslan, N. (2016). Concept creep: Psychology's expanding concepts of harm and pathology. *Psychological Inquiry: An International Journal for the Advancement of Psychological Theory, 27,* 1–17.

Hawton, K., Sutton, L., Haw, C., Sinclair, J., & Harriss, L. (2005). Suicide and attempted suicide in bipolar disorder: A systematic review of risk factors. *Journal of Clinical Psychiatry, 66*(6), 693–704.

Hibbeln, J. R. (1998). Fish consumption and major depression. *Lancet, 351,* 1213.

Hillegers, M. H., Reichart, C. G., Wals, M., Verhulst, F. C., Ormel, J., & Nolen, W. A. (2005). Five-year prospective outcome of psychopathology in the adolescent offspring of bipolar parents. *Bipolar Disorders, 7*(4), 344–350.

Hirschfeld, R. M., Williams, J. B., Spitzer, R. L., Calabrese, J. R., Flynn, L., Keck, K. P. E., Jr., et al. (2000). Development and validation of a screening instrument for bipolar spectrum disorder: The Mood Disorder Questionnaire. *American Journal of Psychiatry, 157,* 1873–1875.

Hoffman, C., Dunn, D. M., & Njoroge, W. F. M. (2017). Impact of postpartum mental illness upon infant development. *Current Psychiatry Reports, 19*(12), 100.

Hollander, M. (2017). *Helping teens who cut: Using DBT skills to end self-injury* (2nd ed.). New York: Guilford Press.

Hooley, J. M. (2007). Expressed emotion and relapse of psychopathology. *Annual Review of Clinical Psychology, 3,* 329–352.

Hooley, J. M., Siegle, G., & Gruber, S. A. (2012). Affective and neural reactivity to criticism in individuals high and low on perceived criticism. *PLOS ONE, 7*(9), e44412.

Ikeda, M., Saito, T., Kondo, K., & Iwata, N. (2017). Genome-wide association studies of bipolar disorder: A systematic review of recent findings and their clinical implications. *Psychiatry and Clinical Neurosciences.*

Insel, T. R. (2009). Translating scientific opportunity into public health impact: A strategic plan for research on mental illness. *Archives of General Psychiatry, 66*(2), 128–133.

Isojärvi, J. I. T., Taubøll, E., & Herzog, A. (2005). Effect of antiepileptic drugs on reproductive endocrine function in individuals with epilepsy. *CNS Drugs, 19*(3), 207–223.

Jacobs, G. D. (2009). *Say good night to insomnia: The six-week, drug-free program developed at Harvard Medical School*. New York: Holt Paperbacks.

Jamison, K. R. (1993). *Touched with fire: Manic–depressive illness and the artistic temperament*. New York: Free Press.

Jamison, K. R. (1995). *An unquiet mind*. New York: Knopf.

Jamison, K. R. (2000a). *Night falls fast: Understanding suicide*. New York: Vintage Books.

Jamison, K. R. (2000b). Suicide and bipolar disorder. *Journal of Clinical Psychiatry, 61*(Suppl. 9), 47–56.

Jamison, K. R. (2005). *Exuberance: The passion for life*. New York: Vintage.

Jamison, K. R. (2017). *Robert Lowell, setting the river on fire: A study of genius, mania, and character*. New York: Knopf.

Jette, N., Patten, S., Williams, J., Becker, W., & Wiebe, S. (2008). Comorbidity of migraine and psychiatric disorders—a national population-based study. *Headache, 48*(4), 501–516.

Jiang, B., Kenna, H. A., & Rasgon, N. L. (2009). Genetic overlap between polycystic ovary syndrome and bipolar disorder: The endophenotype hypothesis. *Medical Hypotheses, 73*(6), 996–1004.

Joffe, H. (2007). Reproductive biology and psychotropic treatments in premenopausal women with bipolar disorder. *Journal of Cinical Psychiatry, 68*(9), 10–15.

Joffe, H., Cohen, L. S., Suppes, T., McLaughlin, W. L., Lavori, P., Adams, J. M., . . . Sachs, G. S. (2006). Valproate is associated with new-onset oligoamenorrhea with hyperandrogenism in women with bipolar disorder. *Biological Psychiatry, 59*(11), 1078–1086.

Joffe, H., Kim, D. R., Foris, J. M., Baldassano, C. F., Gyulai, L., Hwang, C. H., . . . Cohen, L. S. (2006). Menstrual dysfunction prior to onset of psychiatric illness is reported more commonly by women with bipolar disorder than by women with unipolar depression and healthy controls. *Journal of Clinical Psychiatry, 67*(2), 297–304.

John, H., & Sharma, V. (2009). Misdiagnosis of bipolar disorder as borderline personality disorder: Clinical and economic consequences. *World Journal of Biological Psychiatry, 10*(4, Pt. 2), 612–615.

Johnson, S. L., Cuellar, A., Ruggero, C., Perlman, C., Goodnick, P., White, R., & Miller, I. (2008). Life events as predictors of mania and depression in bipolar I disorder. *Journal of Abnormal Psychology, 117*, 268–277.

Johnson, S. L., Murray, G., Fredrickson, B., Youngstrom, E. A., Hinshaw, S., Bass, J. M., . . . Salloum, I. (2012). Creativity and bipolar disorder: Touched by fire or burning with questions? *Clinical Psychology Review, 32*(1), 1–12.

Johnson, S. L., Winett, C. A., Meyer, B., Greenhouse, W. J., & Miller, I. (1999). Social support and the course of bipolar disorder. *Journal of Abnormal Psychology, 108*, 558–566.

Joseph, M. F., Frazier, T. W., Youngstrom, E. A., & Soares, J. C. (2008). A quantitative and qualitative review of neurocognitive performance in pediatric bipolar disorder. *Journal of Child and Adolescent Psychopharmacology, 18*, 595–605.

Joyce, P. R. (1985). Illness behaviour and rehospitalisation in bipolar affective disorder. *Psychological Medicine, 15*, 521–525.

Judd, L. L., Akiskal, H. S., Schettler, P. J., Coryell, W., Endicott, J., Maser, J. D., . . . Keller, M. B. (2003). A prospective investigation of the natural history of the long-term weekly symptomatic status of bipolar II disorder. *Archives of General Psychiatry, 60*, 261–269.

Judd, L. L., Akiskal, H. S., Schettler, P. J., Endicott, J., Maser, J., Solomon, D. A., . . . Keller, M. B. (2002). The long-term natural history of the weekly symptomatic status of bipolar I disorder. *Archives of General Psychiatry, 59*, 530–537.

Katalinic, N., Lai, R., Somogyi, A., Mitchell, P. B., Glue, P., & Loo, C. K. (2013). Ketamine as a new treatment for depression: A review of its efficacy and adverse effects. *Australian and New Zealand Journal of Psychiatry, 47*(8), 710–727.

Kenna, H. A., Jiang, B., & Rasgon, N. L. (2009). Reproductive and metabolic abnormalities associated with bipolar disorder and its treatment. *Harvard Review of Psychiatry, 17,* 138–146.

Kessler, R. C., Adler, L., Barkley, R., Biederman, J., Conners, C. K., Demler, O., . . . Zaslavsky, A. M. (2006). The prevalence and correlates of adult ADHD in the United States: Results from the National Comorbidity Survey Replication. *American Journal of Psychiatry, 163,* 716–723.

Kessler, R. C., Berglund, P., Demler, O., Jin, R., & Walters, E. E. (2005). Lifetime prevalence and age-of-onset distributions of DSM-IV disorders in the National Comorbidity Survey Replication. *Archives of General Psychiatry, 62,* 593–602.

Kim, E. Y., & Miklowitz, D. J. (2002). Childhood mania, attention deficit hyperactivity disorder, and conduct disorder: A critical review of diagnostic dilemmas. *Bipolar Disorders, 4,* 215–225.

Kishi, T., Ikuta, T., Matsunaga, S., Matsuda, Y., Oya, K., & Iwata, N. (2017). Comparative efficacy and safety of antipsychotics in the treatment of schizophrenia: A network meta-analysis in a Japanese population. *Neuropsychiatric Disease and Treatment, 13,* 1281–1302.

Kivilcim, Y., Altintas, M., Domac, F. M., Erzincan, E., & Gülec, H. (2017). Screening for bipolar disorder among migraineurs: The impact of migraine-bipolar disorder comorbidity on disease characteristics. *Neuropsychiatric Disease and Treatment, 13,* 631–641.

Kochman, F. J., Hantouche, E. G., Ferrari, P., Lancrenon, S., Bayart, D., & Akiskal, H. S. (2005). Cyclothymic temperament as a prospective predictor of bipolarity and suicidality in children and adolescents with major depressive disorder. *Journal of Affective Disorders, 85*(1–2), 181–189.

Kocsis, J. H., Shaw, E. D., Stokes, P. E., Wilner, P., Elliot, A. S., Sikes, C., . . . Parides, M. (1993). Neuropsychological effects of lithium discontinuation. *Journal of Clinical Psychopharmacology, 13,* 268–275.

Kyaga, S., Landén, M., Boman, M., Hultman, C. M., Långström, N., & Lichtenstein, P. (2013). Mental illness, suicide and creativity: 40-year prospective total population study. *Journal of Psychiatric Research, 47*(1), 83–90.

Lan, W. H., Bai, Y. M., Hsu, J. W., Huang, K. L., Su, T. P., Li, C. T., . . . Chen, M. H. (2015). Comorbidity of ADHD and suicide attempts among adolescents and young adults with bipolar disorder: A nationwide longitudinal study. *Journal of Affective Disorders, 176,* 171–175.

Leibenluft, E., Cohen, P., Gorrindo, T., Brook, J. S., & Pine, D. S. (2006). Chronic vs. episodic irritability in youth: A community-based, longitudinal study of clinical and diagnostic associations. *Journal of Child and Adolescent Psychopharmacology, 16*(4), 456–466.

Leucht, S., Cipriani, A., Spineli, L., Mavridis, D., Orey, D., Richter, F., . . . Davis, J. M. (2013). Comparative efficacy and tolerability of 15 antipsychotic drugs in schizophrenia: A multiple-treatments meta-analysis. *Lancet, 382*(9896), 951–962.

Levin, J. B., Krivenko, A., Howland, M., Schlachet, R., & Sajatovic, M. (2016). Medication adherence in patients with bipolar disorder: A comprehensive review. *CNS Drugs, 30*(9), 819–835.

Lewinsohn, P. M., Muñoz, R. F., Youngren, M. A., & Zeiss, A. M. (1992). *Control your depression.* New York: Fireside/Simon & Schuster.

Lewinsohn, P. M., Seeley, J. R., & Klein, D. N. (2003). Bipolar disorders during adolescence. *Acta Psychiatrica Scandinavaca, 418*(Suppl.), 47–50.

Lewis, K. J. S., Di Florio, A., Forty, L., Gordon-Smith, K., Perry, A., Craddock, N., . . . Jones, I. (2018). Mania triggered by sleep loss and risk of postpartum psychosis in women with bipolar disorder. *Journal of Affective Disorders, 225,* 624–629.

Lewis, L. (2000). A consumer perspective concerning the diagnosis and treatment of bipolar disorder. *Biological Psychiatry, 48,* 442–444.

Lewis, M. A., & Rook, K. S. (1999). Social control in personal relationships: Impact on health behaviors and psychological distress. *Health Psychology, 18*(1), 63–71.

Lin, P. Y., & Su, K. P. (2007). A meta-analytic review of double-blind, placebo-controlled trials of antidepressant efficacy of omega-3 fatty acids. *Journal of Clinical Psychiatry, 68*(7), 1056–1061.

Linehan, M. M. (1985). The reasons for living inventory. In P. A. Keller & L. G. Ri (Eds.), *Innovations in clinical practice: A source book* (pp. 321–330). Miami, FL: Professional Resource Exchange.

Linehan, M. M., & Dexter-Mazza, E. T. (2007). Dialectical behavior therapy for borderline personality disorder. In D. H. Barlow (Ed.), *Clinical handbook of psychological disorders* (4th ed., pp. 365–420). New York: Guilford Press.

Linehan, M. M., Goodstein, J. L., Nielsen, S. L., & Chiles, J. A. (1983). Reasons for staying alive when you are thinking of killing yourself: The Reasons for Living Inventory. *Journal of Consulting and Clinical Psychology, 51*, 276–286.

Linehan, M. M., & Wilks, C. R. (2015). The course and evolution of dialectical behavior therapy. *American Journal of Psychotherapy, 69*(2), 97–110.

Lish, J. D., Dime-Meenan, S., Whybrow, P. C., Price, R. A., & Hirschfeld, R. M. (1994). The National Depressive and Manic-Depressive Association (NDMDA) survey of bipolar members. *Journal of Affective Disorders, 31*, 281–294.

Liu, H. Y., Potter, M. P., Woodworth, K. Y., Yorks, D. M., Petty, C. R., Wozniak, J. R., . . . Biederman, J. (2011). Pharmacologic treatments for pediatric bipolar disorder: A review and meta-analysis. *Journal of the American Academy of Child and Adolescent Psychiatry, 50*(8), 749–762.

Lobban, F., Taylor, L., Chandler, C., Tyler, E., Kinderman, P., Kolamunnage-Dona, R., . . . Morriss, R. K. (2010). Enhanced relapse prevention for bipolar disorder by community mental health teams: Cluster feasibility randomised trial. *British Journal of Psychiatry, 196*(1), 59–63.

Loebel, A., Cucchiaro, J., Silva, R., Kroger, H., Hsu, J., Sarma, K., & Sachs, G. (2014). Lurasidone monotherapy in the treatment of bipolar I depression: A randomized, double-blind, placebo-controlled study. *American Journal of Psychiatry, 171*(2), 160–168.

Lopez, R., Micoulaud-Franchi, J. A., Galera, C., & Dauvilliers, Y. (2017). Is adult-onset attention deficit/hyperactivity disorder frequent in clinical practice? *Psychiatry Research, 257*, 238–241.

Luby, J. L., & Navsaria, N. (2010). Pediatric bipolar disorder: Evidence for prodromal states and early markers. *Journal of Child Psychology and Psychiatry, 51*(4), 459–471.

Machado-Vieira, R., Manji, H. K., & Zarate, C. A. J. (2009). The role of lithium in the treatment of bipolar disorder: Convergent evidence for neurotrophic effects as a unifying hypothesis. *Bipolar Disorders, 11*(Suppl. 2), 92–109.

MacPherson, H. A., Weinstein, S. M., Henry, D. B., & West, A. E. (2016). Mediators in the randomized trial of Child- and Family-Focused Cognitive-Behavioral Therapy for pediatric bipolar disorder. *Behavior Research and Therapy, 85*, 60–71.

MacQueen, G., Parkin, C., Marriott, M., Bégin, H., & Hasey, G. (2007). The long-term impact of treatment with electroconvulsive therapy on discrete memory systems in patients with bipolar disorder. *Journal of Psychiatry and Neuroscience, 32*(4), 241–249.

Malhi, G. S., Adams, D., & Berk, M. (2009). Medicating mood with maintenance in mind: Bipolar depression pharmacotherapy. *Bipolar Disorders, 11*(Suppl. 2), 55–76.

Malhi, G. S., Bargh, D. M., Coulston, C. M., Das, P., & Berk, M. (2014). Predicting bipolar disorder on the basis of phenomenology: Implications for prevention and early intervention. *Bipolar Disorder, 16*(5), 455–470.

Malhi, G. S., Morris, G., Hamilton, A., Outhred, T., & Mannie, Z. (2017). Is "early intervention" in bipolar disorder what it claims to be? *Bipolar Disorder, 19*(8), 627–636.

Malkoff-Schwartz, S., Frank, E., Anderson, B. P., Hlastala, S. A., Luther, J. F., Sherrill, J. T., . . . Kupfer, D. J. (2000). Social rhythm disruption and stressful life events in the onset of bipolar and unipolar episodes. *Psychological Medicine, 30,* 1005–1016.

Manji, H. K. (2009). The role of synaptic and cellular plasticity cascades in the pathophysiology and treatment of mood and psychotic disorders. *Bipolar Disorders, 11*(Suppl. 1), 2–3.

Manji, H. K., Quiroz, J. A., Payne, J. L., Singh, J., Lopes, B. P., Viegas, J. S., & Zarate, C. A. (2003). The underlying neurobiology of bipolar disorder. *World Psychiatry, 2*(3), 136–146.

Mansell, W., & Pedley, R. (2008). The ascent into mania: A review of psychological processes associated with the development of manic symptoms. *Clinical Psychology Review, 28*(3), 494–520.

Marangell, L. B., Suppes, T., Zboyan, H. A., Prashad, S. J., Fischer, G., Snow, D., . . . Allen, J. C. (2008). A 1-year pilot study of vagus nerve stimulation in treatment-resistant rapid-cycling bipolar disorder. *Journal of Clinical Psychiatry, 69*(2), 183–189.

Martell, C. R., Dimidjian, S., & Herman-Dunn, R. (2010). *Behavioral activation for depression: A clinician's guide.* New York: Guilford Press.

Mayberg, H. S., Lozano, A. M., Voon, V., McNeely, H. E., Seminowicz, D., Hamani, C., . . . Kennedy, S. H. (2005). Deep brain stimulation for treatment-resistant depression. *Neuron, 45*(5), 651–660.

McCrady, B. S. (2007). Alcohol use disorders. In D. Barlow (Ed.), *Clinical handbook of psychological disorders* (4th ed., pp. 492–546). New York: Guilford Press.

McCraw, S., Parker, G., Fletcher, K., & Friend, P. (2013). Self-reported creativity in bipolar disorder: Prevalence, types and associated outcomes in mania versus hypomania. *Journal of Affective Disorders, 151*(3), 831–836.

McIntyre, R. S., Soczynska, J. K., Cha, D. S., Woldeyohannes, H. O., Dale, R. S., Alsuwaidan, M. T., . . . Kennedy, S. H. (2015). The prevalence and illness characteristics of DSM-5-defined "mixed feature specifier" in adults with major depressive disorder and bipolar disorder: Results from the International Mood Disorders Collaborative Project. *Journal of Affective Disorders, 172,* 259–264.

Merikangas, K. R., Akiskal, H. S., Angst, J., Greenberg, P. E., Hirschfeld, R. M. A., Petukhova, M., & Kessler, R. C. (2007). Lifetime and 12-month prevalence of bipolar spectrum disorder in the National Comorbidity Survey Replication. *Archives of General Psychiatry, 64*(5), 543–552.

Merikangas, K. R., Jin, R., He, J. P., Kessler, R. C., Lee, S., Sampson, N. A., . . . Zarkov, Z. (2011). Prevalence and correlates of bipolar spectrum disorder in the World Mental Health Survey Initiative. *Archives of General Psychiatry, 68*(3), 241–251.

Mesman, E., Nolen, W. A., Reichart, C. G., Wals, M., & Hillegers, M. H. (2013). The Dutch Bipolar Offspring Study: 12-year follow-up. *American Journal of Psychiatry, 170*(5), 542–549.

Michalak, E. E., Yatham, L. N., Maxwell, V., Hale, S., & Lam, R. W. (2007). The impact of bipolar disorder upon work functioning: A qualitative analysis. *Bipolar Disorders, 9*(1–2), 126–143.

Miklowitz, D. J. (2010). *Bipolar disorder: A family-focused treatment approach* (2nd ed.). New York: Guilford Press.

Miklowitz, D. J., Alatiq, Y., Geddes, J. R., Goodwin, G. M., & Williams, J. M. (2010). Thought suppression in bipolar disorder. *Journal of Abnormal Psychology, 119*(2), 355–365.

Miklowitz, D. J., Biuckians, A., & Richards, J. A. (2006). Early-onset bipolar disorder: A family treatment perspective. *Development and Psychopathology, 18*(4), 1247–1265.

Miklowitz, D. J., & Chung, B. D. (2016). Family-focused therapy for bipolar disorder: Reflections on 30 years of research. *Family Process, 55*(3), 483–499.

Miklowitz, D. J., & George, E. L. (2007). *The bipolar teen: What you can do to help your teen and your family.* New York: Guilford Press.

Miklowitz, D. J., George, E. L., Richards, J. A., Simoneau, T. L., & Suddath, R. L. (2003). A randomized study of family-focused psychoeducation and pharmacotherapy in the outpatient management of bipolar disorder. *Archives of General Psychiatry, 60,* 904–912.

Miklowitz, D. J., & Gitlin, M. J. (2014a). *Clinician's guide to bipolar disorder.* New York: Guilford Press.

Miklowitz, D. J., & Gitlin, M. J. (2014b). Psychosocial treatments for bipolar disorder. *Focus: Journal of Lifelong Learning in Psychiatry, 12*(3), 359–371.

Miklowitz, D. J., Goldstein, M. J., Nuechterlein, K. H., Snyder, K. S., & Mintz, J. (1988). Family factors and the course of bipolar affective disorder. *Archives of General Psychiatry, 45,* 225–231.

Miklowitz, D. J., Schneck, C. D., George, E. L., Taylor, D. O., Sugar, C. A., Birmaher, B., . . . Axelson, D. A. (2014). Pharmacotherapy and family-focused treatment for adolescents with bipolar I and II disorders: A 2-year randomized trial. *American Journal of Psychiatry, 171*(6), 658–667.

Miklowitz, D. J., Schneck, C. D., Singh, M. K., Taylor, D. O., George, E. L., Cosgrove, V. E., . . . Chang, K. D. (2013). Early intervention for symptomatic youth at risk for bipolar disorder: A randomized trial of family-focused therapy. *Journal of the American Academy of Child and Adolescent Psychiatry, 52*(2), 121–131.

Miklowitz, D. J., Schneck, C. D., Walshaw, P., Garrett, A. G., Singh, M. K., Sugar, C., & Chang, K. D. (2017, August 4). Early intervention for youth at high risk for bipolar disorder: A multisite randomized trial of family-focused treatment. *Early Intervention in Psychiatry.* [Epub ahead of print]

Miller, A. H., Maletic, V., & Raison, C. L. (2009). Inflammation and its discontents: The role of cytokines in the pathophysiology of major depression. *Biological Psychiatry, 65,* 732–741.

Miller, W. R., & Rollnick, S. (2012). *Motivational interviewing: Helping people change* (3rd ed.). New York: Guilford Press.

Millett, K. (1990). *The loony-bin trip.* New York: Simon & Schuster.

Modabbernia, A., Taslimi, S., Brietzke, E., & Ashrafi, M. (2013). Cytokine alterations in bipolar disorder: A meta-analysis of 30 studies. *Biological Psychiatry, 74*(1), 15–25.

Monk, T. H., Kupfer, D. J., Frank, E., & Ritenour, A. M. (1991). The social rhythm metric (SRM): Measuring daily social rhythms over 12 weeks. *Psychiatry Research, 36,* 195–207.

Moreno, C., Laje, G., Blanco, C., Jiang, H., Schmidt, A. B., & Olfson, M. (2007). National trends in the outpatient diagnosis and treatment of bipolar disorder in youth. *Archives of General Psychiatry, 64*(9), 1032–1039.

Morris, C. D., Miklowitz, D. J., Wisniewski, S. R., Giese, A. A., Allen, M. H., & Thomas, M. R. (2005). Care satisfaction, hope, and life functioning among adults with bipolar disorder: Data from the first 1,000 participants in the Systematic Treatment Enhancement Program. *Comprehensive Psychiatry, 46,* 98–104.

Newberg, A. R., Catapano, L. A., Zarate, C. A., & Manji, H. K. (2008). Neurobiology of bipolar disorder. *Expert Reviews in Neurotherapeutics, 8*(1), 93–110.

Newman, C., Leahy, R. L., Beck, A. T., Reilly-Harrington, N., & Gyulai, L. (2001). *Bipolar disorder: A cognitive therapy approach.* Washington, DC: American Psychological Association.

Novick, D. M., Gonzalez-Pinto, A., Haro, J. M., Bertsch, J., Reed, C., Perrin, E., . . . Board, E. A. (2009). Translation of randomised controlled trial findings into clinical practice: Comparison of olanzapine and valproate in the EMBLEM study. *Pharmacopsychiatry, 42*(4), 145–152.

Novick, D. M., Swartz, H. A., & Frank, E. (2010). Suicide attempts in bipolar I and bipolar II disorder: A review and meta-analysis of the evidence. *Bipolar Disorders, 12*(1), 1–9.

Nusslock, R., Almeida, J. R., Forbes, E. E., Versace, A., Frank, E., Labarbara, E. J., . . . Phillips, M. L. (2012). Waiting to win: Elevated striatal and orbitofrontal cortical activity during reward anticipation in euthymic bipolar disorder adults. *Bipolar Disorder, 14*(3), 249–260.

O'Brien, M. P., Miklowitz, D. J., & Cannon, T. D. (2014). A randomized trial of family focused therapy with youth at clinical high risk for psychosis: Effects on interactional behavior. *Journal of Consulting and Clinical Psychology, 82*(1), 90–101.

Occhiogrosso, M., Omran, S. S., & Altemus, M. (2012). Persistent pulmonary hypertension of the newborn and selective serotonin reuptake inhibitors: Lessons from clinical and translational studies. *American Journal of Psychiatry, 169*(2), 134–140.

O'Donnell, L. A., Deldin, P. J., Grogan-Kaylor, A., McInnis, M. G., Weintraub, J., Ryan, K. A., & Himle, J. A. (2017a). Depression and executive functioning deficits predict poor occupational functioning in a large longitudinal sample with bipolar disorder. *Journal of Affective Disorders, 215*, 135–142.

O'Donnell, L. A., Himle, J. A., Ryan, K., Grogan-Kaylor, A., McInnis, M. G., Weintraub, J., . . . Deldin, P. (2017b). Social aspects of the workplace among individuals with bipolar disorder. *Journal of the Society for Social Work and Research, 8*(3), 379–398.

Öhlund, L., Ott, M., Oja, S., Bergqvist, M., Lundqvist, R., Sandlund, M., . . . Werneke, U. (2018). Reasons for lithium discontinuation in men and women with bipolar disorder: A retrospective cohort study. *BMC Psychiatry, 18*(1), 37.

Oldani, L., Altamura, A. C., Abdelghani, M., & Young, A. H. (2016). Brain stimulation treatments in bipolar disorder: A review of the current literature. *World Journal of Biological Psychiatry, 17*(7), 482–494.

Otto, M. W., Reilly-Harrington, N., Sachs, G. S., Knauz, R. O., Miklowitz, D. J., & Frank, E. (1999). *Collaborative care workbook: A workbook for individuals and families.* Boston: Partners Bipolar Treatment Center, Massachusetts General Hospital.

Palmier-Claus, J. E., Berry, K., Bucci, S., Mansell, W., & Varese, F. (2016). Relationship between childhood adversity and bipolar affective disorder: Systematic review and meta-analysis. *British Journal of Psychiatry, 209*(6), 454–459.

Pavuluri, M. N., Birmaher, B., & Naylor, M. W. (2005). Pediatric bipolar disorder: A review of the past 10 years. *Journal of the American Academy of Child and Adolescent Psychiatry, 44*(9), 846–871.

Pavuluri, M. N., West, A., Hill, S. K., Jindal, K., & Sweeney, J. A. (2009). Neurocognitive function in pediatric bipolar disorder: 3-year follow-up shows cognitive development lagging behind healthy youths. *Journal of the American Academy of Child and Adolescent Psychiatry, 48*, 299–307.

Perez Algorta, G., MacPherson, H. A., Youngstrom, E. A., Belt, C. C., Arnold, L. E., Frazier, T. W., . . . Fristad, M. A. (2017, February 26). Parenting stress among caregivers of children with bipolar spectrum disorders. *Journal of Clinical Child and Adolescent Psychology.* [Epub ahead of print]

Perich, T., Ussher, J., & Meade, T. (2017). Menopause and illness course in bipolar disorder: A systematic review. *Bipolar Disorder, 19*(6), 434–443.

Perlis, R. H., Miyahara, S., Marangell, L. B., Wisniewski, S. R., Ostacher, M., DelBello, M. P., . . . STEP-BD Investigators. (2004). Long-term implications of early onset in bipolar disorder: Data from the first 1000 participants in the Systematic Treatment Enhancement Program for Bipolar Disorder (STEP-BD). *Biological Psychiatry, 55*, 875–881.

Perlis, R. H., Ostacher, M. J., Miklowitz, D. J., Hay, A., Nierenberg, A. A., Thase, M. E., & Sachs, G. S. (2010). Clinical features associated with poor pharmacologic adherence in bipolar disorder: Results from the STEP-BD study. *Journal of Clinical Psychiatry, 71*(3), 296–303.

Perlis, R. H., Ostacher, M. J., Patel, J., Marangell, L. B., Zhang, H., Wisniewski, S. R., . . . Thase, M. (2006). Predictors of recurrence in bipolar disorder: Primary outcomes from the Systematic Treatment Enhancement Program for Bipolar Disorder (STEP-BD). *American Journal of Psychiatry, 163*(2), 217–224.

Phelps, J. (2012). The bipolar spectrum. In G. Parker (Ed.), *Bipolar II disorder: Modelling, measuring and managing* (2nd ed., pp. 10–34). Cambridge, UK: Cambridge University Press.

Phillips, M. L., & Swartz, H. A. (2014). A critical appraisal of neuroimaging studies of bipolar disorder: Toward a new conceptualization of underlying neural circuitry and a road map for future research. *American Journal of Psychiatry, 171*(8), 829–843.

Pigott, K., Galizia, I., Vasudev, K., Watson, S., Geddes, J., & Young, A. H. (2016). Topiramate for acute affective episodes in bipolar disorder in adults. *Cochrane Database of Systematic Reviews, 9*, Art. No. CD003384.

Post, R. M. (2007). Kindling and sensitization as models for affective episode recurrence, cyclicity, and tolerance phenomena. *Neuroscience and Biobehavioral Reviews, 31*(6), 858–873.

Post, R. M., Altshuler, L. L., Kupka, R., McElroy, S. L., Frye, M. A., Rowe, M., . . . Nolen, W. A. (2017). More childhood onset bipolar disorder in the United States than Canada or Europe: Implications for treatment and prevention. *Neuroscience and Biobehavioral Reviews, 74*(Pt. A), 204–213.

Post, R. M., & Leverich, G. S. (2006). The role of psychosocial stress in the onset and progression of bipolar disorder and its comorbidities: The need for earlier and alternative modes of therapeutic intervention. *Development and Psychopathology, 18*(4), 1181–1211.

Post, R. M., Leverich, G. S., Kupka, R. W., Keck, P. E. J., McElroy, S. L., Altshuler, L. L., . . . Nolen, W. A. (2010). Early-onset bipolar disorder and treatment delay are risk factors for poor outcome in adulthood. *Journal of Clinical Psychiatry, 71*(7), 864–872.

Rachid, F. (2017a). Maintenance repetitive transcranial magnetic stimulation (rTMS) for relapse prevention in patients with depression. *Psychiatry Research, 262*, 363–372.

Rachid, F. (2017b). Repetitive transcranial magnetic stimulation and treatment-emergent mania and hypomania: A review of the literature. *Journal of Psychiatric Practice, 23*(2), 150–159.

Rasgon, N. L., Altshuler, L. L., Fairbanks, L., Elman, S., Bitran, J., Labarca, R., . . . Mintz, J. (2005). Reproductive function and risk for PCOS in women treated for bipolar disorder. *Bipolar Disorders, 7*(3), 246–259.

Rasgon, N. L, Bauer, M., Glenn, T., Elman, S., & Whybrow, P. C. (2003). Menstrual cycle related mood changes in women with bipolar disorder. *Bipolar Disorders, 5*(1), 48–52.

Rea, M. M., Tompson, M., Miklowitz, D. J., Goldstein, M. J., Hwang, S., & Mintz, J. (2003). Family focused treatment vs. individual treatment for bipolar disorder: Results of a randomized clinical trial. *Journal of Consulting and Clinical Psychology, 71*, 482–492.

Reichart, C. G., & Nolen, W. A. (2004). Earlier onset of bipolar disorder in children by antidepressants or stimulants?: An hypothesis. *Journal of Affective Disorders, 78*(1), 81–84.

Reilly-Harrington, N., & Sachs, G. S. (2006). Psychosocial strategies to improve concordance and adherence in bipolar disorder. *Journal of Clinical Psychiatry, 67*(7), e04.

Reinares, M., Rosa, A. R., Franco, C., Goikolea, J. M., Fountoulakis, K., Siamouli, M., . . . Vieta, E. (2013). A systematic review on the role of anticonvulsants in the treatment of acute bipolar depression. *International Journal of Neuropsychopharmacology, 16*(2), 485–496.

Rosa, A. R., Fountoulakis, K., Siamouli, M., Gonda, X., & Vieta, E. (2011). Is anticonvulsant treatment of mania a class effect?: Data from randomized clinical trials. *CNS Neuroscience Therapeutics, 17*(3), 167–177.

Rosso, G., Albert, U., Di Salvo, G., Scatà, M., Todros, T., & Maina, G. (2016). Lithium prophylaxis during pregnancy and the postpartum period in women with lithium-responsive bipolar I disorder. *Archives of Women's Mental Heath, 19*(2), 429–432.

Rossouw, T. I., & Fonagy, P. (2012). Mentalization-based treatment for self-harming adolescents: A randomised controlled trial. *Journal of the American Academy of Child and Adolescent Psychiatry, 51*(12), 1304–1313.

Roybal, K., Theobold, D., Graham, A., DiNieri, J. A., Russo, S. J., Krishnan, V., . . . McClung, C. A. (2007). Mania-like behavior induced by disruption of CLOCK. *Proceedings of the National Academy of Sciences of the USA, 104*(15), 6406–6411.

Rush, A. J., Trivedi, M. H., Ibrahim, H. M., Carmody, T. J., Arnow, B., & Klein, D. N. (2003). The 16-item Quick Inventory of Depressive Symptomatology (QIDS), Clinician rating (QIDS-

C), and Self-Report (QIDS-SR): A psychometric evaluation in patients with chronic major depression. *Biological Psychiatry, 54*(5), 573–583.

Rybakowski, J. K. (2014). Response to lithium in bipolar disorder: Clinical and genetic findings. *ACS Chemical Neuroscience, 5*(6), 413–421.

Sachs, G. S., Nierenberg, A. A., Calabrese, J. R., Marangell, L. B., Wisniewski, S. R., Gyulai, L., . . . Thase, M. E. (2007). Effectiveness of adjunctive antidepressant treatment for bipolar depression. *New England Journal of Medicine, 356*(17), 1711–1722.

Sachs, G. S., Thase, M. E., Otto, M. W., Bauer, M., Miklowitz, D., Wisniewski, S. R., . . . Rosenbaum, J. F. (2003). Rationale, design, and methods of the systematic treatment enhancement program for bipolar disorder (STEP-BD). *Biological Psychiatry, 53*, 1028–1042.

Sala, R., Axelson, D. A., Castro-Fornieles, J., Goldstein, T. R., Ha, W., Liao, F., . . . Birmaher, B. (2010). Comorbid anxiety in children and adolescents with bipolar spectrum disorders: Prevalence and clinical correlates. *Journal of Clinical Psychiatry, 71*(10), 1344–1350.

Salcedo, S., Gold, A. K., Sheikh, S., Marcus, P. H., Nierenberg, A. A., Deckersbach, T., & Sylvia, L. G. (2016). Empirically supported psychosocial interventions for bipolar disorder: Current state of the research. *Journal of Affective Disorders, 201*, 203–214.

Salisbury, A. L., O'Grady, K. E., Battle, C. L., Wisner, K. L., Anderson, G. M., Stroud, L. R., . . . Lester, B. M. (2016). The roles of maternal depression, serotonin reuptake inhibitor treatment, and concomitant benzodiazepine use on infant neurobehavioral functioning over the first postnatal month. *American Journal of Psychiatry, 173*(2), 147–157.

Schaffer, A., Sinyor, M., Reis, C., Goldstein, B. I., & Levitt, A. J. (2014). Suicide in bipolar disorder: Characteristics and subgroups. *Bipolar Disorder, 16*(7), 732–740.

Scheffer, R. E., Kowatch, R. A., Carmody, T., & Rush, A. J. (2005). Randomized, placebo-controlled trial of mixed amphetamine salts for symptoms of comorbid ADHD in pediatric bipolar disorder after mood stabilization with divalproex sodium. *American Journal of Psychiatry, 162*(1), 58–64.

Scherk, H., Pajonk, F. G., & Leucht, S. (2007). Second-generation antipsychotic agents in the treatment of acute mania: A systematic review and meta-analysis of randomized controlled trials. *Archives of General Psychiatry, 64*(4), 442–455.

Schlaepfer, T. E., Cohen, M. X., Frick, C., Kosel, M., Brodesser, D., Axmacher, N., . . . Sturm, V. (2008). Deep brain stimulation to reward circuitry alleviates anhedonia in refractory major depression. *Neuropsychopharmacology, 33*(2), 368–377.

Schloesser, R. J., Huang, J., Klein, P. S., & Manji, H. K. (2008). Cellular plasticity cascades in the pathophysiology and treatment of bipolar disorder. *Neuropsychopharmacology Reviews, 33*(1), 110–133.

Schneck, C. D., Chang, K. D., Singh, M., DelBello, M. P., & Miklowitz, D. J. (2017). A pharmacologic algorithm for youth who are at high risk for bipolar disorder. *Journal of Child and Adolescent Psychopharmacology, 27*(9), 796–805.

Schneck, C. D., Miklowitz, D. J., Miyahara, S., Wisniewski, S., Gyulai, L., Allen, M. H., . . . Sachs, G. S. (2008). The prospective course of rapid cycling bipolar disorder. *American Journal of Psychiatry, 165*(3), 370–377.

Scrandis, D. A. (2017). Bipolar disorder in pregnancy: A review of pregnancy outcomes. *Journal of Midwifery and Women's Health, 62*(6), 673–683.

Segal, Z. V., Williams, J. M., & Teasdale, J. D. (2012). *Mindfulness-based cognitive therapy for depression* (2nd ed.). New York: Guilford Press.

Seligman, M. E. P. (2002). *Authentic happiness.* New York: Simon & Schuster.

Seligman, M. E. P., Reivich, K., Jaycox, L., & Gillham, J. (1996). *The optimistic child.* Boston: Houghton Mifflin.

Severus, E., Taylor, M. J., Sauer, C., Pfennig, A., Ritter, P., Bauer, M., & Geddes, J. R. (2014). Lithium for prevention of mood episodes in bipolar disorders: Systematic review and meta-analysis. *International Journal of Bipolar Disorders, 2*(15), 1–17.

Shapiro, L. E. (2008). *Stopping the pain: A workbook for teens who cut and self-injure.* Oakland, CA: Instant Help/New Harbinger.

Shim, I. H., Woo, Y. S., Kim, M. D., & Bahk, W. M. (2017). Antidepressants and mood stabilizers: Novel research avenues and clinical insights for bipolar depression. *International Journal of Molecular Psychiatry, 18*(11), E2406.

Singley, D. B., & Edwards, L. M. (2015). Men's perinatal mental health in the transition to fatherhood. *Professional psychology: Research and Practice, 46*(5), 309–316.

Sit, D. K., McGowan, J., Wiltrout, C., Diler, R. S., Dills, J. J., Luther, J., . . . Wisner, K. L. (2018). Adjunctive bright light therapy for bipolar depression: A randomized double-blind placebo-controlled trial. *American Journal of Psychiatry, 175*(2), 131–139.

Smith, L. A., Cornelius, V., Warnock, A., Tacchi, M. J., & Taylor, D. (2007). Pharmacological interventions for acute bipolar mania: A systematic review of randomized placebo-controlled trials. *Bipolar Disorders, 9*(6), 551–560.

Smoller, J. W., & Finn, C. T. (2003). Family, twin, and adoption studies of bipolar disorder. *American Journal of Medical Genetics, Part C: Seminars in Medical Genetics, 123*(1), 48–58.

Solomon, A. (2002). *Noonday demon: An atlas of depression.* New York: Scribner.

Solomon, D. A., Leon, A. C., Endicott, J., Coryell, W. H., Mueller, T. I., Posternak, M. A., & Keller, M. B. (2003). Unipolar mania over the course of a 20-year follow-up study. *American Journal of Psychiatry, 160*, 2049–2051.

Stewart, D. E. (2011). Depression during pregnancy. *New England Journal of Medicine, 365*, 1605–1611.

Strakowski, S. M., DelBello, M. P., Fleck, D. E., & Arndt, S. (2000). The impact of substance abuse on the course of bipolar disorder. *Biological Psychiatry, 48*, 477–485.

Strober, M., & Carlson, G. (1982). Bipolar illness in adolescents with major depression: Clinical, genetic, and psychopharmacologic predictors in a 3–4 year prospective follow-up investigation. *Archives of General Psychiatry, 39*, 549–555.

Strosahl, K., Chiles, J. A., & Linehan, M. (1992). Prediction of suicide intent in hospitalized parasuicides: Reasons for living, hopelessness, and depression. *Comprehensive Psychiatry, 33*, 366–373.

Styron, W. (1992). *Darkness visible: A memoir of madness.* New York: Vintage Books.

Sun, Y. R., Herrmann, N., Scott, C. J. M., Black, S. E., Khan, M. M., & Lanctôt, K. L. (2018). Global grey matter volume in adult bipolar patients with and without lithium treatment: A meta-analysis. *Journal of Affective Disorders, 225*, 599–606.

Suppes, T., Dennehy, E. B., & Gibbons, E. W. (2000). The longitudinal course of bipolar disorder. *Journal of Clinical Psychiatry, 61*, 23–30.

Suto, M., Murray, G., Hale, S., Amari, E., & Michalak, E. E. (2010). What works for people with bipolar disorder?: Tips from the experts. *Journal of Affective Disorders, 124*(1–2), 76–84.

Sylvia, L. G., Hay, A., Ostacher, M. J., Miklowitz, D. J., Nierenberg, A. A., Thase, M. E., . . . Perlis, R. H. (2013). Association between therapeutic alliance, care satisfaction, and pharmacological adherence in bipolar disorder. *Clinical Psychopharmacology, 33*(3), 343–350.

Teasdale, J., Williams, M., & Segal, Z. (2014). *The mindful way workbook: An 8-week program to free yourself from depression and emotional distress.* New York: Guilford Press.

Thase, M. E. (2010). Pharmacotherapy for adults with bipolar depression. In D. J. Miklowitz & D. Cicchetti (Eds.), *Understanding bipolar disorder: A developmental psychopathology perspective* (pp. 445–465). New York: Guilford Press.

Tohen, M., Kryzhanovskaya, L., Carlson, G., DelBello, M. P., Wozniak, J., Kowatch, R., . . . Biederman, J. (2005). Olanzapine in the treatment of acute mania in adolescents with bipolar I disorder: A 3-week randomized double-blind placebo-controlled study. *Neuropsychopharmacology, 30*(Suppl. 1), 176.

Tohen, M., & Vieta, E. (2009). Antipsychotic agents in the treatment of bipolar mania. *Bipolar Disorders, 11*(2), 45–54.

Torrent, C., Bonnín, C. D. M., Martinez-Aran, A., Valle, J., Amann, B. L., Gonzalez-Pinto, A., & Vieta, E. (2013). Efficacy of functional remediation in bipolar disorder: A multicenter randomized controlled study. *American Journal of Psychiatry, 170*(8), 852–859.

Townsend, J., & Altshuler, L. L. (2012). Emotion processing and regulation in bipolar disorder: A review. *Bipolar Disorders, 14*(4), 326–339.

Tremblay, C. H. (2011). Workplace accommodations and job success for persons with bipolar disorder. *Work, 40*(4), 479–487.

Turvill, J. L., Burroughs, A. K., & Moore, K. P. (2000). Change in occurrence of paracetamol overdose in UK after introduction of blister packs. *Lancet, 355*(9220), 2048–2049.

Van Meter, A. R., Burke, C., Kowatch, R. A., Findling, R. L., & Youngstrom, E. A. (2016). Ten-year updated meta-analysis of the clinical characteristics of pediatric mania and hypomania. *Bipolar Disorder, 18*(1), 19–32.

Van Meter, A. R., Burke, C., Youngstrom, E. A., Faedda, G. L., & Correll, C. U. (2016). The bipolar prodrome: Meta-analysis of symptom prevalence prior to initial or recurrent mood episodes. *Journal of the American Academy of Child and Adolescent Psychiatry, 55*(7), 543–555.

Van Meter, A. R., & Youngstrom, E. A. (2012). Cyclothymic disorder in youth: Why is it overlooked, what do we know and where is the field headed? *Neuropsychiatry, 2*(6), 509–519.

Van Meter, A. R., Youngstrom, E. A., Birmaher, B., Fristad, M. A., Horwitz, S. M., Frazier, T. W., . . . Findling, R. L. (2017). Longitudinal course and characteristics of cyclothymic disorder in youth. *Journal of Affective Disorders, 215*, 314–322.

Vesco, A. T., Young, A. S., Arnold, L. E., & Fristad, M. A. (2018). Omega-3 supplementation associated with improved parent-rated executive function in youth with mood disorders: Secondary analyses of the omega 3 and therapy (OATS) trials. *Journal of Child Psychology and Psychiatry, 59*(6), 628–636.

Vieta, E., Salagre, E., Grande, I., Carvalho, A. F., Fernandes, B. S., Berk, M., . . . Suppes, T. (2018). Early intervention in bipolar disorder. *American Journal of Psychiatry, 175*(5), 411–426.

Viguera, A. C., Newport, D. J., Ritchie, J., Stowe, Z., Whitfield, T., Mogielnicki, J., . . . Cohen, L. S. (2007). Lithium in breast milk and nursing infants: Clinical implications. *American Journal of Psychiatry, 164*(2), 342–345.

Viguera, A. C., Nonacs, R., Cohen, L. S., Tondo, L., Murray, A., & Baldessarini, R. J. (2000). Risk of recurrence of bipolar disorder in pregnant and nonpregnant women after discontinuing lithium maintenance. *American Journal of Psychiatry, 157*(2), 179–184.

Viguera, A. C., Whitfield, T., Baldessarini, R. J., Newport, D. J., Stowe, Z., Reminick, A., . . . Cohen, L. S. (2007). Risk of recurrence in women with bipolar disorder during pregnancy: Prospective study of mood stabilizer discontinuation. *American Journal of Psychiatry, 164*(12), 1817–1824.

Walshaw, P. D., Alloy, L. B., & Sabb, F. W. (2010). Executive function in pediatric bipolar disorder and attention-deficit hyperactivity disorder: In search of distinct phenotypic profiles. *Neuropsychology Review, 20*(1), 103–120.

Ward, S., & Wisner, K. L. (2007). Collaborative management of women with bipolar disorder during pregnancy and postpartum: Pharmacologic considerations. *Journal of Midwifery and Women's Health, 52*(1), 3–13.

Weintraub, M. J., Van de Loo, M. M., Gitlin, M. J., & Miklowitz, D. J. (2017). Self-harm, affective traits, and psychosocial functioning in adults with depressive and bipolar disorders. *Journal of Nervous and Mental Disease, 205*(11), 896–899.

Weissman, M. M., Wickramaratne, P., Pilowsky, D. J., Poh, E., Batten, L. A., Hernandez, M., ... Stewart, J. W. (2015). Treatment of maternal depression in a medication clinical trial and its effect on children. *American Journal of Psychiatry, 172*(5), 450–459.

Weobong, B., Weiss, H. A., McDaid, D., Singla, D. R., Hollon, S. D., Nadkarni, A., . . . Patel, V. (2017). Sustained effectiveness and cost-effectiveness of the Healthy Activity Programme, a brief psychological treatment for depression delivered by lay counsellors in primary care: 12-month follow-up of a randomised controlled trial. *PLOS Medicine, 14*(9), e1002385.

Wesseloo, R., Kamperman, A. M., Munk-Olsen, T., Pop, V. J., Kushner, S. A., & Bergink, V. (2016). Risk of postpartum relapse in bipolar disorder and postpartum psychosis: A systematic review and meta-analysis. *American Journal of Psychiatry, 173*(2), 117–127.

West, A. E., Weinstein, S. M., Peters, A. T., Katz, A. C., Henry, D. B., Cruz, R. A., & Pavuluri, M. N. (2014). Child- and family-focused cognitive-behavioral therapy for pediatric bipolar disorder: A randomized clinical trial. *Journal of the American Academy of Child and Adolescent Psychiatry, 53*(11), 1168–1178.

Wilkinson, S. T., Ballard, E. D., Bloch, M. H., Mathew, S. J., Murrough, J. W., Feder, A., . . . Sanacora, G. (2018). The effect of a single dose of intravenous ketamine on suicidal ideation: A systematic review and individual participant data meta-analysis. *American Journal of Psychiatry, 175*(2), 150–158.

Williams, J. B. W. (1988). A structured interview guide for the Hamilton Depression Rating Scale. *Archives of General Psychiatry, 45*, 742–747.

Williams, J. M., Crane, C., Barnhofer, T., Brennan, K., Duggan, D. S., Fennell, M. J., . . . Russell, I. T. (2014). Mindfulness-based cognitive therapy for preventing relapse in recurrent depression: A randomized dismantling trial. *Journal of Consulting and Clinical Psychology, 82*(2), 275–286.

Williams, J. M., Russell, I., & Russell, D. (2008). Mindfulness-based cognitive therapy: Further issues in current evidence and future research. *Journal of Consulting and Clinical Psychology, 76*(3), 524–529.

Williams, M., Teasdale, J., Segal, Z., & Kabat-Zinn, J. (2007). *The mindful way through depression: Freeing yourself from chronic unhappiness*. New York: Guilford Press.

Wurtzel, E. (1994). *Prozac nation*. New York: Riverhead Books.

Yen, S., Stout, R., Hower, H., Killam, M. A., Weinstock, L. M., Topor, D. R., . . . Keller, M. B. (2016). The influence of comorbid disorders on the episodicity of bipolar disorder in youth. *Acta Psychiatrica Scandinavaca, 133*(4), 324–334.

Young, R. C., Biggs, J. T., Ziegler, V. E., & Meyer, D. A. (1978). A rating scale for mania: Reliability, validity, and sensitivity. *British Journal of Psychiatry, 133*, 429–435.

Youngstrom, E. A., Findling, R. L., Youngstrom, J. K., & Calabrese, J. R. (2005). Towards an evidence-based assessment of pediatric bipolar disorder. *Journal of Clinical Child and Adolescent Psychology, 34*(3), 433–448.

Youngstrom, E. A., Frazier, T. W., Demeter, C., Calabrese, J. R., & Findling, R. L. (2008). Developing a 10-item mania scale from the Parent General Behavior Inventory for Children and Adolescents. *Journal of Clinical Psychiatry, 69*(5), 831–839.

Zarate, C. A. J., Brutsche, N. E., Ibrahim, L., Franco-Chaves, J., Diazgranados, N., Cravchik, A., . . . Luckenbaugh, D. A. (2012). Replication of ketamine's antidepressant efficacy in bipolar depression: A randomized controlled add-on trial. *Biological Psychiatry, 71*(11), 939–946.

Zarate, C. A. J., Payne, J. L., Singh, J., Quiroz, J. A., Luckenbaugh, D. A., Denicoff, K. D., . . . Manji, H. K. (2004). Pramipexole for bipolar II depression: A placebo-controlled proof of concept study. *Biological Psychiatry, 56*(1), 54–60.

Zubin, J., & Spring, B. (1977). Vulnerability: A new view of schizophrenia. *Journal of Abnormal Psychology, 86*, 103–126.

Index

Note. *f* following a page number indicates a figure.

About the Author

David J. Miklowitz, PhD, is Professor of Psychiatry at the Semel Institute for Neuroscience and Human Behavior, University of California, Los Angeles, and Senior Clinical Researcher in the Department of Psychiatry at the University of Oxford, United Kingdom. Dr. Miklowitz is the author of two award-winning books for professionals: *Bipolar Disorder: A Family-Focused Treatment Approach* and, with Michael J. Gitlin, *Clinician's Guide to Bipolar Disorder.* He has received Distinguished Investigator awards from the Brain and Behavior Research Foundation, the Depression and Bipolar Support Alliance, the International Society for Bipolar Disorders, and the Society for a Science of Clinical Psychology.